MW00845238

STRAIN–COUNTERSTRAIN

by
Lawrence H. Jones, DO, FAAO
with
Randall S. Kusunose, PT, OCS
Edward K. Goering, DO, DVM, MSHPE

Hardcover Trade ISBN: 0–9645135–0–1
Hardcover Text ISBN: 0–9645135–2–8
Paper Text ISBN: 0–9645135–4–4

Printed in the United States of America

Published by:
Jones Strain–CounterStrain, Inc.
1501 Tyrell Lane
Boise, ID 83706
208/343–4080

CONTENTS

ACKNOWLEDGMENTS

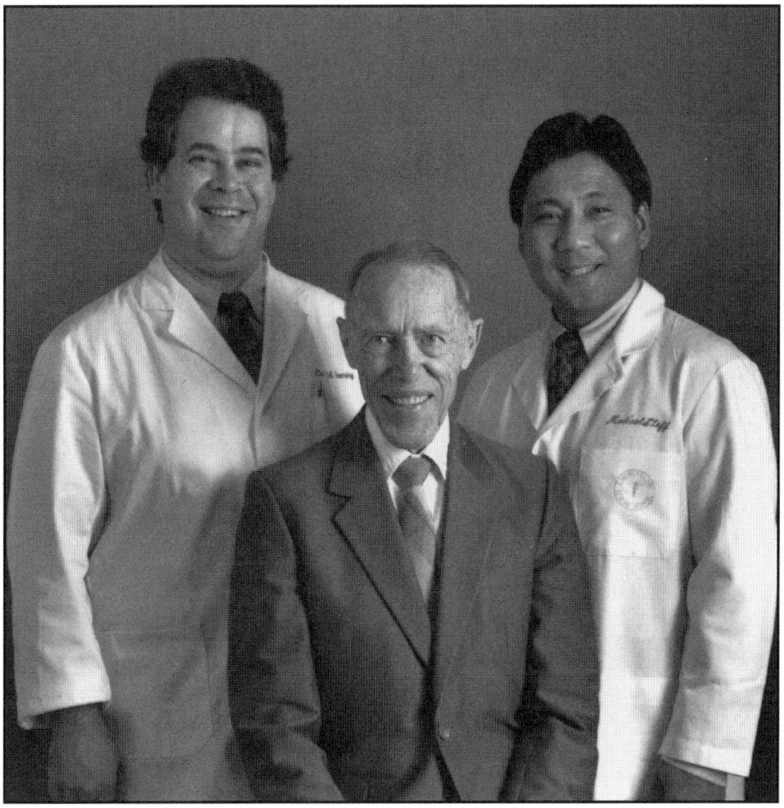

Edward K. Goering, DO **Randall S. Kusunose, PT**
Lawrence H. Jones, DO

This concept could not have been developed nor this book written without aid from several insightful men who advised me, argued with me, instructed me, and encouraged me. Although this list cannot be complete, among those most helpful were: Harry Davis, DO, Perrin T. Wilson, DO, John P. Goodridge, DO, FAAO, Berkeley Brandt Jr., DO, Rollin E. Becker, DO, William L. Johnston, DO, FAAO, George W. Northup, DO, FAAO, John Harakal Jr., DO, FAAO, and Irvin M. Korr, Ph.D.

In addition I owe a debt of gratitude for thousands of hours of selfless effort to R. Rex Conyers, DO, Robert H. Wendorff, DO, Gerald H. Cooper, DO, and Harold R. Schwartz, DO, FAAO, who working both separately and with me, assisted in developing a book that could be understood and used by all our colleagues.

I also wish to thank John Glover, DO, CSP, OMM, John M. Jones, DO, Randall S. Kusunose, PT, OCS, and Edward K. Goering, DO, DVM, MSHPE.

Thanks to Kathy Gaudry, Gail Ward and Tamarack Books, Boise, for their expert guidance and service. Thanks to Kristin Finnegan, Portland, for her beautiful photography.

Lastly, I am indebted to those whose suggested revisions added clarity to the text. This tedious and time-consuming work was done especially by Sarah Sutton, DO, FAAO and Edna Lay, DO, FAAO.

PREFACE

This book has been written in an attempt to pass on to other clinicians the benefits I have been fortunate enough to acquire in fifty-eight years of clinical practice treating joint dysfunctions. It is not a scientific treatise, but the sharing of the experience of one clinician with another.

Especially important and valuable were two phenomena I observed accidentally at different times; each impressed me enough to motivate experimentation with ways to utilize it in treating joint dysfunctions. The first phenomenon provided a unique opportunity to observe the behavior of joints under stress. The second provided a new source of diagnostic information equal to and complementing the knowledge that I had at the time of its discovery.

The hypothesis on the nature of somatic joint dysfunction is derived from an article by Irvin M. Korr, Ph.D.[1] who describes joint dysfunction in a logical manner and provides a scientific basis for understanding it. My observations during some thirty-nine years of using deliberate application of joint strain in treatment bear out the conclusions offered by Korr.

One of the first men in America to put the study of joint dysfunction on a scientific basis was Andrew Taylor Still, a physician living at the time of the American Civil War. He studied the anatomy of the human body diligently, and by reasoning on a physiologic basis he developed manipulative skills, thus greatly improving his capabilities as a physician. Other physicians of his time did not recognize his achievement as beneficial and rejected his ideas concerning the underlying cause of disease. After years of frustration he founded another school of medicine which he called osteopathy. The objective of the school was "to establish a college of osteopathy, the design of which is to improve our present system of surgery, obstetrics and treatment of diseases generally, and place the same on a more rational and scientific basis, and to impart information to the medical profession."[2]

Though the new school served to perpetuate his concepts, it further alienated his contemporaries. Still and the graduates of his school, using manipulative methods, were able to relieve patients of conditions where orthodox medical treatment failed. The rivalry that developed served to discredit the efficacy of joint manipulation in the eyes of orthodox physicians until recent years. It is today considered to be a treatment of choice at many large rehabilitation centers.

Practice of osteopathic medicine in the mid-1930s when I attended the College of Osteopathic Physicians and Surgeons in Los Angeles was not standardized. Many thought that joint stiffness and pain resulted from trauma, which caused joint subluxation or a partial or incomplete dislocation. These practitioners applied a specific thrust to effect a release and restore free and comfortable motion to the painful joint. In most cases they were at least partially successful.

To many of us, however, the nature and etiology of this osteopathic lesion were unclear. At best we had only a skill to relieve a painful syndrome. The evolving concept of somatic dysfunction from that of a mechanical type of structure disorder to that of a reflex neuromuscular dysfunction has proceeded irregularly through the years.

The followers of the traditional concept of joint subluxation reduced by sudden, forceful mobilization have obtained fairly good results in most cases over a long period of time.

William Garner Sutherland, DO,[3] advanced ideas concerning the function of cerebrospinal fluid and the craniosacral respiratory mechanism, areas not touched by any one else I know. One facet that I feel is related to later concepts was his application of slow and very subtle forces applied in the easy direction indicated by the structures he treated. For example, he observed the movements of the skull in the direction it moved most freely. He found that by this approach he could reduce or eliminate asymmetrical limitations of motion.

Harold Hoover, DO, developed a method of treating joint disorders, which he called "functional technique."[4] He learned that the anatomic neutral position for these joints developed asymmetrical muscle tensions. Again his direction of movement of the joint was toward that of least resistance and greatest comfort. He envisioned a position of greatest harmony, in which the tensions all around the joint were equal. He called this position "dynamic neutral." Patients in this position developed a progressive lessening of the need for an eccentric position, until his dynamic position and the anatomic neutral position were the same. He was accused of borrowing from the Sutherland concept, which he explicitly denied. I had studied under him in courses offered by the Academy of Applied Osteopathy on the teachings of Harrison Fryette, DO, and later on his "functional techniques," but I was not yet ready for either method and I returned to the use of low-amplitude, high-velocity thrust-type techniques.

When I published an article in *The DO* entitled "Spontaneous Release by Positioning,"[5] it was suggested that I was borrowing from Hoover's functional technique. I was quick to point out the differences and deprecate the similarities. The position of spontaneous release is in the direction toward immediate ease and comfort—as was his. Whereas his dynamic neutral concept sought a bilateral balance of tension fairly near the anatomic neutral position, the concept of the position of spontaneous release focused on the disorder as unilateral and moved to the position of greatest ease of the abnormally tense side, ignoring the well side. This was always at or close to an actual position of strain.

One of the earliest pioneers, a man with whom I had the good fortune to discuss concepts, was T. J. Ruddy, DO. He developed a very effective method of rapidly repeated active movements against resistance.[6] He explained the benefits in terms of increased blood flow to affected muscles. He called his method "resistive duction." In talking with him, it became apparent to me that he thought of malfunctioning nerves and muscles rather than mechanical disorders. Unfortunately he was already of advanced age and I was unable to follow up on our discussions.

Fred L. Mitchel, Sr., DO, FAAO, the man who developed and taught muscle energy techniques, readily acknowledged Ruddy as the source of his material.[7]

On less self-centered reflection, I am sure that all of these earlier concepts directed my thinking to neuromuscular dysfunction as the basis of joint disorders. What I find heartening and convincing is that on this point, although we each believed that we thought independently, our ideas all converged toward what seems to be a basic truth.

DISCOVERY

FINDING COUNTERSTRAIN

In our fumbling efforts to deal with rheumatic pain, one fact stands out so clearly that it is hard to believe we have been blind for so long.

We all knew that pains were much worse in some positions than in others, but none of us pursued the idea more than to learn to avoid the most painful positions. I treated people for nineteen years without any interest in positions of greater or lesser pain until it was so forcibly impressed upon me I could ignore it no longer.

Yet the pain and tension of every one of these problems is markedly influenced by stretches of the areas involved varying from agony in the worst position to complete comfort in the ideal position. Perhaps we lost interest because we knew that as soon as we returned the patient from his position of comfort, pain would immediately return. As some sage said, "It isn't what you don't know that defeats you. It's what you know that isn't so." A period of only ninety seconds in a position of comfort will have a lasting beneficial effect every time, if we only return from it slowly. It is the most therapeutic thing we can do and almost the easiest.

DEFINITION

1. Relief of rheumatic pain by placing a joint in its position of greatest comfort.
2. Relief of false messages of continuing strain arising in dysfunctioning proprioceptor reflexes, by applying a strain in the direction opposite that of the false messages of strain. This is accomplished by shortening the muscle containing the false strain message so much that it stops reporting strain. The body in normal positions can suffer this pain for years yet have it stopped in ninety seconds of the opposite strain.

DISCOVERY

I have received credit for having the insight to develop this improved way to relieve pain. The truth is that all I supplied was much frustration. I wasn't even trying to treat my patient at the time, but just to help him learn to find a comfortable position that would let him sleep better. The spectacular recovery he had surprised me much more than it did him. It was so unexpected as to be astonishing. I didn't dream that a thing like that could work so well.

My patient was a healthy thirty-year-old man with severe back pain that he had suffered from for four months, a third of it while under my care. I had exhausted all my tricks and didn't know which way to turn before admitting to failure.

He volunteered, "Maybe, I could respond to your treatment if I could just sleep at night. I wake up about every fifteen minutes all night long and try to find a more comfortable position."

By this time I was grasping at straws, ready to try anything no matter how improbable.

I had learned how easy it is to get such a patient addicted to sleeping pills in addition to his other troubles, so I tried to help him find a position of comfort.

I stretched him in some direction and asked him whether he felt less or more pain. I had been trying for twenty minutes before I had much success. By then he was in a wild, grotesque position that looked like he must be in a strain, but he was finally almost completely comfortable. This was the only good thing that had happened to him in four months of treatment and I didn't have the heart to move him back into his position of pain. With a few pillows and a chair, I propped him up to enjoy his comfort while I treated another patient.

When I returned he was still happy and we discussed how he was going to try to find this good position when he went to bed.

When he rose from my table the pain did not return! He stood erect for the first time in four months and almost pain free! He didn't have to stay in his strained position for comfort! We were both delighted, but I was dumbfounded. This impossible problem was greatly relieved just from one position of comfort! Something had happened in his position of comfort that was far more therapeutic for his pain than four month's efforts supplied by three physicians! So far it was lasting. I was suddenly able to reduce my rate of failure from about thirty percent to about five percent. This was so much more effective than any other treatment I knew, I had to try to learn to use it on other problems. Along the way I made many mistakes, but when I did it right it worked on everything. I have been happily devoting the rest of my life to learning to use it and to teaching it to other physicians and physical therapists. It was a lucky accident and nothing more.

As I worked, trying to learn how to use comfortable positions to relieve backpain, I was able to observe many surprising things about how this part of the body behaved. As mentioned before I knew I must return the patient from his position of comfort slowly or his pain would return. My second accidental discovery was the location of the missing tenderpoints. Many of my previous failures, I believed, was because the only reliable diagnosis for me had been the tenderpoints found in the posterior paravertebral area close to the pain site. These, when present, assured a knowledge of where the affected joint was in distress and whether I had succeeded with my treatment. If I had succeeded, the tenderpoint and the pain were both much improved. Unfortunately only about half of the backaches were accompanied by these tenderpoints and other methods of diagnosis were often sketchy in my hands.

My second lucky day occurred perhaps three years after I had begun treating with positions of comfort. A patient I had treated once for a back that couldn't come out of a forward bend was improved enough he was able to hoe in his garden three days later. He called much disturbed that he struck himself in the groin with the end of his hoe handle and suffered agonizing pain. He told me he thought he had caused a "rupture."

When I examined him I found none of the classic symptoms of an inguinal hernia in spite of his sore spot. I reassured him about the hernia. Since he was due back for a second treatment for his back the following day, I suggested we do it while he was in the office to save him another trip.

By this time I had been able to reduce the length of time in the position of comfort to ninety seconds, but while I had him in his position of comfort again, I idly probed his tender groin again. The tenderness was mostly gone! He was pleased, but he set me off on another tangent. Could the missing tenderpoints not found in the posterior paravertebral area be over the front of the body? For the next three years I searched every square inch of the front of the body whenever I needed a tenderpoint and did find them. Half of them are on the front of the body where there is seldom any pain! Now I had a fast and nearly complete ability to make a reliable diagnosis. Partly because of improved ability to diagnose, my rate of success improved remarkably. Again I learned by a lucky accident. These points are not limited to the spinal disorders, but may be found near any joint of the body. Treating extremities involves much greater amplitude of movements than spinal treatment. The methods follow the same principles, but it is easier to observe the responses to motion. An expected strain starting a permanent pain here is hard to reconcile with a permanent damage to tissue. Pain complained of by a patient is a subjective sympton, able to be influenced by the personality of the patient and so considered less reliable. We were schooled to count on objective evidence, that learned first by the doctor. Since tenderpoints were not known by the patient until the doctor demonstrated their presence, they qualified as objective evidence for diagnosis. The tenderpoints in arms and legs were found not in the muscle strained, but in its antagonist! The antagonist had suffered no strain, but only a maximal shortening at the time its antagonist was being strained, followed by a sudden panic type lengthening.

I remembered that patients who knew exactly when their pain started, it was, "when I started to straighten up." Surely the severe unexpected strain, if it were due to damage of the strained tissue would have hurt the most at the moment of greatest strain, not, "when I started to straighten up." If the strained muscle should have healed in a few days, the permanent dysfunction must have been related to the sudden stretch of the antagonist after maximal shortening. From then on it behaved exactly as if it were being strained even when the joint was in a neutral position. The more it was stretched the more it hurt. Effective treatment and immediate comfort was obtained by again maximally shortening the antagonist of the weak painful muscle and restretching the supposedly lesioned muscle. If it had really been lesioned, my stretch would have aggravated the tissue damage. The false message of strain in the antagonist stopped even after months or years of dysfunction when it was made so short it couldn't continue to report in a strain. The fact that the pain and weakness that were felt by the patient were still on the side strained, was enough to insure the "obvious" diagnosis.

The idea of blaming the unstrained antagonist was so illogical no one else ever examined the antagonist.

If this phenomenon occurs in appendicular joints, it would be easy to believe it occurs in all joints.

Working with patients eight hours a day permitted me to observe these functions and dysfunctions of strained joints. The rationale for it all waited for Dr. Korr's article. "Proprioceptors and Somatic Dysfunction."

CASE HISTORIES

The physician is supplied with a source of information from his thousands of patients that is seldom available to scientists. At least occasionally he observes phenomena that offer insight into the nature of the conditions he treats. The following case histories illustrate, among other factors, the time element related to onset of continuing joint dysfunction. Many case histories offer significant information in the development of a particular concept. A case history that illustrates all of the points of a concept is rare; Case 1 is one such history.

<u>CASE 1:</u> The patient, a middle-aged, generally healthy factory worker, had a habit of napping for an hour or so on on his sofa in the living room before dinner. Several times during a nap, while lying supine, he would hang his right arm off the edge of the sofa in marked extension. (For a minute or two this position cannot be considered much of a strain, but for a period of forty-five minutes, it may become one.) His wife, preparing dinner in the next room, would look in on him occasionally. Worried about his position but not wanting to awaken him, she would very slowly and gently raise his arm and lay it over his chest. This performance was repeated several times over the years, with never a twinge in the man's arm when he wakened for dinner.

One day he napped when his wife was out, and, as before, he slept with his arm extended. A phone rang near his head and he awoke with a start, rapidly flexing his overstretched elbow. As he spoke on the phone he became aware of pain in his right biceps. He wasn't a worrier and didn't think much about it, until the pain gradually worsened. There was pain whenever he flexed his elbow, especially against resistance. His work called for much of this at the factory and he was afraid he would lose his job. In time, his biceps actually had become smaller and weaker. Now very concerned, he consulted physicians, who diagnosed strain of the biceps. Surgery was considered but not performed because careful probing did not demonstrate tenderness in the biceps where his pain was.

The man had been suffering for two years when he consulted me. Like the other physicians, I failed to elicit tenderness in the biceps. However, palpation revealed sharp tenderness beside the olecranon process of the ulna. (This is evidence of excessive proprioceptor activity in the triceps.) The triceps had never been overstretched, but had suffered only prolonged overshortening and sudden, panic-type lengthening. Yet, despite location of pain in the biceps, the abnormal myofascial tenderpoint was situated in the triceps.

Treatment consisted of positioning the elbow in hyperextension so that the biceps was put on a stretch and the triceps was allowed to shorten again maximally. If there had been tissue rupture in the biceps, surely this stretch would have aggravated the patient's condition. He was relieved immediately and left the office with half his pain gone. A few more similar treatments brought complete recovery and there was no recurrence. The biceps when I saw him six months later were restored to full size and strength.

The case is unusual only in that it demonstrates the importance of slow return from a strained position. The patient's wife did not know this; she was moving his arm slowly to avoid waking him. Yet her actions had served the purpose of aborting a potential joint dysfunction on possibly a dozen occasions. His pain did not start as long as his wife slowly returned his hyperextended elbow to a neutral position. The pain began because of his sudden flexion of a joint that had been overstretched in extension. Even more surprising, the continuing dysfunction, complete with its tenderpoint, was on the posterior aspect of the elbow where tissues had never been strained. The real strain, the pain, and the apparent weakness were on the front of the elbow and biceps, but the tenderpoint was on the extensor side of the elbow related to the triceps. The atrophy of the biceps had resulted from disuse; it recovered completely. No physician but me ever thought to examine the back of his arm.

CASE 2: A young man was running down some steps with low risers and wide treads, such as are found at the entrance of many public buildings. He ran a little too fast and overstepped with his left foot, so that only his heel landed on the edge of the step. His ankle was sharply and painfully strained or sprained in extension. There was residual pain and a weakness in lifting his foot. He scuffed his toes and occasionally stumbled, and he learned to raise the left knee higher than the right. The affected foot was strong enough for him to stand well, and he could even hop on it, but he couldn't lift his foot when he walked.

An orthopedist advised surgery for torn ligaments. The patient, not wishing to bear the substantial costs surgery would incur, consulted me. My examination revealed no tenderness in the anterior ankle. Sharp tenderness was found by palpation beside the attachment of the Achilles tendon. Treatment incorporated positioning of the ankle in hyperextension, which allowed hypershortening of the gastrocnemius muscle, holding the position for ninety seconds, and slowly returning to the neutral position. Two additional treatments were sufficient for lasting comfort. The tenderpoint and evidence of excessive proprioceptor activity were again on the opposite side from the real strain, the pain, and apparent weakness. Again my treatment stretched the area of supposedly torn ligaments.

CASE 3: A middle-aged businessman arrived home a little early for lunch one spring morning, so he squatted down and pulled a few weeds in the flower garden while he waited. He was still at it forty-five minutes later. Finally, his wife called him, and he arose suddenly and felt a low-back pain, which prevented him from standing erect. Examination revealed a myofascial tenderpoint in the psoas muscle. Treatment included marked thoracolumbar flexion until the tenderness subsided, holding the position for ninety seconds, then slowly returning to normal. Although the pain was in the back, there was no posterior tenderpoint. Assuming that forty-five minutes of squatting constitutes a strain for a businessman, the strain surely must have been in the posterior part of the spine. Apparently the only injury the psoas muscle had suffered was prolonged shortening and sudden lengthening. Just one treatment was needed because the patient sought treatment promptly.

CASE 4: A lady of seventy years sometimes, while seated, would nod off, then awaken with a start and raise her head off her chest. After one particularly long doze with her head down, followed by an abrupt awakening, she was unable to hold her head up, because of severe lower cervical pain radiating across the top of her shoulders. No tenderness was found posteriorly where the pain was located, but there was sharp sensitivity in the suprasternal notch, indicating dysfunction at the level of the first thoracic intervertebral joint. With the patient seated, and with her hands clasped over the top of her head, it was easy to attain marked cervico-thoracic flexion at that level. Ninety seconds of holding this position and slow return to neutral relieved her pain. She continued to have recurrences for several months. I assumed that this was because she was repeating the original strain, nodding off and jerking up on waking. No cure.

Far from being rare, this type of scenario is so standard as to become almost predictable. In many cases I examine the area near the pain just because a patient expects it. He is impressed at my finding a sharp tenderpoint where he has no pain, but he would be disappointed if I didn't examine the site of the pain.

Except for the ankle case, these histories follow a similar course—that of prolonged strain and sudden recovery. Regardless of the type of strain, whether prolonged or sudden and violent, successful treatment follows the same pattern.

RATIONALE OF TREATMENT

In my early years in practice, among other frustrating things about our treatment of rheumatic pain, was the fact that we didn't know just what the malady was or how our treatment influenced it. We had believed that a strain produced some sort of a mechanical disorder in the joint itself, not a complete dislocation, but a subluxation. We knew that once the strain had happened, the joint couldn't come all the way back from its position of strain without pain. It could move passively in the same direction as the strain without pain. If we had been thinking clearly, this fact alone should have made us suspicious of our belief in this problem as one of overstrained tissues. It now hurt to go into the opposite direction. We envisaged something lodged tightly enough it couldn't move back because of a bind or impingement in the joint.

A skilled pathologist did postmortems on several patients who had had longstanding back pain before death. He did macroscopic and microscopic studies of all joint tissues shortly after death and found no evidence of impingement and no limitation of motion. That left only muscles chronically contracted until death let them relax again until rigor mortis set in.

He disproved our concepts of joint impingement and subluxation. With evidence against overstrained tissues and subluxation we were in limbo, but he made a great contribution to the understanding of rheumatic pain. By the time I wanted to write about him I was unable to learn his name.

LESION OR DYSFUNCTION

The approach to disease has for a long time been oriented toward finding a lesion. There must be something that can be demonstrated by x-ray, ultrasound, computerized tomography or magnetic resonance—a real something to which we could point. To my knowledge none of them can show a dysfunctioning reflex.

For many patients suffering rheumatic pain we are often hard put to demonstrate any lesion, yet thought of a lesion is so compelling that thousands of patients suffering severe pain have been told by their physician that their pain was psychosomatic, because it was impossible for him to demonstrate a lesion. After a few physicians agree on this diagnosis, a patient may accept the idea that his pain is mental. Unless he finally finds relief, he now suffers from an iatrogenic neurosis as well. Several patients I have relieved have been as glad to prove their pain had been real as to get the relief of pain.

The history of these problems, remitting and exacerbating indefinitely but not healing, didn't fit any concept of a lesion so much as some ongoing process. It wasn't in any strain at time of examination, but it behaved exactly as it would, if it were in a strain. The response to changes of position was exactly what one would expect of a person really in a strain. If it wasn't real, at least that part of the body behaved as if it were real. Osteopathic physicians began to accept the idea of dysfunction or malfunction outside the joint proper—some kind of a sensation of continuing strain. An ongoing neuromuscular reflex would not show as any lesion.

We have thought "back strain" for so long that it is heresy to suggest that the source of all the pain and weakness is not on the side of the muscle that was strained and still hurts to contract, especially against resistance. It must have suffered permanent damage—a "strain that never heals," but there is no palpable evidence of strain or any kind of laceration in the muscle actually strained.

It was strained. It has been weak ever since and hurts to contract. But, the correct position of comfort doesn't shorten it; it strains it again! Our only logical conclusion must be false. For consolation this provides a surprising short cut. Stretch the painful muscle! Passive shortening aggravates the pain. When we say this couldn't be just backstrain, because it would have healed from any strain short of frank laceration within a few days instead of persisting through life, this makes our point. This has been proven millions of times by responses to treatment, and can be proven any time in the future, yet it seems so illogical, many are still unable to accept it. Thousands of patients have escaped surgery for "torn ligaments" because the surgeon could find no objective evidence at the site where the tear "obviously" was. So far as I have ever learned, none of them ever thought to probe on the opposite side of the joint where they would have easily found tenderness.

CONCLUSIONS AND POSTULATE

WORK OF IRVIN M. KORR, Ph.D.

All the previous observations don't explain what ongoing process this is or what kind of a dysfunction. How did it get there and why is it in the antagonist of the muscle strained? Just what is dysfunctioning? This was finally revealed in a paper by Irvin M. Korr, Ph.D., a physiologist, in his article "Proprioceptors and Somatic Dysfunction," *Journal of The American Osteopathic Association,* March 1975, Volume 74, No. 7.

Korr said, "To a physiologist it seems much more reasonable that the limitation and resistance to motion of a joint that characterizes an osteopathic lesion do not ordinarily arise within the joint, but are imposed by one or more of the muscles that traverse and move the joint."

The article provided a brief revue of proprioceptor reflexes and how they function normally. He described Rufini, Golgi, and especially blamed the primary or annulospiral proprioceptor reflexes in the muscle spindle. His hypothesis blames the rise in the exciting gamma outflow in response to the momentarily silent proprioceptor input from the spindle of the hypershortened antagonist muscle, causing an inappropriate "gain" in the primary proprioceptor reflexes in its muscle spindle. When it is restretched, it overreacts and reports strain before any real strain is reached.

Due to my long experience with the necessity of a slow return to a neutral muscle length from my position of comfort, I was especially excited by an earlier paragraph:

"One distinction may be worth mentioning. Although both types of (proprioceptor) endings are, more or less proportional to length, the primary (annulospiral) ending has the additional feature that, its frequency of firing during a stretch is in proportion to the rate of change. That is, the secondary ending reports length at any moment, but the primary ending reports velocity of stretch (hence joint motion) and length (hence joint position)."

CONCLUSIONS, MY POSTULATE

Although my early observations taken alone did not point in any useful way, in the light of Korr's revelation, they began to add up.

1. This is not a lesion, but an ongoing noxious process.

2. For success the hypershortened muscle must return to neutral length slowly.

3. In spite of subjective pain and weakness in the strained muscle objective evidence (tenderness, contraction, edema) were in the antagonist of the painful muscle.

4. Position of comfort and lasting relief come with maximum shortening of this antagonist and a repeated stretch of the painful muscle, followed by a slow return to neutral lengths. Slow return does not restart the dysfunction.

How does this continuing strain message begin? The primary proprioceptor in the antagonist is suddenly changed from maximal shortening to panic type lengthening so fast as to report strain before ever reaching its neutral length. From then on it reports strain where there is none and the joint behaves as if in strain. Continuing strain behavior is irritating and painful.

Counterstrain treatment again brings maximal shortening to the proprioceptor reporting strain so well it cannot continue to report strain. The false strain message is stopped and with it the irritation and pain.

If not somehow stopped, like other continuing irritations and inflammations, it ends in degeneration. So the inflammation and any degeneration are lesions, resulting not from the injury but from prolongued behavior as if in strain. Treatment itself does not cure; it only stops this irritation, finally permitting the body to cure itself. Stopping the irritation causes healing to begin. Maintaining it stopped gives the body opportunity to use its ability to heal itself for this problem too.

My postulate differs only slightly from Korr's revelation.

PHYSIOLOGY

PHYSIOLOGY OF MANIPULATION

By Edward K. Goering, DO, DVM, MSHPE

Before establishing the technique in your mind you must first understand the physiology involved in the creation of the osteopathic somatic lesion. This "lesion" has qualities that we can all appreciate. Tissue texture changes, asymmetry, changes in the range of motion of certain muscles and joints and tenderness that is manifested through the palpation of the patient's body. All of these fundamental changes are the physiologic manifestation of the somatic dysfunction. These somatic dysfunctions are detectable through the physiologic manifestations we recognize as tenderpoints. It is through the appreciation of this internal concept that we are able to perform the maneuvers of strain-counterstrain.

REVIEW OF THE ANATOMIC STRUCTURES

Joint capsule innervation. Table 1.1 is after neurohistologic studies that enable the visualization of these joint receptors (Wyke and Polacek, 1973[1] and 1975; Freeman and Wyke,[2] 1967; Vrettos and Wyke, 1979[3]). Each of these receptors will play an important role in this somatic dysfunction that is manifested with the tenderpoint of strain-counterstrain.

MECHANORECEPTORS

TYPE I—These receptors are thinly encapsulated, slow adapting, with small myelinated nerve pathways. These receptors will result in the inhibition of nociceptive

Table 1.1. Morphologic and functional characteristics of articular receptor symptoms (Wyke, 1979b; Freeman and Wyke, 1967)

Type	Morphology	Location	Source Nerve Fibers	Behavioral Charactertistics	Function
I	Thinly encapsulated globular corpuscles (100 um x 40 um) in clusters of 3–8	Fibrous capsulae of joint (superficial layers)	Small myelinated (6–9 um)	Static and dynamic mechanoreceptors: low threshold, slowly adapting	Tonic reflexogenic effects on neck, limb, jaw, and eye muscles. Postural and knesthetic sensation. Pain suppression
II	Thickly encapsulated conical corpuscles (280 um x 100 um) singly or in clusters of 2–4	Fibrous capsulae of joint (deeper layers). Articular fat pads	Medium myelinated (9–12 um)	Dynamic mechanoreceptors: low threshold, rapidly adapting	a) Phasic reflexogenic effects on neck, limb, jaw, and eye muscles. b) Pain suppression
III	Fusiform corpuscles (600 um x 100 um) usually singly, also in clusters of 2–3	Ligaments, also in related tendons	Large myelinated (13–17 um)	Mechanoreceptor: high threshold, very slowly adapting	
IV	Three-dimensional plexus of unmyelinated nerve fibers	Entire thickness of fibrous capsulae of joint. Walls of articular blood vessels. Articular fat pads	Very small myelinated (2–5 um), and unmyelinated	Nociceptor (pain-provoking): high threshold, nonadapting	a) Tonic reflexogenic effects on neck, limb, jaw, and eye muscles. b) Evocation of pain. c) Respiratory and cardiovascular reflexogenic effects

(pain) pathways at the level of the spinal cord. These are static and dynamic mechanoreceptors with a low threshold and slow adapting which function in the tonic reflexogenic effects on neck, limb, jaw, and eye muscles. They also participate in postural and kinesthetic or proprioceptive sensation.

TYPE II—These receptors are thickly encapsulated, rapidly adapting, with medium myelinated nerve pathways. These are suppress pain input. The Type II function as dynamic mechanoreceptors, with low threshold, and are rapidly adapting and are found in phasic reflexogenic effects on neck, limb, jaw, and eye muscles.

TYPE III—These receptors are fusiform corpuscles with large myelinated nerve pathways. These mechanoreceptors are high threshold, very slow adapting and are found located in ligaments and tendons. Their form resembles the ligamentous receptors of the golgi corpuscles and it can be assumed that they have a similar function. These slow adapting receptors have an inhibitory effect on motor neurons (Freeman and Wyke, 1967).[4]

NOCICEPTORS

TYPE IV—These receptors are high threshold, non-adapting three dimensional plexus of unmyelinated nerve fibers found in the entire thickness of the capsules of the joint capsule, within the walls of the articular blood vessels and in the articular fat pads. They can be stimulated with constant pressure, as with narrowing of the intervertebral disk, dislocation of articular joints, or by chemical irritation of tissue metabolites or a chronic inflammatory process. These receptors have very small mylenated and unmyelinated fiber pathways. These are involved in the function of tonic reflexogenic effects on neck, limb, jaw, and eye muscles.

Joint capsule innervation is a balanced interaction between mechanoreceptors and nociceptive input. It has been demonstrated in the dorsal horn of the spinal cord that mechanoreceptors require much less stimuli to fire than do nociceptors in normal physiologic situations. This relationship requires an increased rate of firing in the nociceptors to overcome the dampening effect of the mechanoreceptors. This relationship is demonstrated in Figure 1.2 (Wyke, 1979).

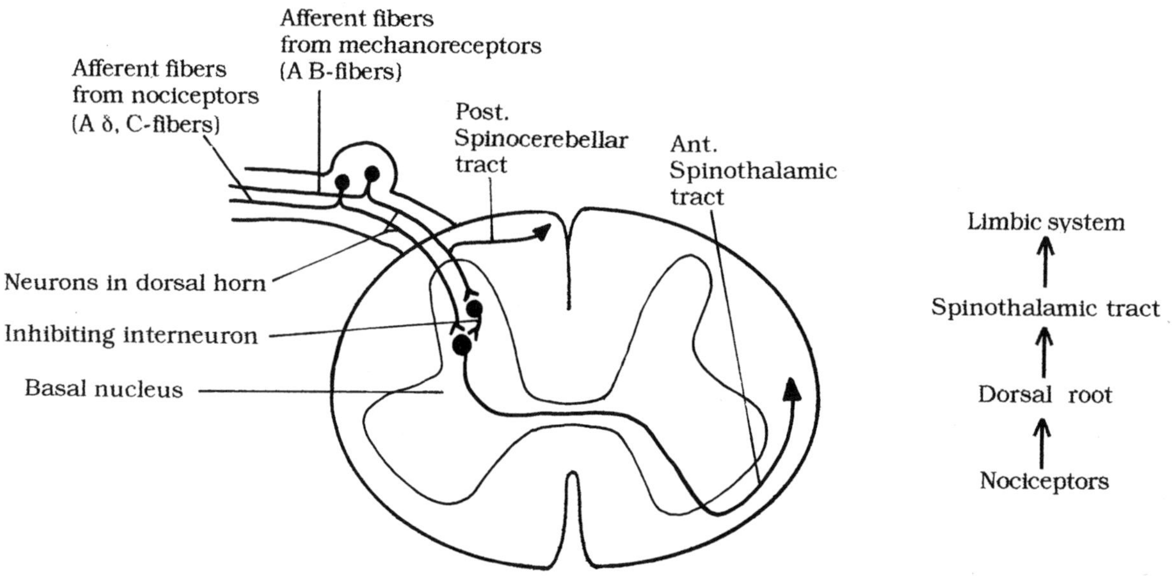

Figure 1.2 **Fibers of nociceptors and mechanoreceptors in the region of the posterior horns (after Wyke, 1979)**

The perception of pain requires the perceptual input to travel through the basal nuclei (basal spinal nucleus or lamina IV and V after Rexed). The mechanoreceptors provide a dampening effect on the nociceptive input through the interneuron. This effectively blocks the transport of information to the spinothalamic tract and the limbic system (Wyke, 1979[5]; Bonica and Albe-Fessard, 1980[6]). These interneurons are believed to have their inhibitory effect through an endogenous enkephalin which serves as an inhibiting neurotransmitter. Stimulation of the Type II mechanoreceptors leads to a depot like storage increase in the levels of enkephalins in the dorsal horn (Wyke, 1983[7]). Perhaps it is through these same mechanisms that the opioids have their pain inhibiting effects.

Wyke showed that much less voltage is required to stimulate the mechanoreceptor input than that required to stimulate the nociceptors. Sato (1975)[8] made similar observations. Based on clinical observations, a relationship between soft tissue changes, segmental (somatic) dysfunction and diseases of internal organs have been observed (Beal and Dvorak, 1984[9]; Larson, 1976[10]).

Korr[11] and Denslow discovered and documented the relationship between the somatic dysfunction and the sympathetic nervous system which has become an accepted concept within the osteopathic community. This altered neurologic relationship, called a "facilitated segment," is perhaps the best way to understand how the tenderpoint is created. The tenderpoint is a manifestation of the facilitated segment, which in turn is the expression of the somatic dysfunction which often is detectable by changes in tissue texture, asymmetry, alteration in the range of motion and tenderness both at the site of dysfunction as well as in the referred tenderpoint of strain-counterstrain. Chronic pain can induce long term changes in the tissue involved.

Table 1.3. Characteristics of slow twitch and fast twitch muscle fibers.

Flexion	Slow Twitch (I)	Fast Twitch (II)
Function	tonic (postural)	phasic
Twitch speed	slow	fast
Metabolism/enzymes	oxidative	glycolytic
Myosin ATPase	low activity	high activity
Fatigability rate	slow	rapid
"Color"	red	white
Capillary density	high	low
Spindle number	high	moderate
Innervation	a_2-motor neuron	a_1-motor neuron
Reaction to functional disturbance	shortening	weakening

MUSCLE PHYSIOLOGY AND NEUROLOGIC WIRING

Human muscles are of two types. Each of these types has inherent characteristics as seen in the Table 1.3.[12] Each of these make up various proportions of the overall muscles. This proportion is determined primarily by the type of exercise and function these muscles perform. Postural muscles, also known as tonic muscles have a greater proportion of slow twitch (Type I) fibers. Phasic muscles have a greater proportion of fast twitch (Type II) fibers. The physiology of the individual muscles is determined to a large extent by the function.

Fast twitch fibers are high in glycolytic enzymes as well as myosin ATPase activity and depend on anaerobic metabolism. These fibers accumulate lactic acid and tend to fatigue much more rapidly than the postural muscles. Postural muscles on the other hand are high in oxidative enzymes and are low in glycolytic enzymes. Energy is derived for these muscles through aerobic mechanisms, utilizing fat and glycogen as the primary source. This metabolic process produces very little lactic acid.

These slow twitch fibers in contrast to the fast twitch are resistant to fatigue and have the endurance required by the postural muscles. Vascular and nerve supply varies as well. The slow twitch fibers have a more extensive capillary bed than do the fast twitch fibers and are innervated by alpha-2 fibers with a very high concentration of spindle fibers. Fast twitch fibers are innervated by alpha-1 fibers and have relatively few muscle spindles (Richmond and Abrahams, 1979[13]). This disparity in the number of muscle spindles is believed to be a reflection of the function of the muscles. These physiologic and anatomic differences result in different responses to irritation. The slow twitch respond by shortening and the fast twitch fibers respond by weakening.

We see that these changes have an interesting implication when understanding counterstrain. Phasic muscles involved with counterstrain tenderpoints are frequently seen to have weakness on exertion. Postural muscles with tenderpoints are seen to manifest themselves with shortening that is treated by shortening the offended muscle.

Afferent input from the muscles is via one of five receptors. These are muscle spindles, golgi tendon organs, pacinian corpuscles, free nerve endings (nociceptors, Type IV), and mechanoreceptors (Type III). When trying to understand the physiology of manipulation it is imperative that one becomes familiar with the function of the muscle spindle and the golgi tendon organs which function as tension monitoring receptors.

Muscle spindles are very sensitive to changes in length and when stretched sufficiently will induce reflex contraction of the same muscle and help in the process of reciprocal inhibition of the antagonistic muscles. These specialized fibers are intimately involved in the facilitated segment of osteopathic medicine. Muscles responsible for fine and precise movement have a significantly higher concentration of spindles than those muscles that must accomplish more gross movement. The small sub occipital muscles have approximately 150–200 muscle spindles per gram of muscle tissue, whereas the rectus femoris muscle has only 50 muscle spindles per gram of muscle tissue (Richmond and Abrahams, 1979[14]). An exceptionally high level of muscle spindles is found in the paraspinal musculature. As much as 200–500 spindles per gram of tissue. This concentration of spindles tends to be around the slow twitch fibers.

Once again the relationship between somatic dysfunction and clinical experience is validated. Postural muscles shortening with over stimulation and the phasic muscles become weaker.

The muscle spindle is composed of three to eight slender, specialized muscle fibers, referred to as intrafusal fibers. Muscle spindle intrafusal fibers are embedded in a network in the body of each muscle. These individual spindles line up in parallel with groups of muscle fibers, concentrated heavily around the slow twitch fibers. These intrafusal fibers are surrounded by the balance of skeletal muscle tissue called extrafusal fibers. The overall apparatus includes the annulospiral nerve endings (Ia afferent nerve endings), the flower spray nerve endings (II afferent nerve endings), the alpha and gamma motor efferents, and the intrafusal fibers, Figure 1.4. The spindle apparatus monitors stretch and rate of change.

The golgi tendon organs (type Ib afferent nerve endings) are imbedded in the musculotendinous area at the distal ends of the muscles. These receptors measure muscle tension and are more sensitive to stretch during contraction. Sufficient impulses from the golgi tendon organs will result in inhibition of the muscle innervated and its synergists and facilitate the antagonists (Granit, 1955, 1975, 118–119[15,16]).

MUSCLE SPINDLE FUNCTION, THE ALPHA-GAMMA COACTIVATION

The complex muscle spindles interspersed among skeletal fibers, offer the most important sensory feed back from the muscles (Figure. 1.4). One large sensory annulospiral afferent nerve (Ia fiber) has fibers that entwine around each muscle spindle (intrafusal muscle fibers). A second afferent nerve fiber (Ib fibers), the flower spray ending is located near the extremities of the spindle apparatus. These fibers communi-

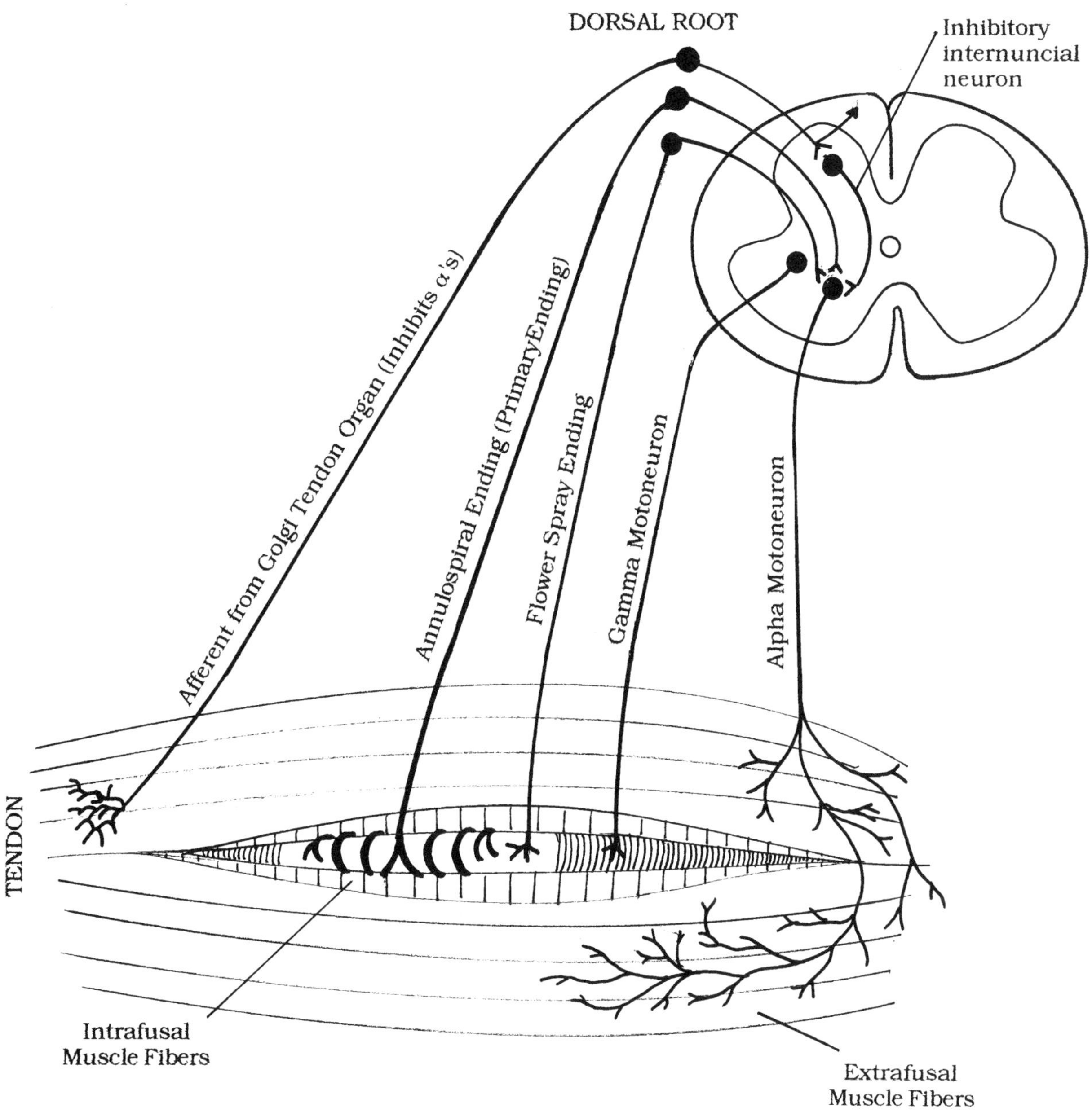

Muscle Spindle Apparatus (after E. K. Goering, DO)

Figure 1.4

cate information about fiber length (contraction magnitude) in respect to the amount of stretch. These same nerve endings are able to communicate about the rate of stretch (velocity). This is the function of alpha-gamma coactivation through which the afferent receptors are able to enter into the circuit and excite a feedback stretch reflex that produces contraction of the muscle of origin. It also causes reciprocal inhibition of the antagonists. Examining Figure 1.5 by Hassler will allow the reader to understand the intricacies of this elegant design (Hassler, 1981[17]).

Stimulation of the gamma-2 efferent neurons will result in the contraction of the

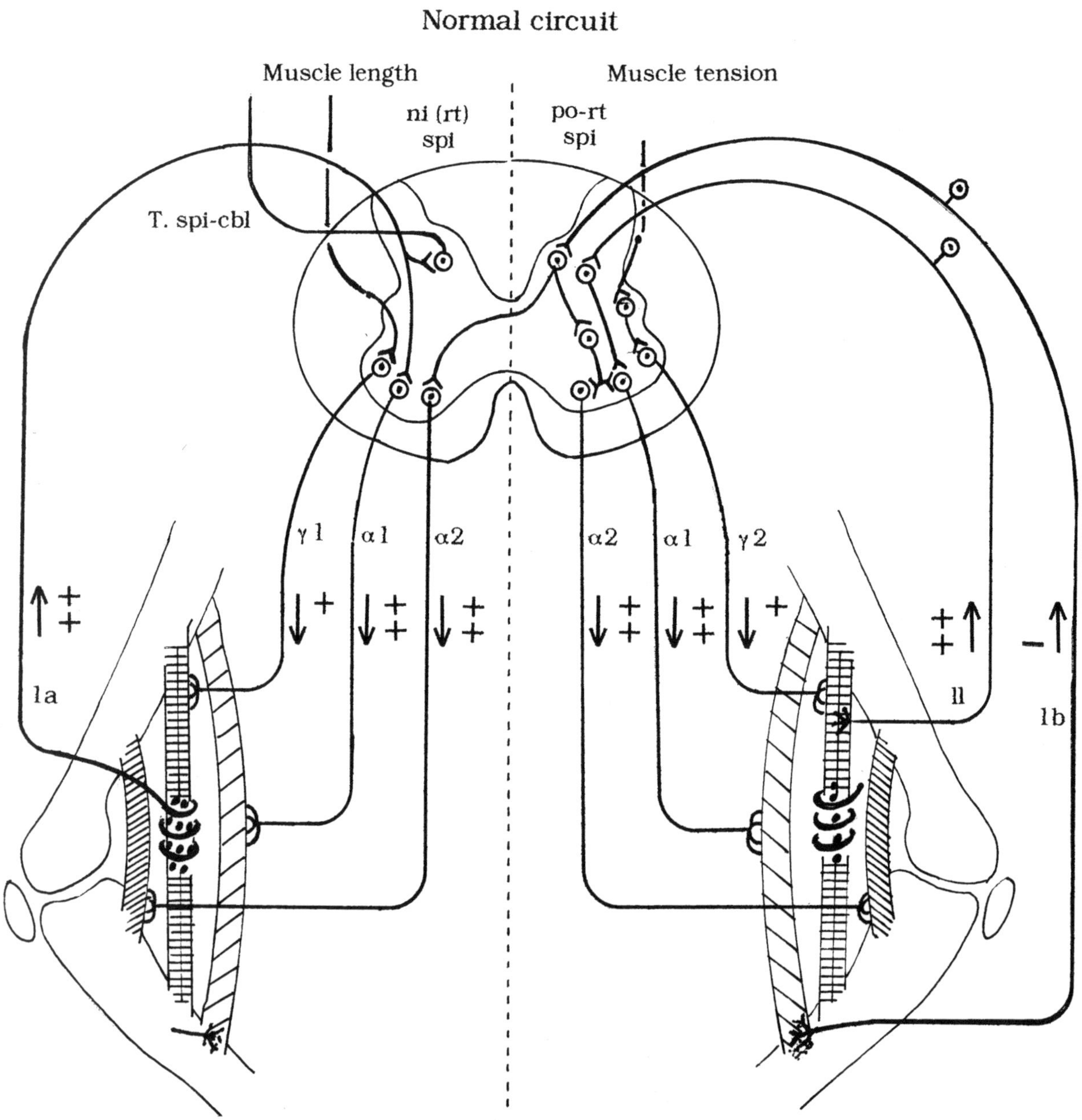

Control of muscle length (circuit on the left) and muscle tension (right) with the appropriate reflex arc (after Hassler)

Figure 1.5

intrafusal fiber. This tension is conveyed via the type II afferent fibers to the spinal cord where there is activation of the alpha-efferent fibers which will increase tone in the phasic muscles primarily and via the alpha-2 efferent fibers which exert their influence on the postural muscles. The length of the muscles is maintained as long as the nuclear chain fibers are kept at the same length by the influence of a tonic stimulus from the gamma-2 efferent neurons. This input is derived from higher brain centers. Contraction of the extrafusal fibers will relax or induce a flaccid state in the spindle reducing the rate of firing from the annulospiral endings which in turn will reduce the strength of contraction, creating a fine balance that may control velocity as well as distance in movement. Stretch applied to both elements will result in contraction of the extrafusal fibers increasing the tone in both postural and phasic muscles with the expected results: weakness in the phasic muscles and increased tone with spasm in the postural muscles.

Safeguarding the anatomic integrity of the structure is the golgi tendon apparatus which produces a marked inhibitory effect on the alpha-1 and alpha-2 fibers when the amplitude of the stretch becomes too severe. This is sometimes referred to as a "Relief Reflex."

The final analysis is that muscle tension is under the influence of two control mechanisms, the spindle apparatus and the secondary relief reflex that help regulate the tension and control movement.

From studies involving a single muscle annulospiral ending, as well as from studies from the entire root portion, the following observation was made: tetanic stimulation of a single muscle spindle or gamma-efferent caused an increased discharge pattern at the respective annulospiral ending. A shortening of the spindle led to a decrease in the discharge (Dvorak, Dvorak, 1990[18]). This in turn would result in a decrease in the positive feedback that occurs between the spindle apparatus and the extrafusal muscle fibers.

In work done with the phenomena of sensitization, habituation and fixation (spinal memory) are described (Groves, et al, 1968[19], 1970[20]; Patterson and Steinmetz, 1986[21]). With this theory some movements, such as an inappropriate step might result in a slight strain, or even more severe muscle trauma that would disrupt this balance that exists between these proprioceptive mechanisms and the higher levels of the CNS and the interplay that occurs at the level of the spinal cord. This research in conjunction with that of Korr and Denslow (reviewed 1975[22]), demonstrates the increase level of firing of the sympathetic nervous system at the level of the somatic dysfunction. This increased muscle tone associated with that phenomenon demonstrates in part how the somatic dysfunction is created and in turn maintained. We should now turn our attention to yet another factor that seems to be playing an important role in the development and maintenance of the somatic dysfunction, the nociceptive input.

NOCICEPTIVE INPUT AND MUSCLE TONE

We have previously described the innervation of the muscle tissues. Ia afferent provides input from the primary muscle spindle apparatus and Ib afferents provides input from the golgi tendon organs. The Type II afferents innervate the distal ends of the intrafusal fibers and also report tension of the spindle apparatus. There are also three dimensional free nerve endings called nociceptors. There is less known about these fibers. They are believed to serve the purpose of registering actual tissue damage or toxic stimuli. Mense (1977)[23] discovered that the nociceptors of the muscles are not a uniform group. They can be activated by chemicals (bradykinen, potassium, serotonin, and hypoxia) and mechanically (firing in the presence of prolonged muscle contraction or ischemic changes which may indeed be due to metabolite buildup. In Figure 1.6 Schmidt, et al. (1981)[24] demonstrated that stimulation of the small fiber muscle afferents, nociceptive input (Type III and IV),

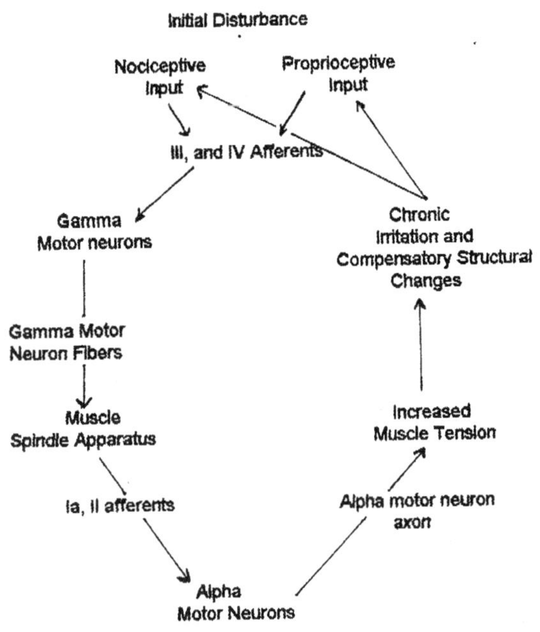

Modified after Schmidt et al. (1981)

Figure 1.6

had direct input to the alpha and gamma fibers. This input was shown to be with significant intensity. From this data we can surmise that the small caliber afferents can have a dramatic impact on the duration, location, and intensity of muscle tone. Findings from these animal studies illustrate that stimulation of these receptors by pain induction and chronic irritation of the small fiber afferents (Type III and IV), and the direct input they have on the alpha-gamma loop will create as well as maintain the somatic dysfunction.

Examining the input we have accumulated thus far, we realize the increased tone of the somatic dysfunction is initially created in many ways. Visceral pain, viscerosomatic nociception, may cause an increase in the rate of sympathetic firing with an increase and perhaps maintained increase in muscle tone at the level of the segment involved. Generalized anxiety of the patient can result in marked increase in the sympathetic tone that may not cause the specific alteration in the alpha-gamma loop but certainly provides an environment that predisposes for that outcome. The understanding of the habituation and sensitization theory can allow one to understand how a short term alteration in the alpha-gamma loop may be created and in the proper environment, may be maintained through the positive feedback of the positive nociceptive increase in tone and the associated pathology that exists with this situation. Finally trauma that initiates and maintains the changes in the tone are easily accepted on clinical experience as well as a research basis.

This positive feedback mechanism is illustrated in Figure 1.6. The primary disturbance: a misstep, a visceral disease process (myocardial infarction, irritable bowel disease), a severe muscle strain with inappropriate care or the acute nociceptive input that deranges the normal alpha-gamma loop initiates the process with stimulation of the nociceptors. This in turn induces increased firing rates to the gamma motor neuron which then induces increased tension in the spindle. This increased tension causes an increased rate of firing in the Ia and II afferents with an increase in firing of the alpha motor neuron. This increase in firing rate will cause the extrafusal fiber tone to be increased with the long term changes of chronic irritation and somatic dysfunction to ensue which in turn perpetuates the pathologic state. Fassbender (1980)[25] reported the changes of regressive muscle damage caused by a chronic myotendinosis (localized muscle spasm).

The "Nervous Misinformation" of Schmidt's (1981)[26] positive feedback loop results in the myotendinotic changes described by Fassbender (1980). These changes are well described in *Manual Medicine,* Dvorak and Dvorak, 1990.[27] Segmental dysfunction will lead to the stimulation of mechanoreceptors and nociceptors. This in turn affects the reflexes of the CNS with the misinformation output inducing the myotendinosis seen clinically.

A variety of scenarios then ensue. Long

term increase in muscle tone will overload the tendons and impair an already marginal circulation. This will result in localized lack of oxygen at the cellular level leading to progressive degenerative tendon changes.

What then is the role of manipulation in the correction of the somatic dysfunction? An ideal model would find a body in correct anatomic position. This would reflect normal pressures and tension in the myofascial tissues. The mechanoreceptors would have their proper dampening effect on the nociceptive input of the tissues and the normal resting tone would be present in the myofascial tissues, with a dynamic equilibrium present between the antagonists, synergists. and agonists. This would be the normal pain free state. These painfree states are also found clinically with only anatomically palpable changes including those of the tenderpoints of strain-counterstrain. Wyke[28] demonstrated that nociceptors had a much higher threshold than did the pain inhibiting mechanoreceptors. With sufficient mechanoreceptor (Type II primarily) stimulation the nociceptive input may/can be inhibited presynaptically delaying the time it may become consciously perceived. This delay is a function of the enkephalins from internuncial inhibiting cells in the substantia gelatinosa of the spinal cord.

In the correction of the somatic dysfunction, we are pressed to examine where in the model our input occurs. The abberrant reflexogenic state causes the myotendinous changes previously described that induce changes that are found acutely and chronically. These are supplemented with additional impulses, mechanical and chemical, and if sufficient nociceptive input is present to overcome the dampening of the mechanoreceptors pain will be perceived through the spinothalamic tract and the limbic system. Counterstrain corrects the aberrant alpha-gamma loop misinformation as well as other mechano-receptor misinformation and restores the normal tone to the tissues. The severity, acuteness, chronicity, and emotional investment of the injury will all determine the length of treatment required for resolution of the lesion.

ROLE OF THE MUSCLE

Figure 1 Figure 2 Figure 3

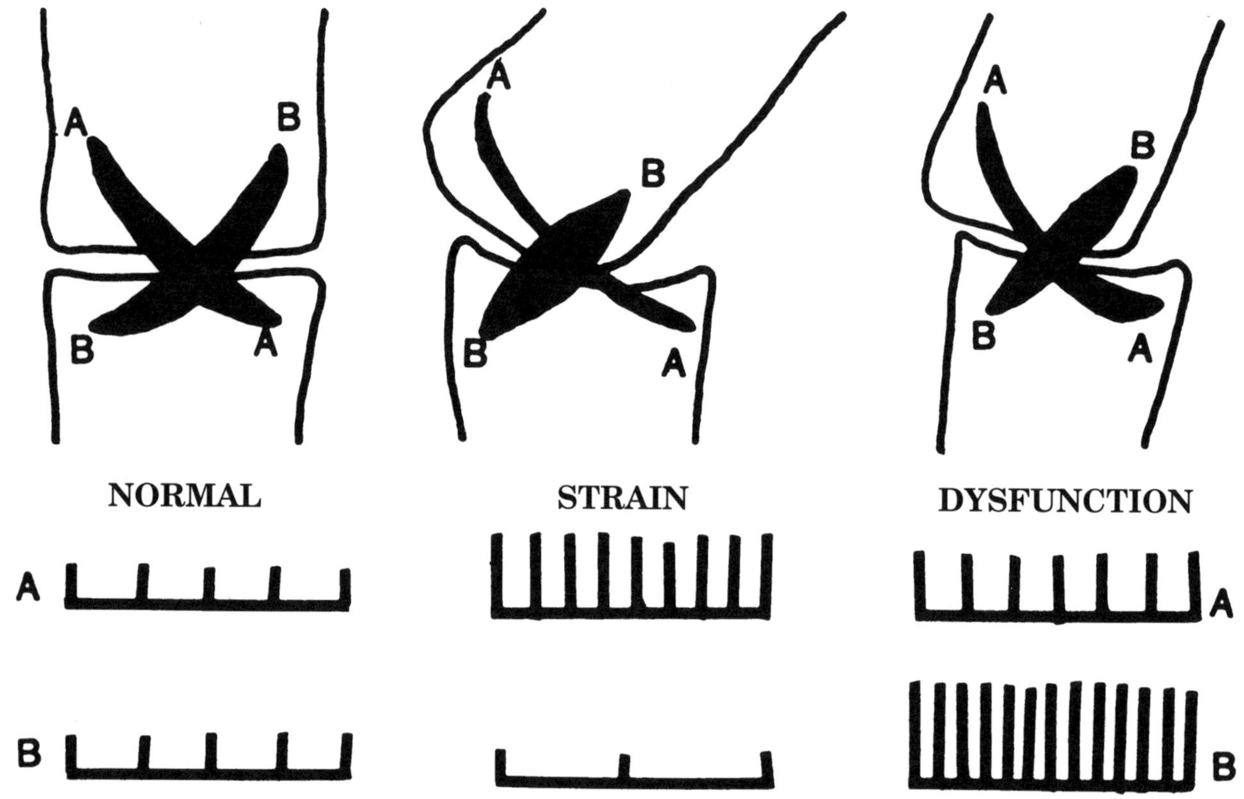

SOMATIC MODE AND PROPRIOCEPTOR ACTIVITY

This is a schematic representation of the reactions of muscles around a joint that goes through a strain and a successful counterstrain treatment.

In Figure 1, the joint is a neutral position. Both muscles are in a state of mild tonic tension, ready for whatever demands the brain and nervous system put on them. Proprioceptor activity is shown to be present, but low and equal in both antagonistic muscles. This is just normal physiology.

Figure 2 shows a severe strain of the joint; one of the muscles shows a great increase in proprioceptor activity due to stretch, while the other which has been abnormally shortened, shows almost a complete drop to zero. This is still not a dysfunction, just normal physiology of the neuromuscular reflexes doing their work. This joint can still be moved slowly directly back into its neutral position with no pain and no beginning dysfunction. All effects will disappear in a few days.

If this were a deliberate strain and return, this would be the story, but this is an unexpected and painful experience, probably involving a panic tensing of the strained muscle to protect the body from permanent injury. This sudden powerful contraction of the strained muscle probably comes from an overriding nociceptor reflex. It results in an equally sudden lengthening of its antagonist, muscle B, from its condition of maximal shortening and almost zero proprioceptor activity, except for possible gain from the ever watchful gamma outflow. This nociceptor override and the panic response serves to lengthen the maximally shortened muscle so fast that it starts reporting itself in a strain before ever reaching its neutral length. Now the proprioceptor in the antagonist is dysfunctioning and the joint cannot return further toward neutral length. Even though shorter than neutral length, it is reporting strain, so the treatment will be to return the joint and its muscles to their original position of strain. This will again hypershorten the antagonist to make it stop reporting strain even after years of dysfunction. Then after holding it there for ninety seconds a slow return to neutral will not cause the pain to return. The dysfunction has stopped.

PRACTICE OF COUNTERSTRAIN

POSITION OF MAXIMUM COMFORT

Despite all the sophisticated diseases listed in the *Merc Manual,* two thirds of all human body pain comes from one poorly understood malady—rheumatic pain. It is almost universal in one form or another and is uniquely everlasting, because it is seldom cured or even correctly diagnosed.

Modern medicine alone isn't effective in treating it, because it isn't a medical problem, but a physical problem, a malfunctioning neuromuscular reflex reporting continuous strain where there is none.

This malfunction can be stopped with a simple body stretch to a position of maximum comfort which shortens the muscle supposedly in strain enough that it now reports no more strain. After only ninety seconds in this stretch, it may be returned slowly to a neutral position and still remain pain free.

A novice can succeed with this method on his first attempt just by trying different positions and repeatedly asking the patient whether he is more or less comfortable. If he finds comfort for the patient, he will relieve the pain. A physician skilled in feeling the changes in the tenderpoints that accompany all of these pains can relieve two thirds of all body pains with a success rate of ninety-five percent, which is much higher than with most other methods. With good patient cooperation, by repeatedly turning off this malfunction. he can produce a permanent cure in eighty-five percent, tremendously higher than with most other methods.

The physician only stops the malfunctioning of the strain reflex and its continuous irritation, enabling the body to heal what it couldn't heal before. Patient cooperation is extreme avoidance of painful positions or efforts for a few weeks. These painful positions and efforts can easily restart the malfunctioning of the strain reflex and stop the healing.

As the inflammation subsides, the danger of causing a pain (and a return of the false strain reflex) gradually becomes much less until healing is complete. That is a cure that will last a lifetime. Once tissues have healed, a severe new strain of the joint will be necessary before a recurrence will take place.

The skill most necessary is learning to feel tissue tension of the tenderpoints and the changes in them in response to positioning of the patient's body. This seems frightening to most beginners, because they don't believe that they can learn to feel these changes. Simple practice will increase palpatory skills manyfold. Almost everyone who tries can learn to feel all that is necessary. The author learned to feel more in two years practicing with counterstrain than in the previous nineteen years he had practiced with thrusting techniques. Anyone able to feel a pulse can develop enough ability. This involves fine tuning the position to its ideal degree, because a surprising part of the relief occurs within a positional change of less than two degrees.

Until he has developed some palpatory skill, he can proceed by trying some position and asking his patient whether he is better or worse. Patients will be found to be very certain of the ideal relief. Later when he is able to find the ideal position by monitoring the changes with his finger tips, it makes his work much faster and more accurate. It even brings him to the level where he can be confident of a good position even when a patient is still saying, "It hurts." These patients will agree they are comfortable thirty seconds later. This pain started after a strain or sprain, although patients usually have forgotten the original strain by the time they seek help. Exacerbations of pain usually occur after relatively slight strains. "I just bent over to pick up a piece of paper!" The pain may subside for several days or weeks after injury, but this isn't recovery, just a partial and temporary remission. An exacerbation at the same site is almost certain sometime in the future. Most will progress to a state of chronic continuous pain.

TENDERPOINTS

These are points of hypersensitivity found with almost all of these pains. They are beneath the skin, smaller than a finger tip and are about four times normal in tenderness to finger probing; they are enough to make a patient flinch from a pressure not at all painful to normal tissue. They are valuable for diagnosis and the changes in tension that can be felt for monitoring the success of the treatment. Each is specific for one joint dysfunction and nearly always for the position that will relieve it. This fact serves to reduce any "complex pain" to its causative elements.

A patient presents with what he thinks of as "a pain." In reality, by the time he has arrived at the office, this pain is often composed of three or four elements of irritation, making both diagnosis and treatment confusing. Each tenderpoint is specific for one source of irritation, so the physician needs to search for the tenderpoints of all likely areas to learn the location of all of the sources of "a pain." By noting the different degrees of tenderness he can schedule his treatments and treat the most severe first. This serves to take the guesswork out of treatment and reduces the likelihood of having a new pain develop while he is treating another nearby. He will feel tissue tension and swelling. When position of comfort is found, there is a rapid relaxation felt at the tenderpoint. During the ninety seconds before he starts to return the body to a neutral position, he can feel further softening thought to be due to resorption of edema. Surprisingly the point is often found where the pain is not. When a physician is skilled in finding, feeling, and monitoring the changes in these points, he can check for about six spots for tenderness each minute with each hand and make a comprehensive diagnosis of all the causes for any "pain" in two minutes or less. During treatment he rests his finger lightly over the tenderpoint to aid his ability to feel changes, probing occasionally to be certain the patient agrees that tenderness is subsiding, as he feels the tension subside under his finger tip. This patient feedback is what "coaches" him in learning palpatory skill.

Until one develops confidence in his ability to feel these changes, he can treat them and say, "walk around a little. Do you still hurt?" "Yes, right here." "Then get back on the table." It is there to be had every time.

ANTERIOR TENDERPOINTS

Originally we knew only of tenderpoints in the posterior, paravertebral areas of the spine. When present these provided enough information that we could check the point for tenderness before and after treatment to be sure of success. If treatment was sucessful, tenderness was much reduced. Unfortunately only about half the pains were accompanied by these points and we were called upon to depend on some other form of diagnosis, which for me was much less reliable. I longed for the other tenderpoints, because most of my failures were in cases with inadequate tenderpoints. This was resolved for me again with no credit to myself, because it was another accident.

A few days before I had treated a patient who had stood humped over forward until after treatment. He was relieved well enough three days later that he was able to hoe his garden.

While hoeing he struck a root with his hoe deflecting it enough that he hit himself in the groin with the end of the hoe handle, causing excruciating pain. He called on the phone that he had ruptured himself. When I examined him he did have a terribly tenderpoint, but none of the classic signs of hernia and I was glad to reassure him. Since his appointment for the next treatment of his back was to be the next day, I treated him one day early. By this time I had learned to hold the position for just ninety seconds. In his treatment he lay supine and I raised his legs and rotated them to one side. When he was comfortable I had nothing to do for ninety seconds, but hold him there. Just for idle curiosity I probed his "rupture" again—gently at first and then firmly and still elicited no pain! Could all the other much needed tenderpoints be on the front of the body? Surely not. My patients didn't complain of front pain, just back pain. But I was off on a new tangent. For three years I searched every inch of the front of the bodies where I needed a tenderpoint and did find them all! The missing half of the tenderpoints are on the front of the body. Now I have a full complement of the tenderpoints that, to me, spell the difference between knowing what I am doing half the time and all the time.

Ninety-five percent of the tenderpoints needed are shown in illustrations in the book, but they are not visible, and must be found by probing for them. Pressure of the probing finger is less than the amount that would cause pain in a normal spot. Five percent the physician will have to find for himself, but after many hours of using the ones shown, he will be able to locate almost any one he needs and monitor its changes.

Development of this skill requires hours a day of hands on effort to find the tenderpoints and to produce the necessary positions on patients, working with real problems. Fortunately, there is no shortage of real problems to practice on.

Practice on a healthy subject in order to learn ideal positions is a waste of time, because the operator is not guided by patient feedback.

Time required to develop necessary skills does not depend so much on aptitude as dedication. Eight hours of effort a day for two years is enough to become highly competent and effective with it. During all of this practice he is rewarded by successfully relieving pains and so building his confidence. Skills continue to improve as long as he practices. The author, with nothing to go on, but one accidental success, devoted eight years to practicing the method, and nearly always felt well rewarded for his efforts. By this time he was so delighted with his successes he wanted to share his good fortune with his colleagues.

If a student adopts a half-hearted, occasional attempt to use this method, his skills will never become adequate and his results will not be much better than with other methods. Fortunately, while he is learning, there need be little danger of doing his patient harm, if he just observes three simple rules of procedure:

1. Stretch the affected joint passively into its position of greatest comfort;
2. Return him slowly enough that his pain doesn't return; and
3. Always avoid any sudden return, even if the position is painful. Usually here it is best just to back off a little and wait a few seconds and then proceed slowly again.

Before skills are acquired, almost all failures are due to a lack of skill, rather than inadequacy of the method itself.

Once a physician is skilled, he never abandons this form of treatment for any other method. He is too pleased with his new ability.

STRAIN AND COUNTERSTRAIN IN THE MANUAL MEDICINE ARMAMENTARIUM

By Randall S. Kusunose, PT, OCS

The therapeutic uses for strain and counterstrain range from acute injuries to the chronic pain patient, infant torticollis to the fragile osteoporotic, post-operative pain to secondary tone in the neurologically involved patient. It is gentle and atraumatic and therefore enjoys a broad application for patients with somatic dysfunction. It is "user friendly" and equally gentle on the operators. It is most easily performed in an office on a Hi-Lo treatment table but can be easily modified to the inpatient hospital setting or home treatment setting. It can be used as a sole treatment procedure or as an adjunct to other manual medicine techniques.

It is the treatment of choice with the acute patient because it is so gentle and atraumatic. The patient's body is moved slowly in nonpainful directions to positions that are non-threatening and readily within their limited range of motion. The operator is guided by local decrease in tissue tension and relief of palpatory tenderness to find the optimal position of release. Dramatic changes can be made in relief of subjective pain complaint, diminished muscle guarding spasms, and reduction of congested inflammatory fluid. Treating the neuromuscular component to the acute condition facilitates improved circulation and promotes the body's ability to heal the injured or damaged tissue.

The gentleness of strain and counterstrain makes it safe and effective for treating pain conditions related to the fragile elderly patient (i.e., arthritis, osteoporosis), pregnant patient, and infants. Pain associated with primary joint or bone disease can be eased with simple positioning that feels good to the patient. Pain reduction then facilitates the introduction of exercise and other rehabilitation techniques to increase patient's function. Sacral and pubic pain associated with pregnancy can be helped tremendously. The effect is sometimes temporary owing to the constant load on the musculoskeletal system but home treatment positioning can be taught which supports the office treatment and assists in maintaining a comfortable status. Postural deviation and pain seen with infant torticollis is managed with positioning that exaggerates the postural deviation. Moving in the direction of comfort and ease the infant is taken willingly to a posture that imitates and is only slightly more extreme than the posture that he/she came in with. Often dramatic results are seen in a singular treatment. Infant cooperation is far greater when the treatment does not hurt.

The strain and counterstrain approach is valuable with chronic patients for two reasons. First, a scan evaluation for tenderpoints provides a quick assessment that allows the operator to uncover the areas of major dysfunction contributing to the pain complaint. Proper treatment sequencing can then be done. Second, the treatment will overcome the aberrant flow of afferent impulses in the involved musculature which have fixated joint motion maintaining longterm dysfunction. Restoring the normal neuromuscular reflexes balances the muscular forces that effect joint function. Increased range of motion, relief of pain, and improved joint function results.

Patients with severely restricted range of motion (i.e., adhesive capsulitis, spondylosis, post-operation) find strain and counterstrain helpful to reduce pain and secondary muscle guarding. Positions of comfort are easily found but within the available ranges which will be in lesser degrees of motion than in patients with full range of motion. Measurable gains in range and quality of motion can be made. Reduction of pain and muscle guarding facilitates the effectiveness of direct mechanical mobilization and rehabilitative exercise. The integration of these techniques is valuable to regain maximum range of motion and function.

The neurologically involved patient with aberrant tone can also receive benefit from positional release. Reduction of aberrant tone is accomplished by maximally shortening the involved muscle. The skilled operator is guided less, by a decrease in palpable tenderness and more by tissue tension changes. The operator is able to guide the unwinding with a motion hand in the involved tissue until optimum softening occurs. For example, this approach can diminish the flexor tone in the painful stroke shoulder facilitating functional activities or reposition the subluxed stroke shoulder by reducing the tone in the latissimus dorsi.

Strain and counterstrain can make a significant contribution when integrated with other manual medicine procedures. Combining strain and counterstrain with direct action techniques (i.e., muscle energy, direct myofascial release) for joint dysfunction that presents with neuromuscular and mechanical components (i.e., capsular adhesions, ligamentous fibrosis) often brings about the best therapeutic outcome.

Strain and counterstrain and muscle energy technique can be combined with effective results. Re-establishing the normal neuromuscular reflexes prior to contraction and stretching of mechanically restricted tissues enhances the effectiveness of this direct technique. Muscle energy done carefully and slowly does not reinstate the abnormal reflex response.

Strain and counterstrain used before direct myofascial release reduces the neurophysiologic barriers allowing myofascial release to break down biomechanical barriers between the muscle and fascia with far greater ease.

Strain and counterstrain treatment is valuable diagnostically when ruling out inflammatory conditions (i.e., tendonitis, bursitis, fasciitis, costo-chondritis). Subjective pain complaint from extremity tenderpoints can mimic inflammatory pain. Corresponding tenderpoint placement in many cases is over the painful tendon or bursa etc. and when palpated illicits an exquisite pain. For example, tenderpoints over the long head or short head of the biceps tendons can mimic bicipital tendonitis. Tender points over the subacromial or trochanteric bursas can mimic bursitis. A tenderpoint over the plantar aspect of the anterior calcaneus will mimic plantar fasciitis and tenderpoints over the costocartilage immediately adjacent to the sternum can mimic costo-chondritis. Similar presentations can be seen with tenderpoints over the infra-patella tendon, achilles tendon, and radial head for lateral epicondylitis. A true inflammatory process can be ruled out by placing the injured area in the strain and counterstrain treatment position. If the palpable tenderness over the affected tendon/bursa etc. is completely relieved and is no longer tender when returned to the neutral posture, the source of the pain was probably not an inflammatory process but neuromuscular dysfunction. If it is a true inflammatory problem, treating the neuromuscular component with strain and counterstrain reduces the muscular tension which helps relieve the inflammatory fluid congestion and facilitates the body's healing processes. Extremity pain caused by tenderpoints in contractile tissue does not usually test positive to resistive isometric testing unlike inflammatory conditions.

PRINCIPLES OF TREATMENT SEQUENCING

By Randall S. Kusunose, PT, OCS

Second only in importance to an accurate diagnosis in the effective management of the painful patient is the proper treatment sequencing of tenderpoint dysfunctions. Out of sequence treatment limits the neurophysiologic response and dooms the patient to recurrence of the same tenderpoints. Unknowing operators do not understand why they are treating the same dysfunctions over and over again with seemingly little long term effect. Areas of pain complaint are often not where treatment is initiated. A scan evaluation for tenderpoints will identify the major areas of dysfunction. Once the tenderpoints have been identified, a treatment plan is then formulated, applying the general rules of treatment sequencing.

1. Treat proximal tenderpoints before distal tenderpoints.
2. Treat the most sensitive or "hottest" tenderpoints first.
3. Treat areas of highest accumulation of tenderpoints first.
4. When tenderpoints are in rows (i.e., over transverse processes or spinous processes), treat the one in the middle.

Correct treatment sequencing reduces the clinicians' work load by as much as fifty percent. Effective proximal treatment will often dissipate distal tenderpoints. Treatment of the most sensitive tenderpoints will improve or dissipate less sensitive tenderpoints and treating tenderpoints in the middle of a row will produce multiple results as tenderpoints above and below dissipate.

Other indicators that help with treatment sequencing can be:

1. Direction of ease versus bind. For example: a patient presents with anterior cervical tenderpoints that would be eased with flexion and posterior cervical tenderpoints that would be eased in extension. Range of motion testing demonstrates mild painfree flexion restriction and moderate painful extension restriction. Flexion would be the direction of greater ease or comfort and treatment would be sequenced by initiating techniques for the anterior tenderpoints. Extra care must be taken when tenderpoints are on both sides of a single vertebral level. Initiating a flexion position to treat an anterior tenderpoint can irritate a posterior tenderpoint. Careful positioning permits the clinician to effectively treat the anterior tenderpoint without posterior irritation.
2. Postural deviations. For example: a flattened forward curve or accentuated backward curve can suggest a major area of posterior tenderpoints. An accentuated forward curve or flat backward curve can suggest a major area of anterior tenderpoints. A lateral shift can suggest tenderpoints more lateral to midline. Treatment would be sequenced by initiating techniques in positions that would exaggerate the postural deviations.
3. Specific pain versus diffuse pain. A pain complaint that is specific in posterior location suggests posterior tenderpoints in the area of pain complaint and would support posterior initiation of treatment. A posterior pain complaint that is diffuse, or in a large area suggests anterior tenderpoints and would support anterior initiation of treatment.

The primary indicator that supports the treatment sequence is success in relieving tenderpoints. If the practitioner chose wrong and did not sequence in the correct order, the results will be temporary. In that scenario, tenderpoints continually reoccur and the operator finds himself treating the same "Hot" tenderpoints at each session.

Following the general rules for treatment sequencing is key to long term resolution of tenderpoints. Treatment out of sequence is the most common mistake made by both beginner and experienced clinician when tenderpoints continually recur.

OTHER COMPLAINTS THAT SUGGEST DYSFUNCTION

These are a small part of our efforts to help people, yet because of exaggerated claims of cures of almost everything from manipulation offered by some unscrupulous manipulators, they inspire much resentment in practitioners of orthodox medicine. I don't blame them. These claims have done my credit in the world much harm.

These complaints and tenderpoints were all first found from reports of patients who had been treated for something else. They told me of things I hadn't expected to relieve. I have personally verified their validity many times repeatedly in practice. I use them as complementary to orthodox treatment, not as an alternative.

HEADACHE

Frontal, in or behind the eye or with photophobia—First cervical or occipitomastoid areas.

Periorbital—Second cervical level; occipitomastoid, squamosal, infraorbital, and nasal areas.

Occipital area to vertex—Fourth cervical level.

EARACHE

Third cervical, posterior auricular, zygomatic, masseter, and occipitomastoid areas.

TINNITUS

Third cervical, posterior auricular, zygomatic, occipitomastoid areas and temporomandibular dysfunctions, especially affecting the internal pterygoid muscle.

VERTIGO

Third cervical and occipitomastoid areas.

MAXILLARY SINUS

Infraorbital and second cervical areas.

DENTAL NEURITIS

Upper—Squamosal, sphenoid, and lateral canthus areas;

Lower—temporomandibular joint.

NECK PAIN

Tenderpoint may be anterior one or two thoracic. The top two move with the neck.

COUGH (nonproductive, throat tickle)

Anterior fifth, sixth, or seventh cervical levels found on the trachea. May also help in treatment of some productive coughs.

PRECORDIAL PAIN

Anterior third, fourth, fifth, or sixth thoracic ribs or interspaces. In any case with evidence of myocardial infarct I suggest especially mild and gentle treatment, because of the possibility of aggravation of heart function during a period of reaction to treatment. I have had two episodes of exacerbation in almost sixty years practice and that is enough.

HEARTBURN

Anterior fifth thoracic level.

FATIGUE (especially on awakening)

Fifth, sixth, or seventh thoracic areas, especially anterior.

EPIGASTRIC PAIN, GASTRITIC or DUODENAL ULCER

Anterior seventh or eighth thoracic area (augments medical treatment).

UMBILICAL PAIN

Anterior ninth or tenth thoracic area.

DIARRHEA or CONSTIPATION

Anterior ninth or tenth thoracic area.

CYSTITIS (noninfectious, interstitial)

Anterior eleventh thoracic and fourth lumbar areas, especially anteriorly.

SHOULDER PAIN:

Steady—Upper five thoracic levels and ribs;

With arm movement—Dysfunction around the acromio-clavicular and humeral joints and upper five thoracic levels and ribs.

Pain or numbness in entire arm—Top five thoracic and rib areas. I have been disappointed in efforts on the brachial plexus.

Pain, numbness in fingers—Sixth, seventh, or eighth cervical and first thoracic levels.

ELBOW PAIN

Without stiffness—Tenderpoint high on the lateral epicondyle—first thoracic or rib level; tenderpoint high on medial epicondyle- fourth thoracic or rib level.

With stiffness on pronation—Radial head and tip of epicondyle of humerus (epicondylitis).

With pain or stiffness on suppination—Pronator.

On extension—Coronoid areas.

On flexion—Olecranon areas.

WRIST PAIN (local)

Local area, also check elbow.

CARPAL TUNNEL SYNDROME

Many so diagnosed can be relieved by flcxion and rotation of the wrist. Must be because of incorrect diagnosis.

THUMB PAIN AND WEAKNESS

First carpo-metacarpal area and radial wrist flexion; also check radial head.

PAIN AND WEAKNESS IN GRASP

Dorsal carpo-metacarpal area.

GROIN PAIN

Inguinal ligament.

LOW-BACK, HIP, and THIGH PAIN

Lower four thoracic, all lumbar, sacroiliac, and enarthrosis areas (the latter often are influenced markedly by position changes of the femur).

COCCYGODYNIA

A large proportion of these conditions is related to a sacro-iliac dysfunction, with ilium high in back and flared out above.

REACTIONS TO TREATMENT

This treatment is almost completely atraumatic. The doctor just finds the most comfortable position. It feels good right away. Before he leaves, warn him that he has about one chance in three of becoming temporarily worse by the next morning.

Because the treatment was atraumatic, any aggravation of pain alarms the patient more than a traumatic treatment would. He should be warned there is about a thirty percent probability of temporarily aggravated pain.

If it does occur, the physician can reassure the alarmed patient by reminding him he was forewarned. He still hurts as much now, but is not frightened.

It is surprising to doctors and patients how much worse a patient can feel after a treatment limited to positions of comfort.

If you can say, "Remember I told you you may be worse for a day or two," he does remember and is reassured. If you had been using traumatic techniques destined to "pop" some joints loose as I was when I started this work, and he is sore next day, he is not surprised. You are not surprised. But we all are surprised to see how much increase of pain we can produce just from the changes we produced with our completely atraumatic treatment, if we don't warn him.

Patients with a history of myocardial infarction may suffer another episode the day after a traumatic or an atraumatic treatment. This occurred twice in my sixty years of practice. Neither caused death, but I learned to start with a *partially* effective treatment for the first two treatments. By this time, the danger of producing a new episode of myocardial insufficience is much reduced. The spinal segments important here are the 3rd, 4th, 5th, and 6th thoracics and their ribs.

SELF TREATMENT

Most manipulating physicians I have known have accumulated a fund of joint dysfunctions in their own bodies. So why don't we ask our colleague to care for us? Usually, we don't want to bother him except in dire need, because he is so busy. Treatment with thrust to cause joints to "move" relies in part upon the element of surprise. The patient may have a fairly clear idea of what will happen to him, but he will not be aware of the exact moment of thrust. This advantage to the physician is lost in any attempt at self-treatment. It is impossible to surprise oneself. For treating oneself, a slow search for a comfortable position of stretch that releases muscle tension around a joint and restores normal motion, requiring only a slow return from the stretch, is much more effective and our body coaches us all the way.

With the counterstrain approach to self-treatment, we are aware of greatest comfort. We are also able to detect our own tender-point becoming less tender. There is often a tendency for us to produce the stretched position voluntarily with the muscles of the area treated. We need to ask ourselves, "Is this really a passive stretch?" If not, we stop and wait or maybe back up until we can feel ourselves relax. To keep it passive often requires varying the technique from that used upon another person. Anyone with chronic pain is motivated to persist till he finds his ideal position. Especially in neck treatment, he must be alert to a guarding tension developing in his neck. It doesn't trust him. With careful observation of the body's responses, he can get it to where it does trust him. The author has been able to relieve almost every pain he has ever found on his own body by passive stretches and slow returns. In recent years he has aggressively searched for minor ailments that could be easily ignored. By eliminating these, he has achieved a high level of well-being and almost complete freedom from any real pains. There must be many more subclinical than clinical problems. Preventative maintenance is effective prophylactic treatment.

PROPHYLACTIC STRETCHING

Perhaps many physicians dream of some procedure that would clean up most accumulated ailments—some kind of exercise or sauna or something. I too hoped to devise some method of restoring suppleness and comfort to the entire body by use of the principles described above.

Putting each joint in its position of greatest comfort was impractical timewise. What seemed necessary was to devise a method that would affect large numbers of joints at one time. Possibly the entire spine could be stretched at one time, if we just broke down the stretches into one element at a time, such as right sidebending. This wouldn't produce many ideal positions, but maybe putting all the spinal joints into the important parts of all stretches would be useful. I tried stretching my whole spine actively in six directions: flexion, extension, sidebending both ways and rotation both ways. I would begin by moving into an extreme position so that further effort didn't produce more movement. I borrowed from the work of Dr. T.J. Ruddy and made the active pushes at intervals of two a second. With my previous positioning these efforts just produced little twitches. I took pains to do them in ways that would not require overcoming gravity to return, just relaxation. I did two hundred of each, and afterward told myself that I did feel much more supple. The next morning I was sore all over and I hoped it was just reaction to treatment. In three days I was all right and tried it again. From then on, no more reactions and I did feel much better. I seemed to have reached a peak after a while and didn't feel any further improvement, so I stopped after about three months of biweekly stretches. Little by little I realized I was slipping back into my previous state. So I resumed my stretches and soon improved again. Now I just do them after some stressful experience like a long flight.

It was a big disappointment to me that most people weren't interested, but those who did follow my suggestions reported considerable general improvement. With all the dedication to exercise, I guess I'll just have to wait for my turn. I know a lot of people who would feel much better, if they would mix in some stretches with their aerobics or even as an alternative to their aerobics.

FINE TUNING FOR POSITION OF MOBILITY

During the process of searching for the position of ideal comfort for a pain, one might expect a steady reduction of muscle tension as one moves toward a position of comfort, but relief and relaxation at the tenderpoint change in relation to how strongly the reflex is reporting strain. Let's assume we are at a relatively neutral position and move in the wrong direction. At first, tension increases slowly. Then as we get into the area of severe strain, tension changes become so much faster and more powerful as to be unmistakable. Returning toward the relatively neutral position retraces the responses. Moving in the right direction also makes small changes at first, improving until an abrupt and marked relaxation occurs. Within a positional change of less than two degrees, relaxation changes from about two thirds to almost complete. Go beyond it and tension immediately returns. The sudden relaxation and retensing is easy to feel, once a skilled operator is alerted to it. At this small amplitude of change the tenderpoint can be felt to become almost completely flaccid, immediately tensing again with any slight move away in any direction. This is so profound that tissues appear often to be moving with any slight change in position as if nothing in the body is so relaxed as our previously tense joint area. Detecting these changes needs no unusual talent, just practice. Succeeding in finding and using this phenomenon changes a fairly good treatment into an excellent treatment. For the few patients who don't feel relief for thirty seconds, once the physician feels this point of flaccidity, he is certain to be succeeding. The patient will always agree within thirty seconds. The illustration for this also shows the proprioceptor input to agree with the changes in muscle tension. New students fear they can't learn this, but almost all who try can learn. Here again the body feedback coaches the operator, always rewarding him everytime he does something right.

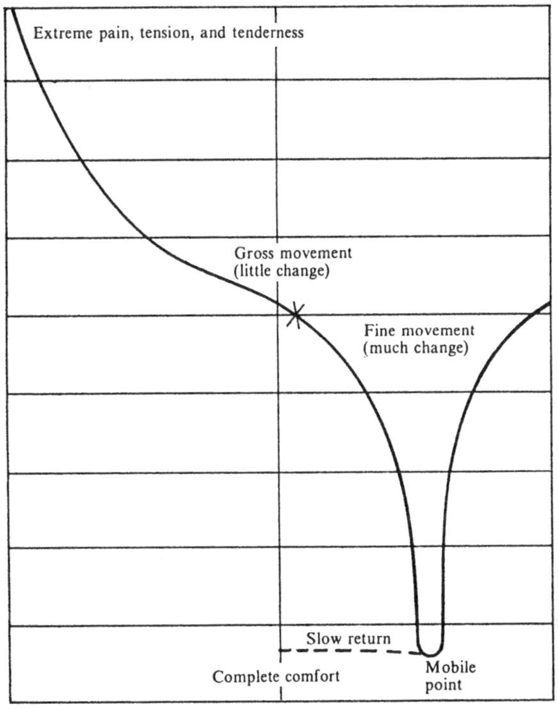

Fig. 2. **Modus operandi for ideal positioning for comfort.**

CONFLICTING DYSFUNCTIONS

Before I paint too rosy a picture, there is often a situation that may be confusing. The pain, as mentioned before, may well be a combination of pains close enough together as to be lumped together as one pain by the patient. This can be especially confusing when the positions of comfort for some of these sources of pain are markedly different from others. If their positions of relief are opposite in direction, we have a dilemma. What one joint likes, makes another hurt worse. This isn't as impossible as it might seem. There is a great tendency to treat the first thing we find without taking the time to make a complete diagnosis. Here is a situation where a comprehensive knowledge of all parts of the pain is important. If we know all the sources of this pain and their relative intensity, we can start with the worst and progress down through the rest of the troubles. Usually this is enough to avoid much conflicting pain. If we still aggravate one element while treating another, the second pain is usually tolerable with a little adjustment, so we can continue in spite of the second pain. Remember, if we return slowly from any stretch, we don't cause any lasting trouble even if our position is wrong. What we have accomplished is a good trade-off, a lasting benefit for a temporary irritation. Then we immediately ease the conflicting one. Sometimes there isn't much relief of the first until the second is also eased. Then both are better. These conflicting problems can arise all in one joint. Mechanically as we used to think, it can't be sidebent right and left at the same time. True, but it can have two conflicting strain messages, both of which are abnormal.

RELIEF OR CURE

Many of my colleagues through the years have told me they could provide relief but, of course, no cure. For years I didn't know that a cure could be achieved. Most patients have a history of long-time suffering from months to many years with exacerbations and remissions. They have had many disappointments and consult me just for relief of their incurable pain. Despite all evidence to the contrary, I believe most of these conditions can be cured. My records go back many years. Any patient who had suffered no relapse in fifteen years was cured. There could have been many more who were cured.

A few patients were relieved, but continued to return with the same pains. For some reason they could not heal their inflammed tissues. I searched for systemic ailments that were complicating their ability to heal. I referred many to internists, but none received any benefit. I, too, tried to find an answer, but with meager success. A few were unable to absorb vitamin B^{12} by mouth and were spectacularly aided by intermuscular injections. Some responded better after clearing up old allergies. Some seemed to have some chronic, low-grade viral or similar infection which would not respond to antibiotic treatment.

My college days were before use of sulfa drugs was widespread. In my pre-sulfa experience in the hospital, I remembered fair success in tertiary syphilis by means of hyperpyrexia by diathermy. One hundred four degrees for four hours produced partial remissions when we had nothing better. It was abandoned in the rush into sulfas and antibiotics. I tried baths hot enough to raise body temperature three degrees, with the patient covered up after and kept warm for two hours. This did raise temperatures three degrees and help some patients to recover.

By far the most effective means of keeping this dysfunction turned off turned out to be the simplest. I could get them into a position of comfort easily, but they could get it into the same trouble again easily too. After a few weeks to a few years, it became so facilitated in its dysfunction as to recur on very slight provocation. By this time they had had to endure pain so long they expected it. Their recurrences came from mild strains or other painful efforts that caused pain, but no more than they were used to. I taught them to think of their problem in two ways. Their dysfunction was the cause of their trouble. It was a continuing irritation. Turning it off was not a cure, just a stopping of an irritation. To achieve a cure they must continue to have no irritation until their bodies could heal. This was almost impossible to accomplish during the first few days. No matter how careful they were they would need to return to have the pain turned off again. If they did work hard to avoid pain, they would soon become more successful.

This success was due to decreasing inflammation in these much abused tissues. This did not need to be a malady that the body could not cure. If the irritation could be turned off and kept turned off, they could heal. The next step was to convince them that a cure was many times as wonderful as some temporary relief. With their best cooperation I was surprised how few recurrences they had. This one device has proven more useful than all the others combined. It is not a permanent sentence, because as they succeed in reducing their inflammatory state, they become less and less likely to have any recurrences. Most can progress far enough in three weeks that they are noticeably less susceptible to pain on slight provocation.

Relieving the irritation was easy for me, but any painful effort easily returned its irritation. It was facilitated in its dysfunction so much as to return it with just a hard sneeze.

Complete healing may require three or more months of comfort, but after the first week or two without a relapse patients become much less vulnerable to relapse. Healing is a cure. Once healed they will not have further pain here unless they have a new injury about as severe as the original one. Tolerating pain because they thought they were doomed to it was one of the things that made them incurable.

Rheumatoid arthritis is not cured by this method, but its pain is considerably reduced by an occasional atraumatic treatment. Its pain must be partly reflex dysfunction too. Osteoarthritic patients can get painfree or nearly so and maintain good comfort levels.

RESTORING STRENGTH

Most of what students in my courses have been taught in their medical training is excellent. Some of them have been taught things that, if what I have learned is true, must be wrong.

A fit body is a healthy body, so exercise. Right. Build the body to its prime condition of fitness. Right. No pain—no gain. For muscle development, right. To cure a disease, wrong. Chronic rheumatic pain is a disease.

If a simple stretch in a position of ideal comfort is enough to stop a chronic dysfuntion, then a simple painful effort is sufficient to restore the dysfunction. Exercise this dysfunction with pain, restore rheumatic pain, no gain!

After inflammation has had a few weeks to subside, the patient gradually becomes more able to engage safely in usual occupations, including strenuous physical effort. By this time there will have been considerable recovery in strength, because weakness was part of the disease. During the period of recovery, exercise strong enough to cause pain will restart the dysfunction.

If this places me in conflict with precepts still taught in some medical schools of starting painful exercise early in treatment, I still cannot retreat from it. If it accelerates increased strength, which I doubt, it will do so at the expense of restoring chronic rheumatic disease. Some of the things we have accepted as true, must be false.

TECHNIQUES

STRAIN-COUNTERSTRAIN

ABBREVIATIONS

A	=	Anterior
C	=	Cervical
CRUC	=	Cruciate
HIFO	=	High Ilium with Flareout
L	=	Lumbar
Lat	=	Lateral
Med	=	Medial
Men	=	Meniscus
P	=	Posterior
PC	=	Post Cervical
Pect	=	Pectineus
PL	=	Posterior lower
PSIS	=	Posterior superior iliac spine
T	=	Thoracic
TM	=	Temporo-Mandibular
TP	=	Tenderpoint
Troch	=	Trochanter
●	=	Force applied inward
➤	=	Arrow indicates direction of force

CERVICAL SPINE

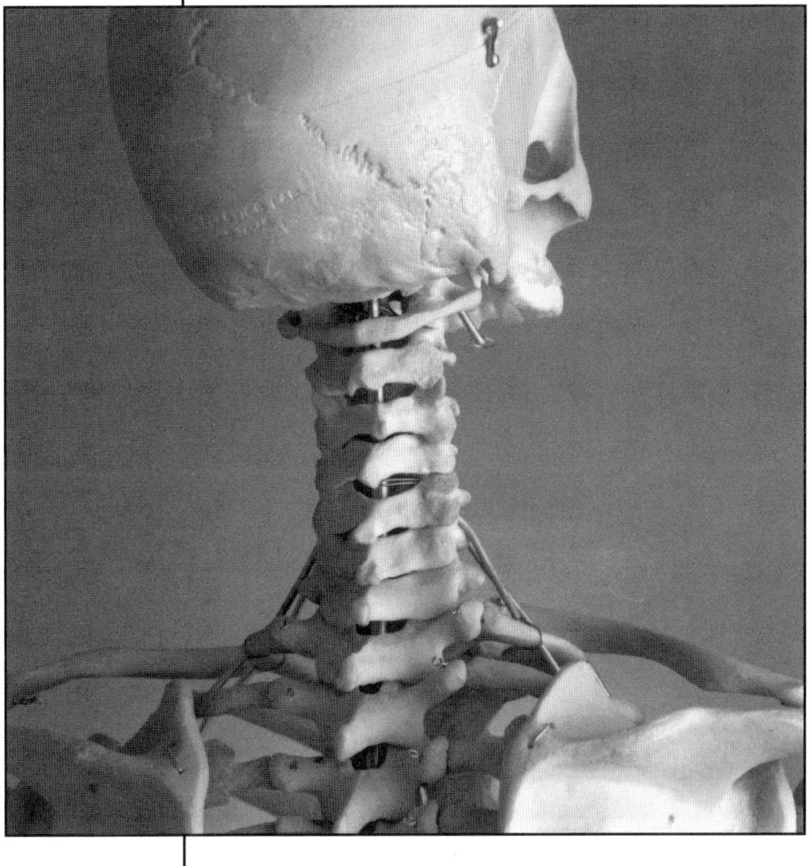

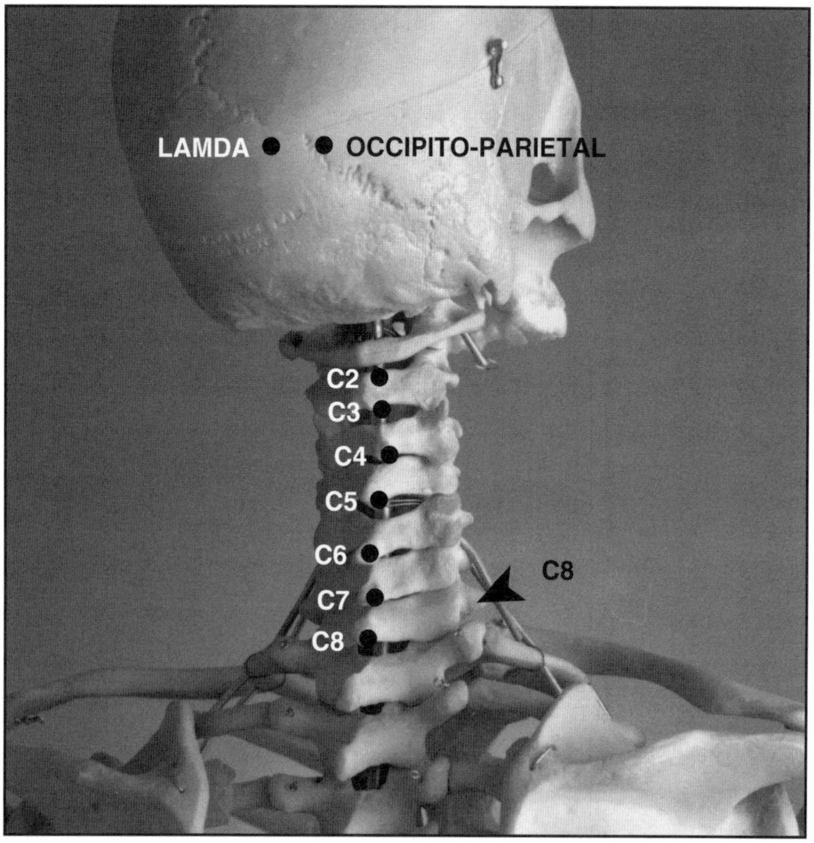

GENERAL

Because the upper two thoracic segments tend to move with the neck, any painful limitation of motion at that level may be interpreted by patients as neck pains. Observe where they show you where their pain is. Some will be found to be in the top two thoracic segments.

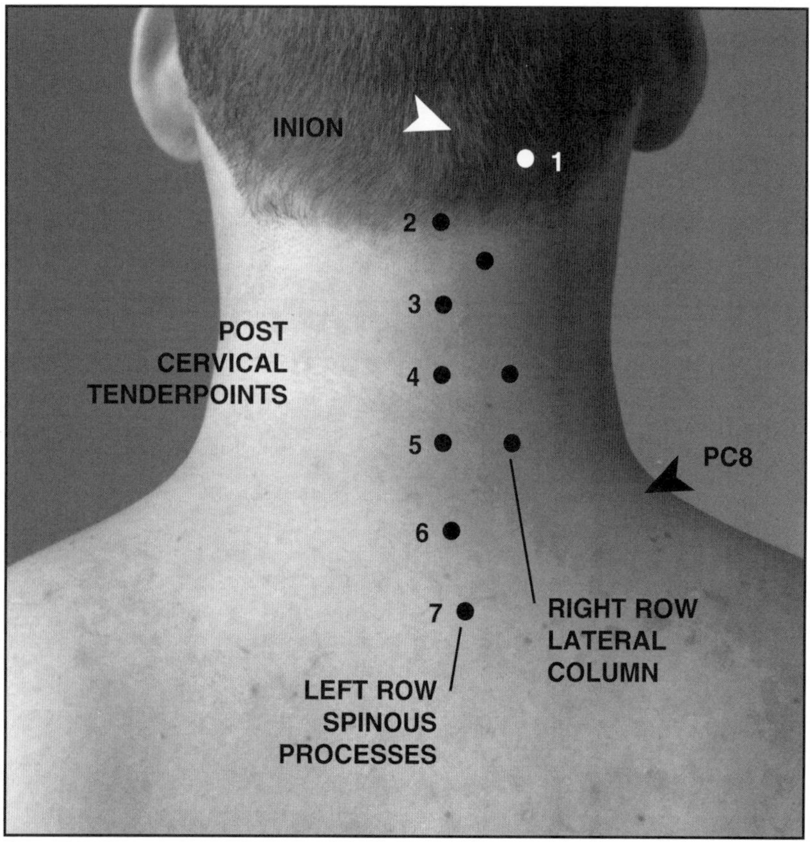

POSTERIOR CERVICAL TENDERPOINTS

Tenderpoints on spinous processes are most often a little to one side, half a centimeter or less from the midline indicating right or left trouble.

ON SPINOUS PROCESSES

Posterior C1–Since the spinous process of the first cervical is not palpable on most persons, we use the tenderpoint for the trouble in the first cervical joint on a point found low on the occiput two centimeters lateral to the main muscle mass at the back of the neck. Pain is often in or around the eye. It is treated in extension with patient supine, by caudad pressure high on the occipital bone. In order for this to succeed, the patient must first permit some extension of his upper neck before pressure is applied or this force will just produce compression instead of extension. This puts the action right under the skull where it is needed. Rotation and sidebending are slight. Similar to posterior C2, see page 40.

ANTERIOR CERVICAL TENDERPOINTS

Tenderpoint AC1 is located on the posterior surface of the ascending ramus of the mandible. Tenderpoints AC2-AC6 are on the anterior surface of the tips of the tranverse processes. Tenderpoint AC7 is found on the superior surface of the clavicle midway between the two heads of the sterno cleido mastoid muscle. Tenderpoint AC8 is located on the medial end of the clavicle, in the suprasternal notch, pushing in a lateral direction.

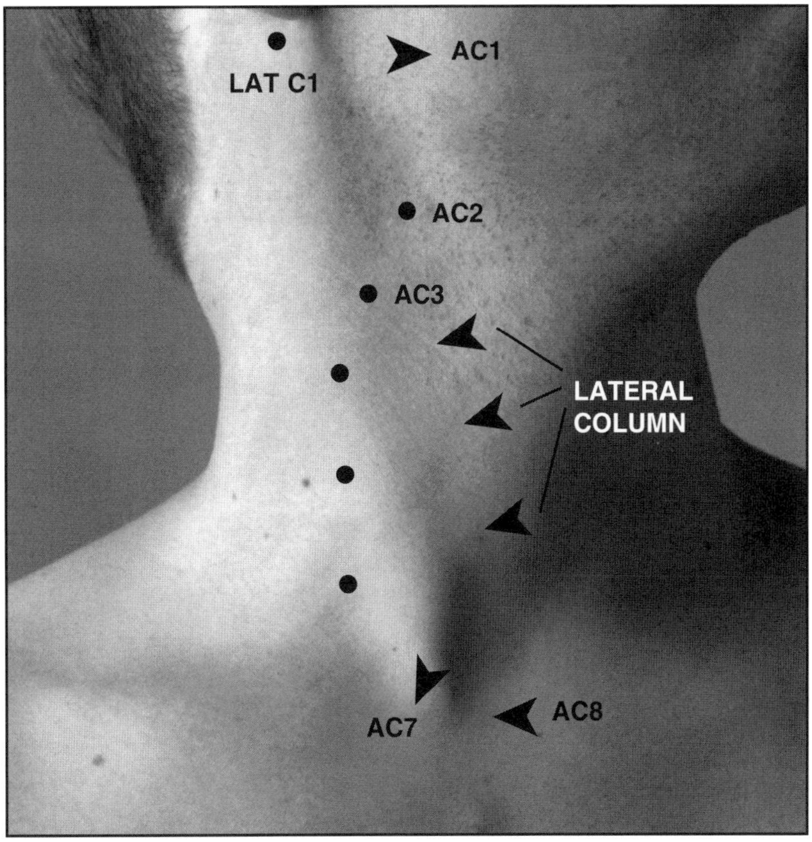

INION

Another dysfunction (probably of the C1 joint) has a tenderpoint on the medial side of one of the main muscles at the back of the skull. It has been named inion for the knob on the back of the occiput which serves as a landmark for finding several tenderpoints. This point is an inch below the knob. It is relieved by marked forward bending of the head on the neck, with greatest flexion applied right under the skull.

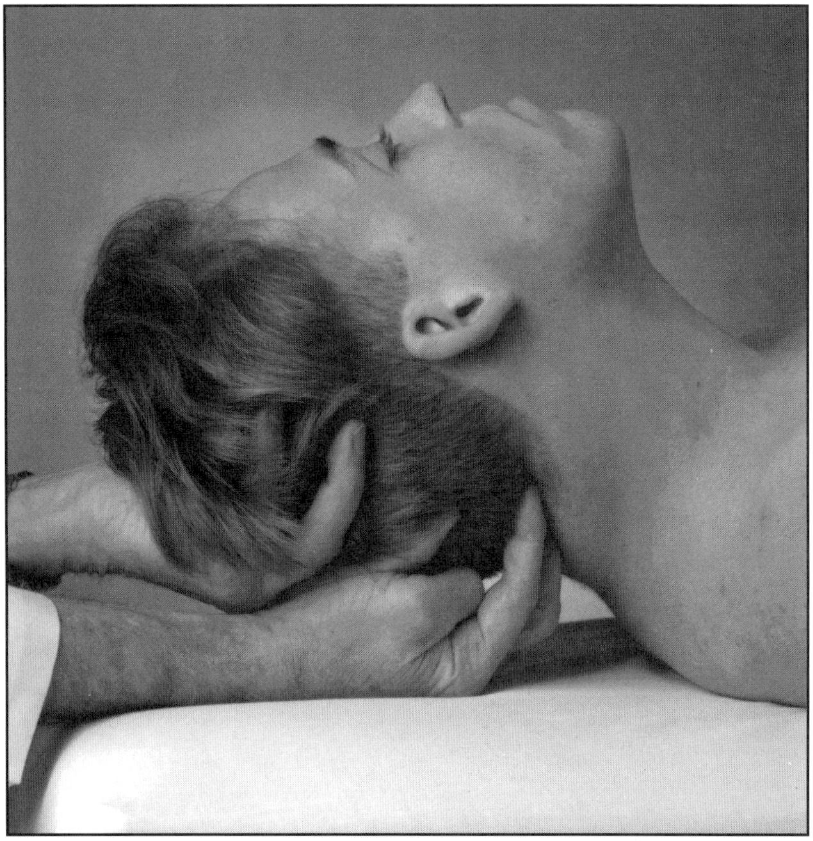

Posterior C2—The top spinous process you are likely to be able to feel is the large one of the second cervical vertebra. The tenderpoint for the second joint is on the superior surface of the spinous process or in the muscle mass itself at that level. Treatment is the same as for the posterior first cervical joint and symptoms are similar. They seem to work as a team.

Tenderpoint for the first cervical is on the low occiput 3/4 inches lateral to main muscle in back of head.

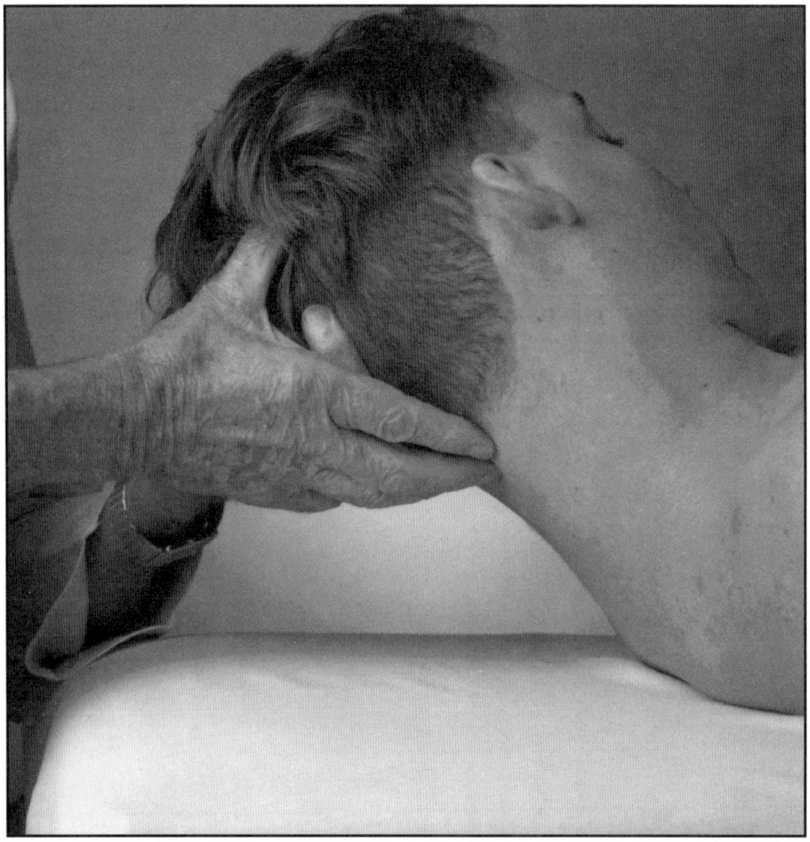

Posterior C3—Tenderpoints found at the inferior surface of the spinous process of the second cervical vertebra indicate a disturbance at the level of the third cervical joint. Treatment for this third cervical problem is flexion about forty-five degrees, sidebending and rotation away from the side on which the spinous process is tender. Commonly found in cases with vertigo.

Posterior C4—This is one of the most commonly missed cervical problems, because the spinous process of the third cervical vertebra is much more recessed than that of the second. Especially in this extension type problem, it can be easy to move over it without feeling it. Flex the neck to be sure to expose the spinous process to your probing finger. Tenderness on this spot goes with a pain that radiates up the back of the head. It is also often found in patients suffering from trouble in the temporo-mandibular joint. Treatment is done with the head hanging over the end of the table. Action is placed at the right level by using a light pressure on the top of the occiput much less than that used for the C1.

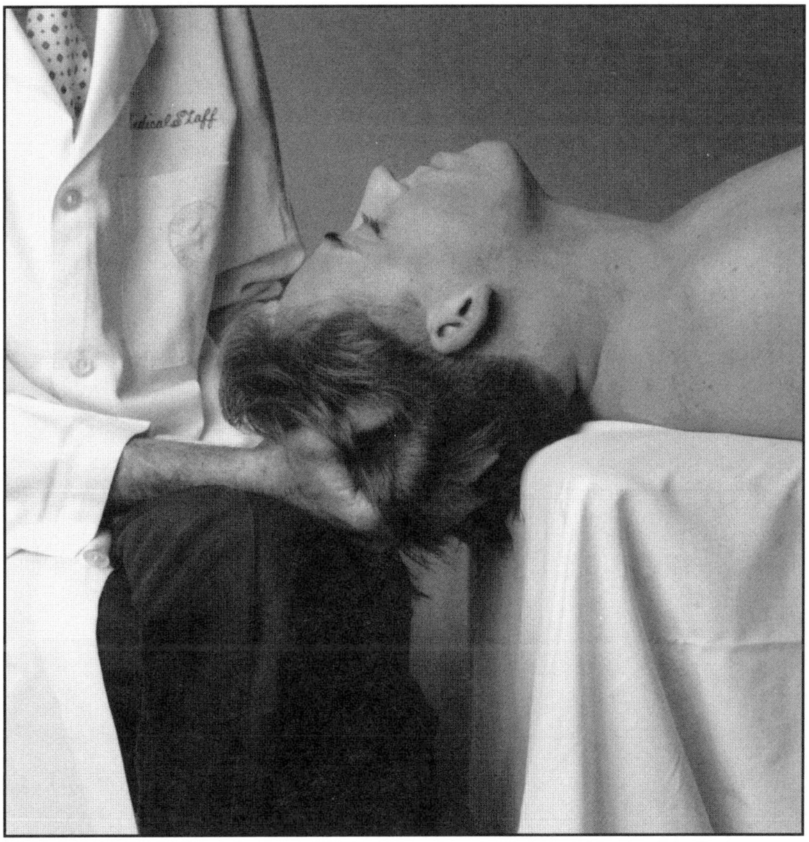

Posterior C5—Tenderness on the spinous process of the fourth vertebra indicates a problem at the fifth intervertebral joint. With this the headaches are more all over the head than in any one area.

Posterior C6, 7, and 8—These dysfunctions give rise just to neck pain and stiffness. Treatment is again with the patient supine with the head and neck suspended over the end of the table, supported by the operator. Neck is stretched back and both rotated and sidebent away from the tender side. As extension increases these lower joints are involved. There is an alternative tenderpoint for the eighth cervical joint on the transverse process of the seventh cervical vertebra which is often more tender than that on the spinous process. It is found at the side of the neck probing deeply in front of the trapezius, with the finger aimed to push forward against the posterior surface of the transverse process.

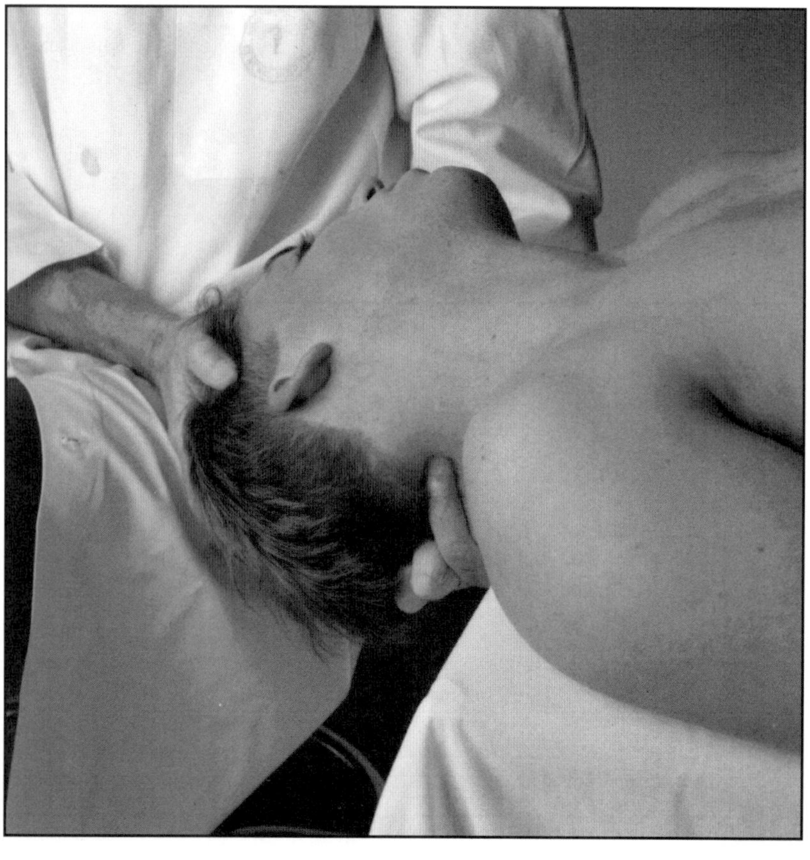

ON POSTERIOR LATERAL COLUMN OF THE VERTEBRA

On posterior surface of the lateral columns of the neck, 3/8 inch lateral to the midline may be found other tenderpoints with a different set of positions of comfort. These are relieved by neck extension, rotation away from the sore side, and usually but not always sidebending a little toward it.

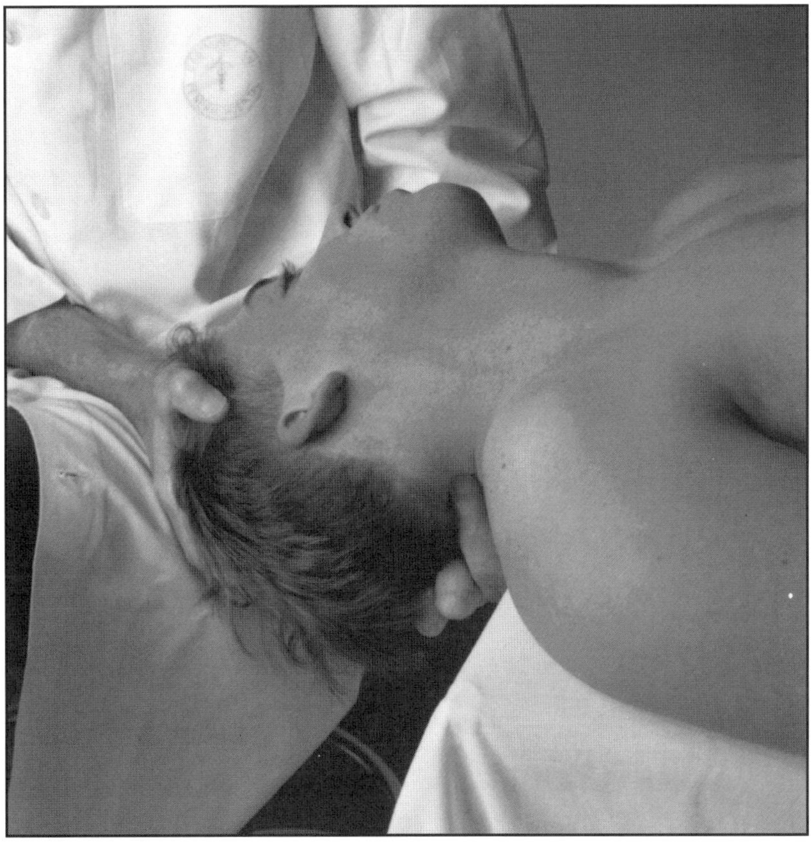

ANTERIOR CERVICAL

Anterior C1—As it is behind, the anterior first cervical or occipito-atlantal joint tenderpoint is atypical. It is found high on the posterior edge of the ascending ramus of the mandible at the lobe of the ear. Since this is so close to the temporo-mandibular joint, many of these have been mistaken for TM problems, yet they are relieved by simply rotating the skull away from the tender side, often nearly ninety degrees. No treatment involving the TM joint is necessary.

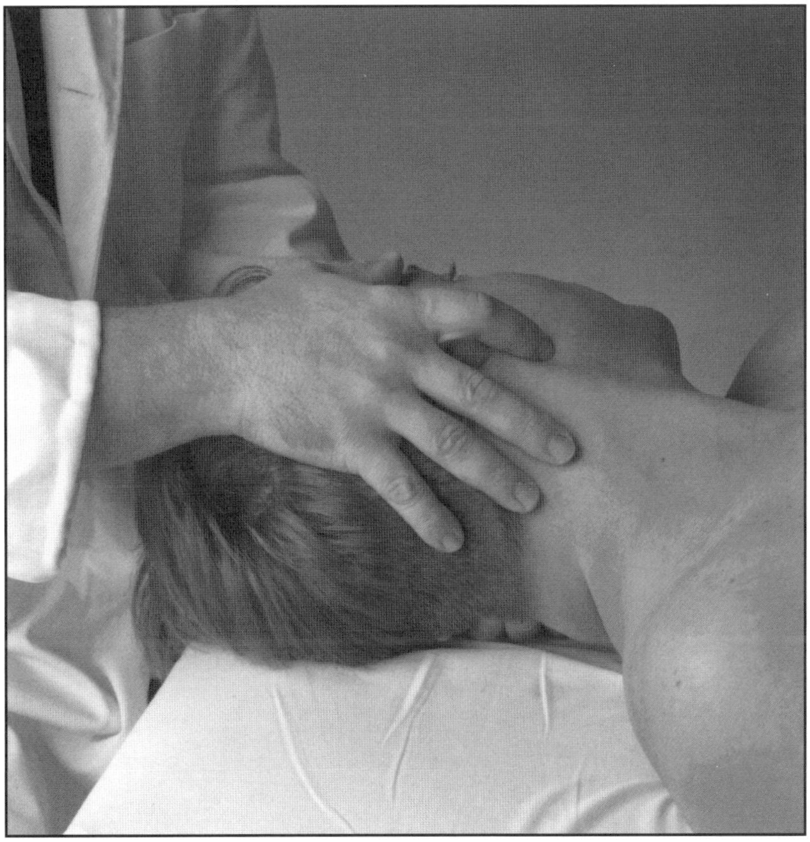

Anterior C2, 3, 4, 5, and 6—These points are found on the anterior surface of the tips of the the transverse processes of the cervical vertebra and easily felt after a little practice learning to feel through the sterno mastoid muscle which crosses over them by probing the side of the neck. Treatment for these dyfunctions is flexion of neck and head (about forty-five degrees with equal amounts of sidebending and rotation away from the tender side).

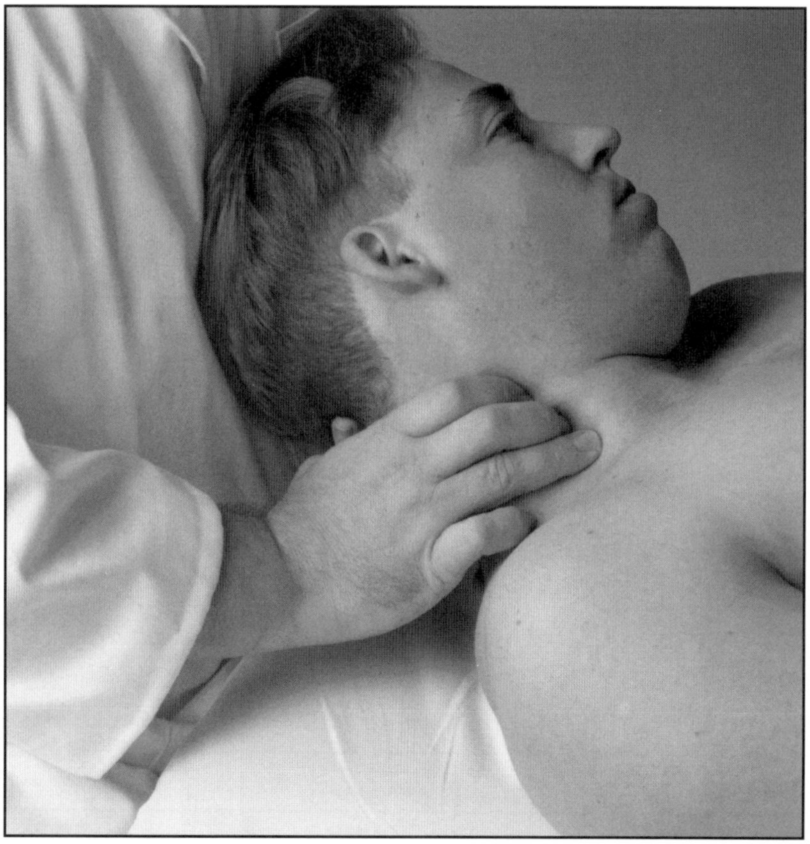

Anterior C7—This is a very common and important anterior cervical dysfunction. The tenderpoint and treatment both seem to relate to the sternomastoid muscle. The tenderpoints are two to three centimeters lateral to the medial end of the clavicle on its superior surface, where part of the origin of the sternomastoid muscle is located. Treatment is a strong flexion force applied by the web of the operator's thumb to the middle of the back of the neck. One of the common mistakes of beginners is to press instead on the head or upper neck, causing a strain in upper cervical joints before achieving enough force to affect the seventh joint. The weight of the head is supported by the palm of the hand, but this is not used to influence the seventh joint. Treatment includes sidebending toward and rotation away (which will maximally shorten the sternomastoid muscle).

This picture appears to show much sidebend. The right position is markedly flexed and slightly sidebent.

Anterior C8—This uncommon and easily managed dysfunction has its tenderpoint on the medial end of the clavicle on the side of the suprasternal notch. Treatment is like that for the C2, 3, 4, 5, and 6.

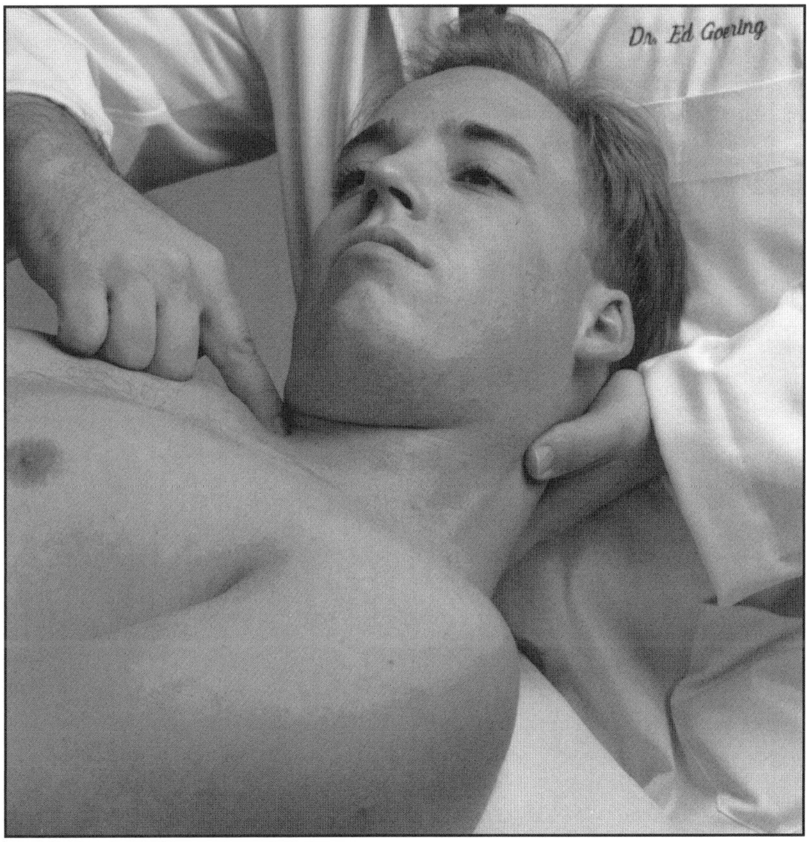

LATERAL FIRST CERVICAL

This joint is unique also as it may have evidence of a lateral strain. This is found by pinching the tips of the mastoid processes between index fingers and thumbs of both hands and permitting the finger tips to move down and more deeply medial, to feel the tips of the transverse processes of the vertebrae just below. This area can be tender. If so, it is often possible to observe that the relationship between the two bones is not the same on both sides. The atlas bone appears to slide away from the side of lateral convexity of the strain and the distance between the mastoid tip and transverse process of the vertebra will be different on the two sides. As with any other deformity of the structure of the body, treatment (sidebending the head on the neck) is aimed at temporarily increasing this deformity to release a muscle contraction guarding against a reported strain. Tenderness is not always on the side of the lateral convexity. Remember the only indication for treatment is tenderness. Never attempt to correct an observed deformity unless there is evidence of irritation! These are relatively uncommon, but occasionally important.

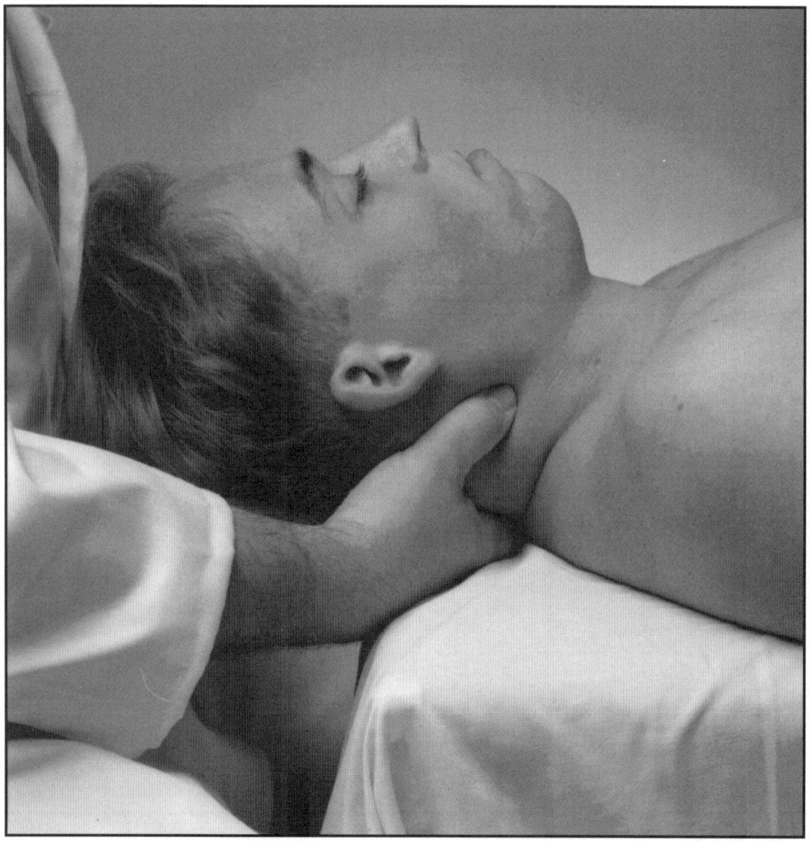

ANTERIOR LATERAL COLUMNS

These same segments may present tenderpoints in the throat on the anterior surface of the lateral columns. Here I like to use caution to avoid prolonged pressure over the internal carotid artery and its plexuses of nerves. This way I am able to avoid causing the abrupt loss of consciousness that had happened to me while under treatment from my sophomore fellow-classmate in college. (Perhaps because of my caution I have never done to a patient what the sophomore did to me.) These points can be surprisingly sensitive. Typical treatment, similar to posterior lateral column points, is marked flexion of the head and neck and rotation away, but usually sidebending slightly toward the tender side. These are again new since the original book and with a different set of positions of comfort.

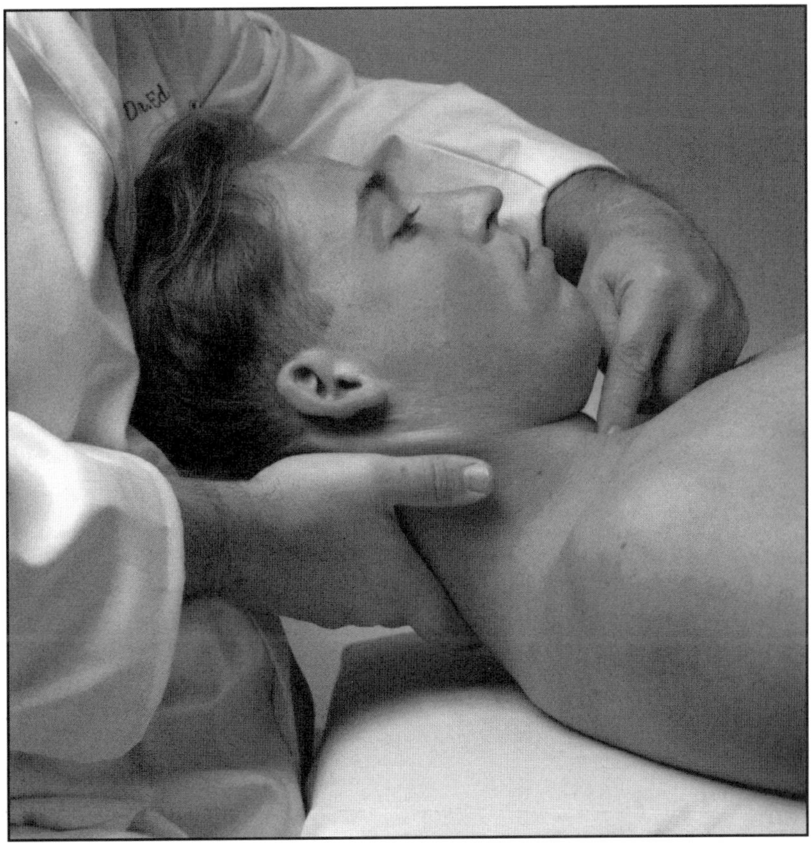

CHRONIC UNPRODUCTIVE
(and sometimes productive) **COUGH**

This is included here because we are in the area. There are many people with chronic unproductive cough. Usually they have come to me with a diagnosis of chronic bronchitis. Like many other things I have learned to treat on the body, this was reported to me by a few of my patients following anterior cervical treatments. "You stopped my bronchitis!" In addition to the other tenderpoints mentioned, I examined the trachea and usually found tenderpoints, mostly near the bottom, but a few higher in the throat. Many of these I learned to ease just by treating anterior cervical problems, but some seemed to need something done to the trachea itself. The technique still is not complete, but usually I am able to press on the opposite side of the trachea and relieve a tenderpoint. Whenever I succeed the "bronchitis" is decreased. For years I had used it only in unproductive coughs (those that don't cough up anything) until I was treating a patient, who had developed a pneumonia which wasn't responding well to treatment. Her coughing was violent enough to exhaust her. I found some tracheal tenderpoints and managed to reduce the coughing markedly and accelerate her recovery. These problems can complicate other body disorders and may, when relieved, make an evident improvement in recovery over medical treatment alone.

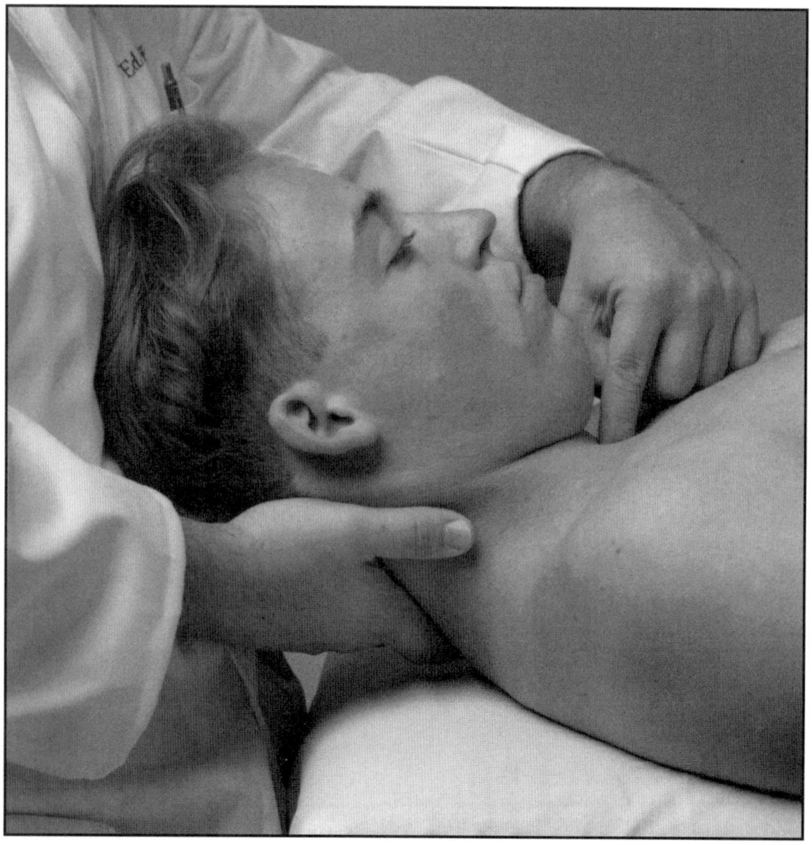

THORACIC SPINE

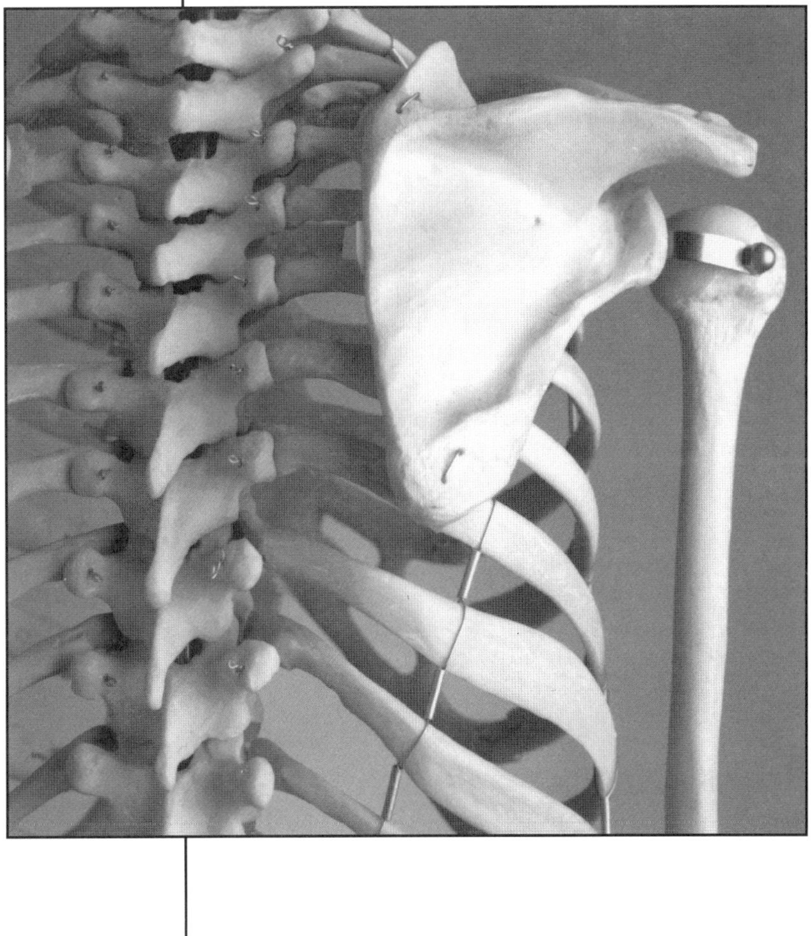

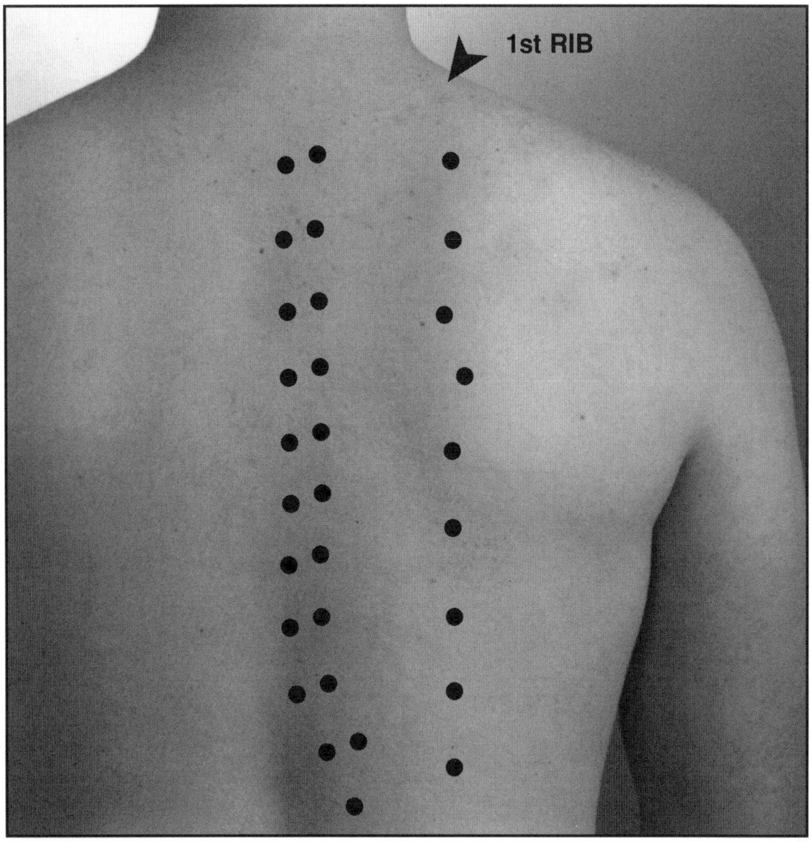

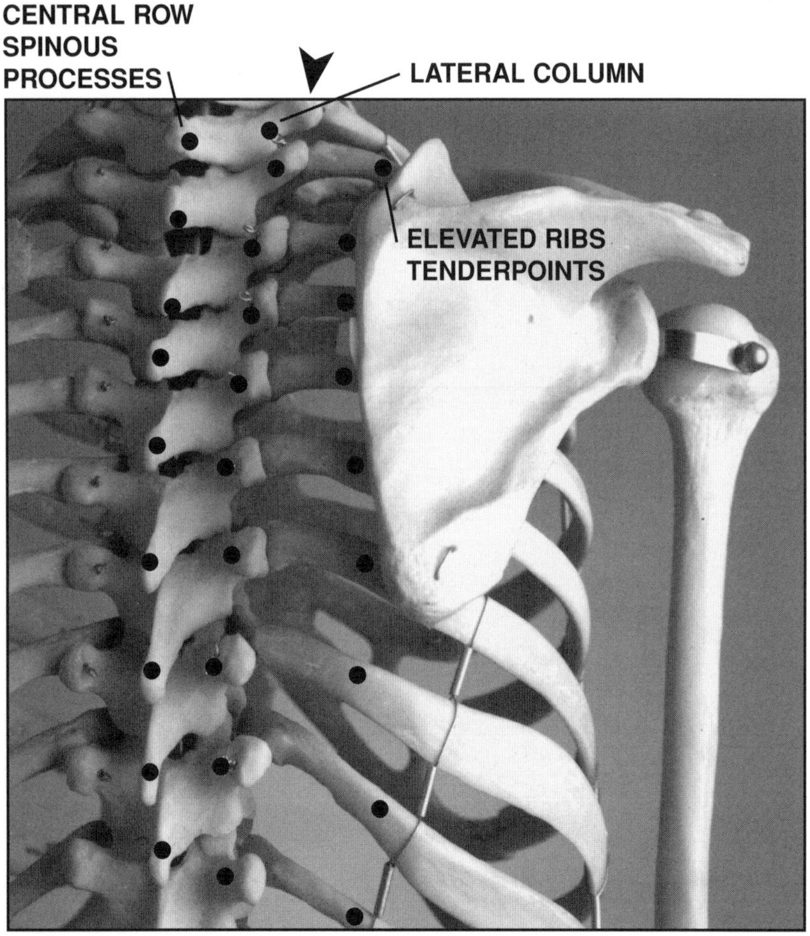

GENERAL

Although the tenderness can usually be found with the patient in the prone position, any time there is any doubt as to the presence or absence of tenderness on these points, central or lateral, for some reason they show up much more definitely if the patient lies supine and the operator reaches under him to probe for tenderness. This is especially valuable in upper and mid thoracics.

ON SPINOUS PROCESSES

Posterior T1, 2, and 3—Patient lies prone with arms hanging over the sides of the table. As with the spinous processes of the cervical area, the point of greatest tenderness is very close to and may be on the midline. The head is supported by cupping the point of the chin in the hand so as to avoid too much pressure on the point of the chin. Force is applied straight back and does not include any force cephalad, which would cause the effect to be greatest up in the neck rather than in the thorax. The back of the operator's hand is often close enough to the surface of the table so that he can rest his hand on it. Rotation and sidebending are slight and most often are away from the sore side. Occasionally when the upper of the two spinous processes related to the joint is not deviated toward the sore side, it may be necessary to reverse the rotation, not the sidebend.

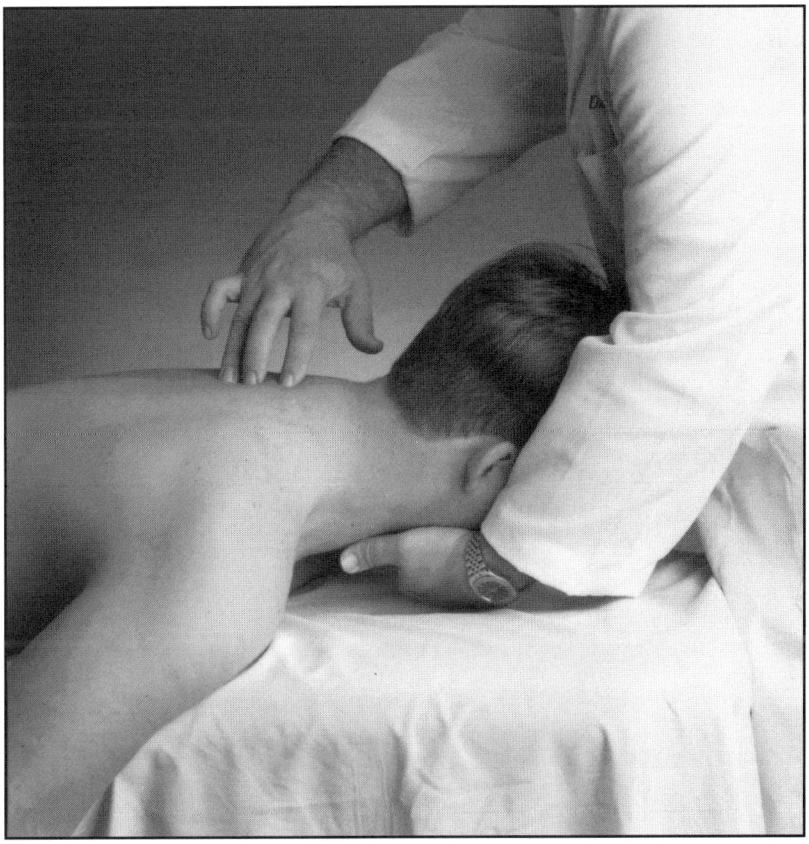

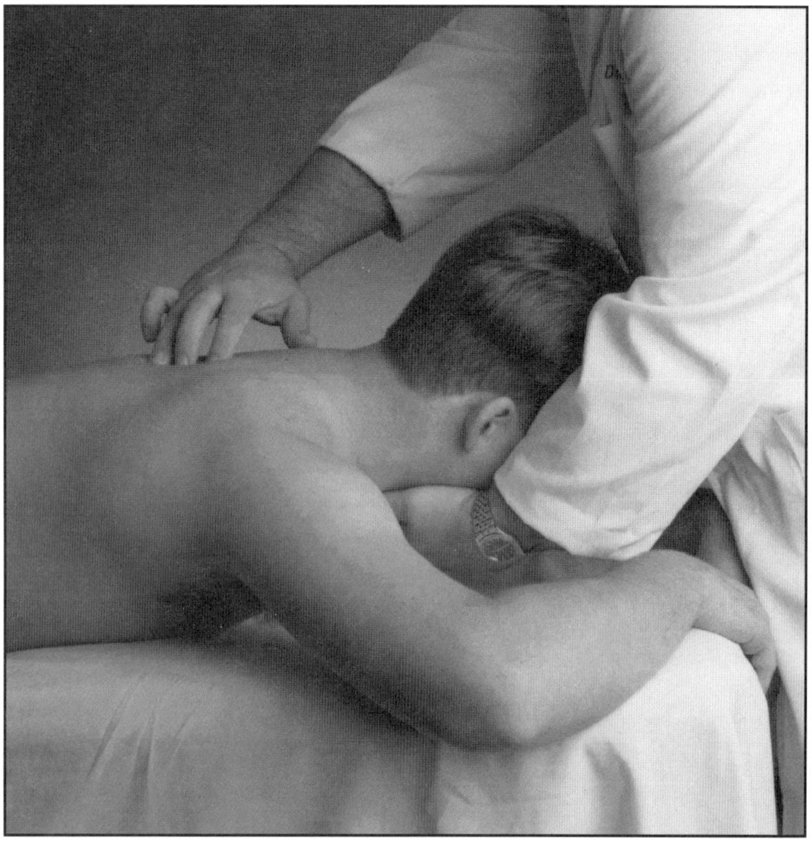

Posterior T4, 5, and 6—Treatment is the same except now the arms of the patient should be on the end of the table near his head. This brings the action of the stretch down into these segments.

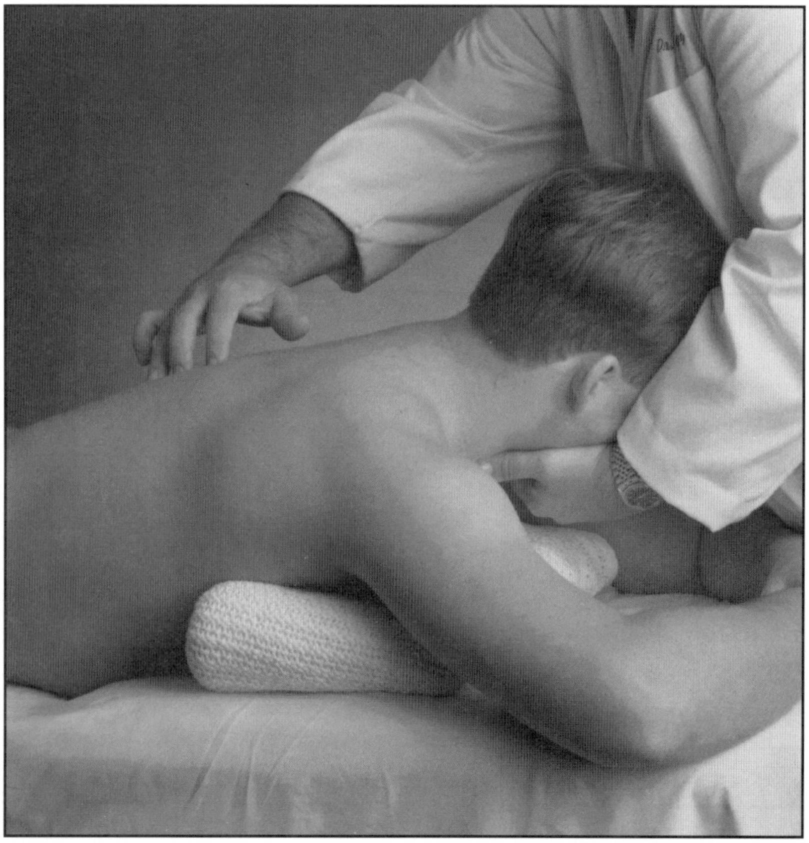

Posterior T7, 8, and 9—Treatment at this level may require something to aid the neck stretch to get the action down to the necessary level. This, on a flat table, can be done with a rolled up bath towel placed under the top of the chest as patient lies prone.

Posterior T10, 11, 12, and L1—At this level, spinous process tenderness indicates a need for a combination of extension and rotation. Again on a flat table there needs to be something under the upper chest to provide some extension. This alone will reduce the tenderness somewhat. The rotation is provided by grasping the pelvis around the anterior superior spine and rotating the pelvis about forty-five degrees. The easiest way for the operator to learn which way to twist is to use the thumbs and index fingers of both hands to pinch the two spinous processes to see what deviations he can find. Whatever he finds he will exaggerate. Occasionally there is so little obvious deviation of the two spinous processes, he may still guess wrong. If he does, the tenderness will not be further relieved, but aggravated. So he reverses his rotation stretch by pulling on the other side of the pelvis. This type of dysfunction at this level is not so common as others.

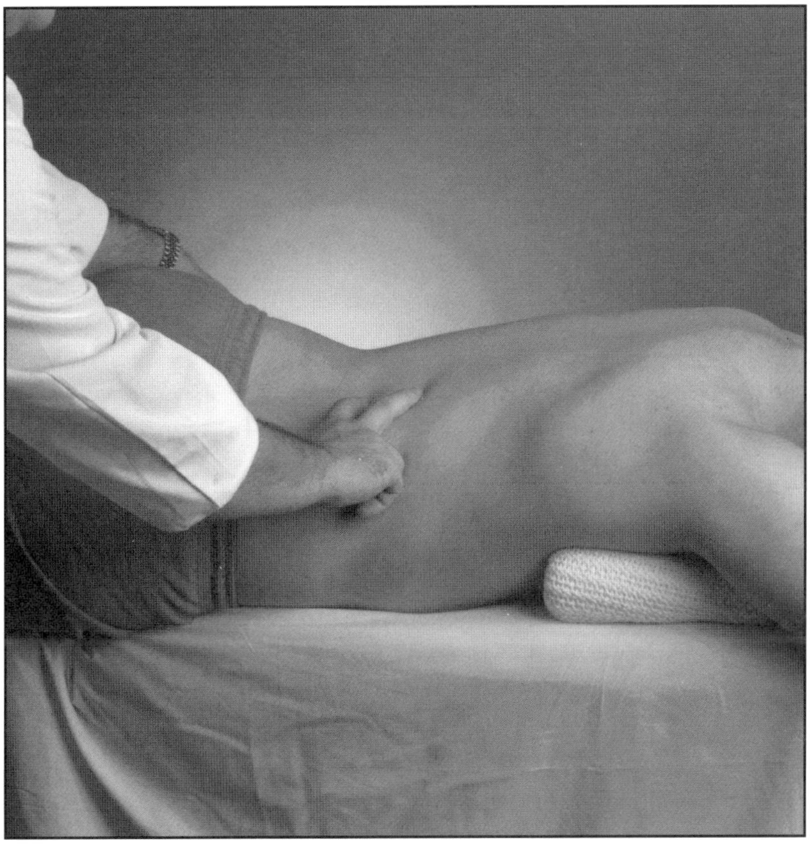

POSTERIOR THORACIC WITH MARKED DEVIATION OF SPINOUS PROCESSES

These are rare but must be treated differently. The shoulder away from the side of the deviation will be pulled caudad and the upper body is also rotated away.

Midthoracic dysfunctions with marked deviation of the spinous process aren't very common, but knowing how to deal with them will be very useful occasionally. They are different in the marked deviation to the side of the spinous process. They are relieved on a prone patient by grasping the shoulder away from the side of the deviation, pulling it caudad and rotating backward. Once more we don't treat any joint that doesn't have any pain and tenderness, no matter how deviated it appears.

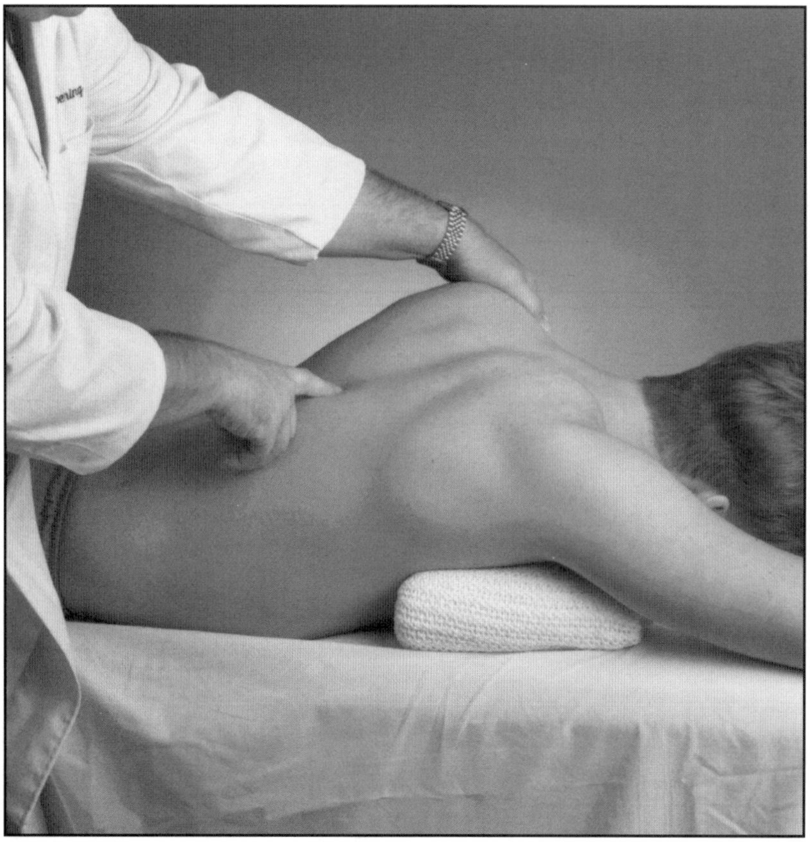

LATERAL POSTERIOR THORACICS

These are any dysfunctions where the greatest tenderness is not on the spinous process but more off to the side, between it and the transverse process or on the transverse process itself. This varies from less than an inch at the upper levels to as much as two inches at the level of the lower thoracics and upper two lumbars.

Posterior T1 to L2—We have here a treatment that with only slight modifications will treat any and all dysfunctions of this type at once. Patient lies prone with the arm of the affected side up beside the head. The action is markedly sidebending the body away from the sore side with a slight rotation toward it. The face is turned toward the sore side. To deal with problems involving the upper thoracic joints, the neck and head must be sidebent away from the sore side too. The patient is just asked to move the head back as far as is comfortable. The operator grasps the arm by grasping both sides of the axilla to hold and pulls cephalad. Most of the mistakes I see in beginners using this stretch is that they use too much rotation and not enough sidebending. Pain for these problems is strongly on one side of the body and especially at lower levels the patient may complain of a side ache rather than a backache. Occasionally I see operators confusing rib tenderpoints and these lateral intervertebral tenderpoints. They are far apart. We are interested in elevated second through sixth ribs. Their tenderpoints are on the angles of the ribs which are about two and a half inches lateral to the midline. Intervertebral lateral tenderpoints at that level are about one inch out from the midline.

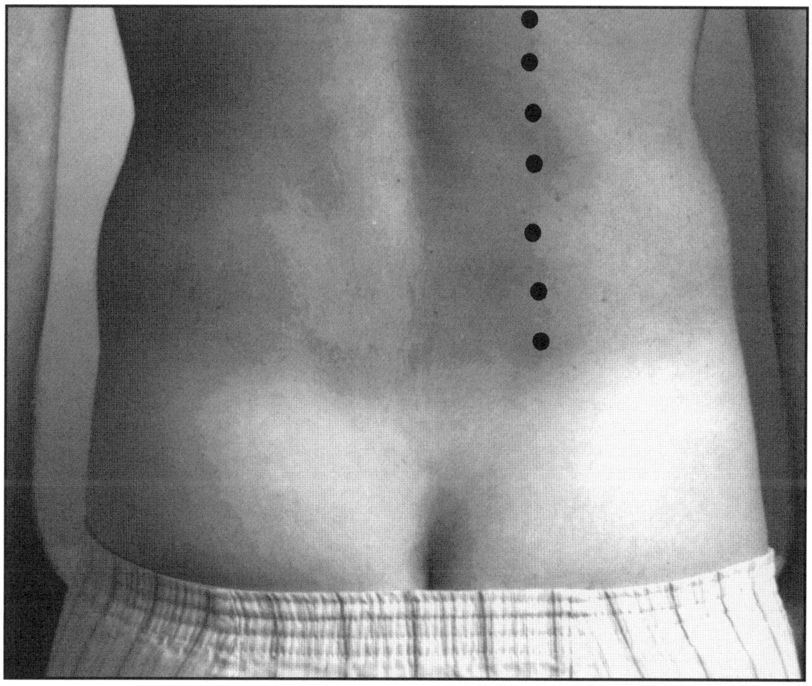

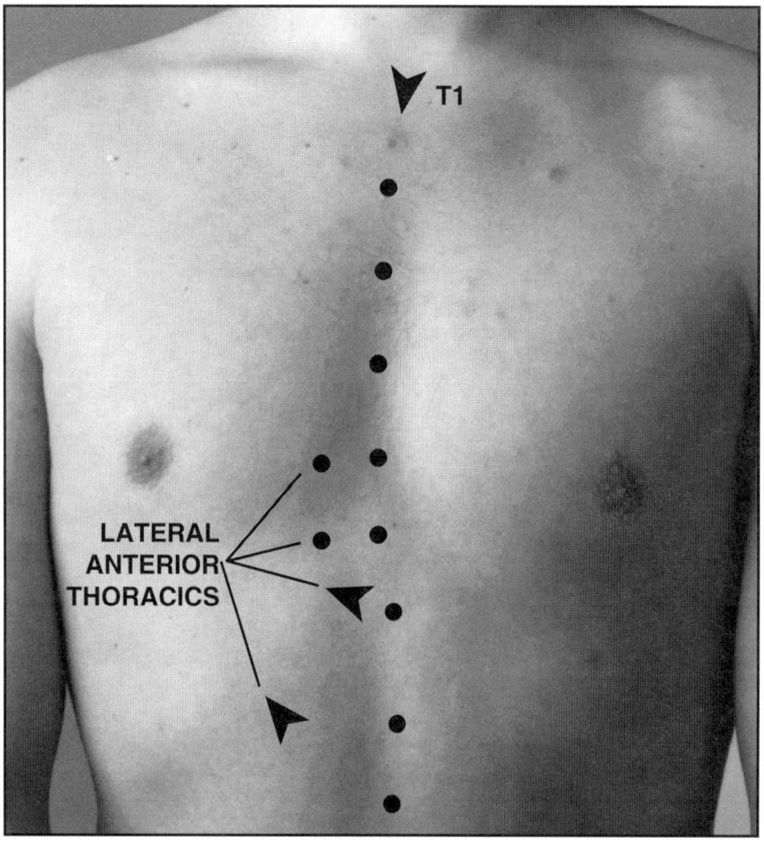

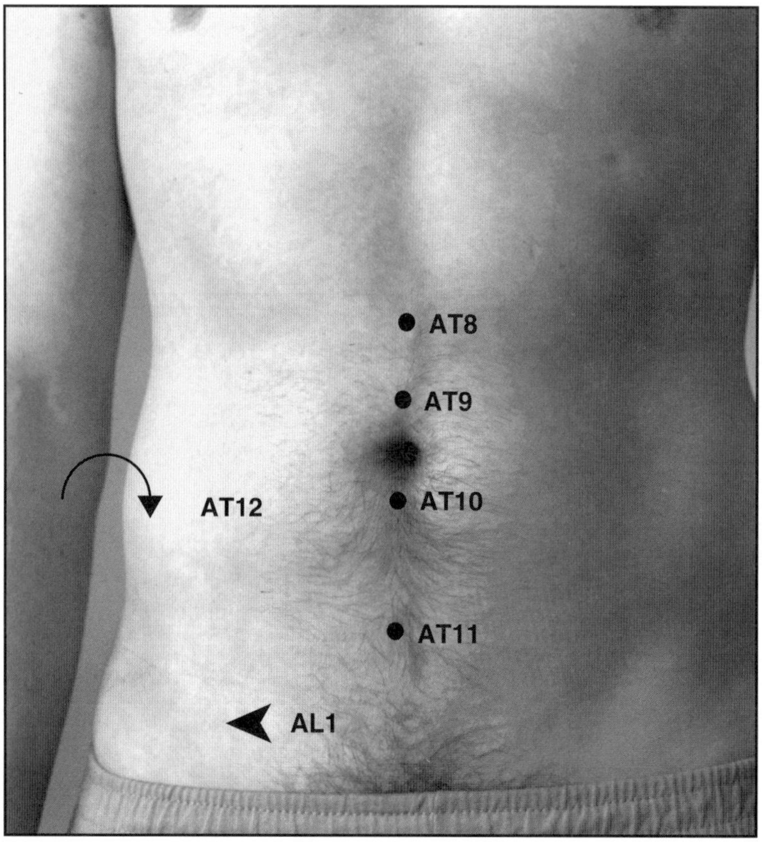

ANTERIOR THORACIC

These points indicate intervertebral dysfunctions too, but are located on the front of the body fairly close to the midline rather than near the spine. The upper seven are on or close to some part of the sternum, usually in the midline. When palpatory skills are developed, this apparently bare bone can be felt to have reducing tension and swelling. Starting with T8 through T11, tenderpoints are best found deep in the abdomen, near the midline.

For the novice this brings up another concern that he isn't skilled enough to differentiate abdominal tenderpoints for intervertebral dysfunctions from actual lesions of abdominal organs. The author solved this difficulty simply by applying flexion and observing the marked reduction in tenderness. An abdominal lesion will not be relieved by body positioning, so a definite relief of tenderness insures the fact that tenderness is due to a joint dysfunction. To be doubly certain the operator should at first recheck for tenderness after returning his patient to a neutral position. If relief continues, (most common), he knows that he is the expert, not the surgeon. Any doubt does indicate need for a consultation. The points for T12 and for the AL1 are more on the side, so less suspect.

All are treated with mostly marked flexion with the attempt to put flexion into the segment involved. In spite of all our discussion of the nature of this dysfunction and inapproprate strain input from a muscle, it is apparent that good success requires flexion of the dysfunctioning segment, not just shortening the long flexors of the spine.

Anterior T1 and T2—The tenderpoint for the first is in the bottom of the suprasternal notch pushing down from above (cephalad). That for the AT2 is on the front of the manubrium of the sternum. They both respond nicely to marked flexion of the neck while sitting crossway on the table with patient's fingers locked over his head. Operator stands behind with his forearms under the patient's arms, monitoring the tenderpoints with his fingers. He asks the patient to lean back on his chest and slides him down enough to achieve the necessary amount of flexion. There is a tendency for the patient to want to take over the process of righting himself after this stretch, so he must be forewarned to permit the operator to return him to neutral.

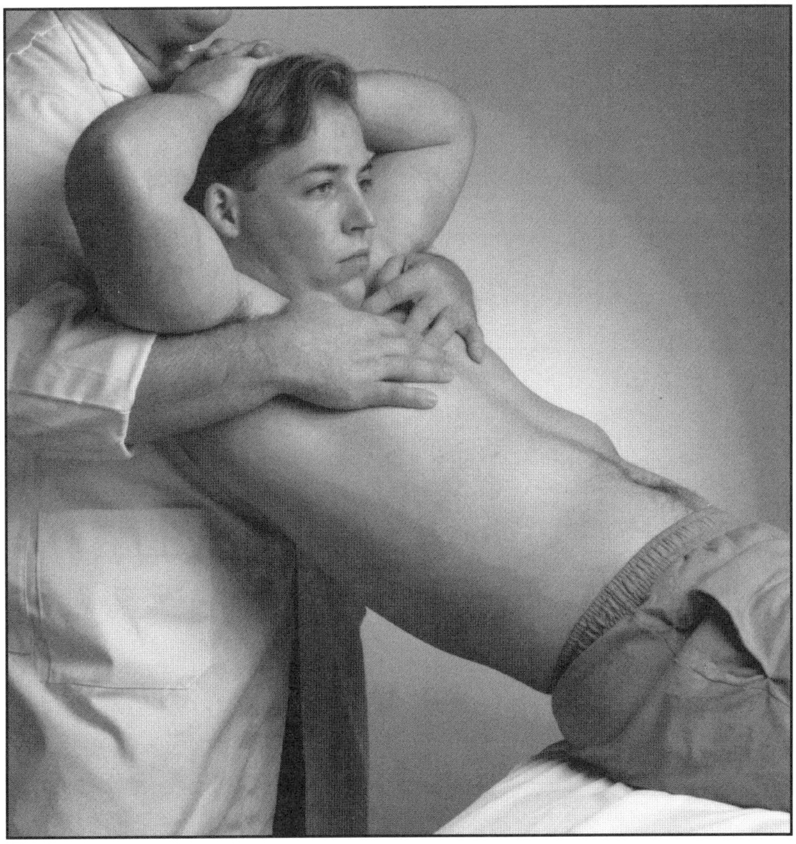

Anterior T3 and T4—These and the balance of these upper anterior thoracic tenderpoints are found at the level of the corresponding costal cartilage. Again the operator stands behind the patient, whose arms this time are hanging behind him. Operator reaches onto the medial side of the wrists of both arms in order to apply some pronation (or internal rotation) to them along with traction toward the floor. Operator's chest pushes against patient's upper thoracic spine, both to increase upper thoracic flexion and to give patient a sense of security. Although we are at this time too busy with both hands to monitor the success of this operation, it is routinely effective and easy.

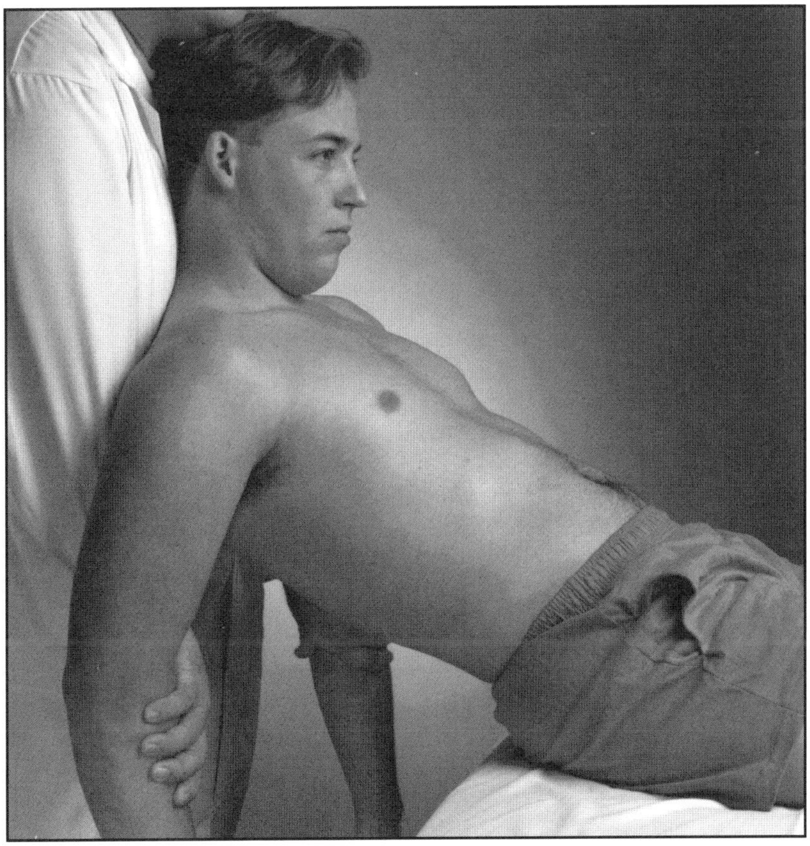

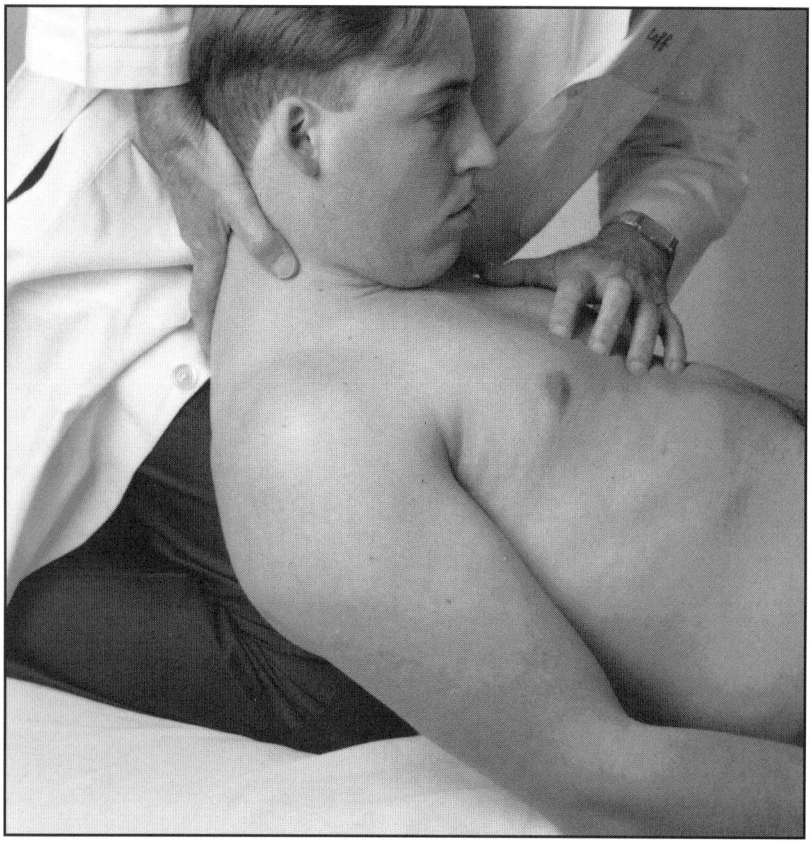

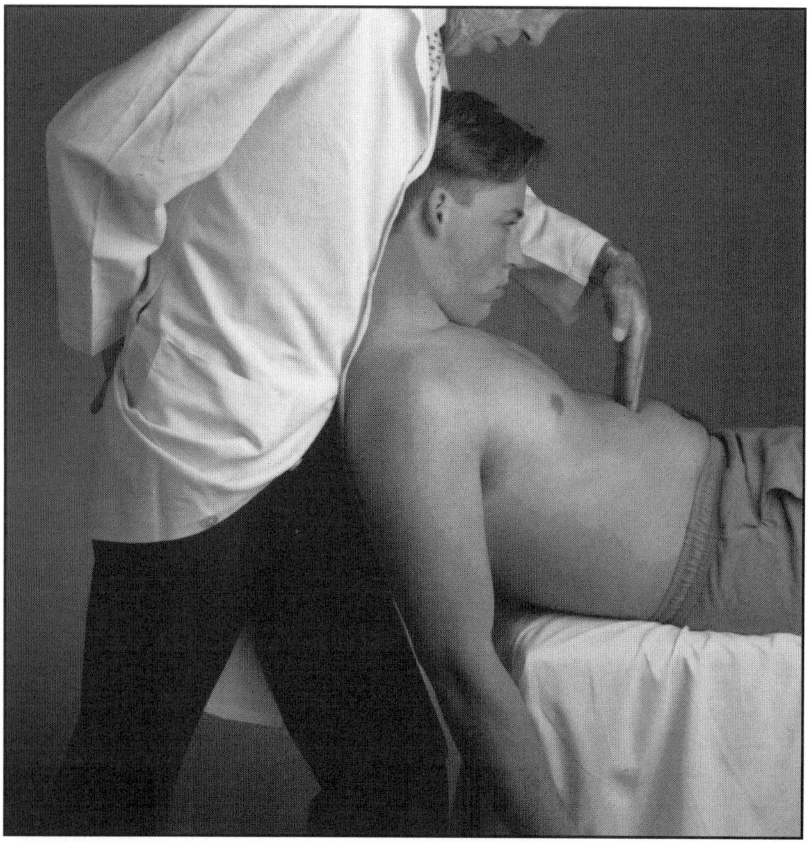

Anterior T5, T6, T7, and T8—Now we are getting into an area requiring considerable force to achieve enough flexion to make correction. At the time of the publication of the first book I was not satisfied with my ability here with any techniques I had been able to devise. I soon got some help from students who learned more effective techniques than I had learned. They will be presented here.

The first was Harold Schwartz, DO, FAAO, who later wrote an article on how to apply my office techniques to acute cases in hospital beds. His method called on the patient to lie supine on his thigh after he had placed one knee beneath the patient's mid thoracic area. By applying force against the upper thoracics from the front of his thigh, he achieved enough flexion to succeed.

Another was a physician from England practicing in Canada, Dr. Douglas Longdon, who pulled his supine patient far enough off the table that he was able to apply strong force by pushing against the upper thoracics with the side of his femur and hip. Because he had an ability to raise the shoulder area higher than possible with the Schwartz Technique, his way seemed especially useful at the level of the seventh and eighth thoracics. Tenderpoint for the AT5 is about an inch above the xiphoid junction, AT6 is at the xiphoid junction, AT7 is at the tip of the xiphoid, and AT8 is about one and a half inches below it, all close to the midline.

ANTERIOR LATERAL 5, 6, 7, AND 8 THORACIC DYSFUNCTIONS

These are a different kind of dysfunction from those requiring little more than straight flexion. Tenderpoints for these are found on the costal cartilages at these levels, close to the side of the sternum for T5 and T6 and off an inch or more to the side of the xiphoid process on the medial, inferior surfaces of the costal cartilages for the seventh and eighth thoracics. (See page 56.)

These are very important dysfunctions as they are responsible for much epigastric pain. They actually contribute remarkably in treatment of gastric or duodenenal ulcer. Also along with central AT5, AT6, AT7, and AT8, they are a likely culprit for chronic fatigue, especially when the complaint includes the statment, "I wake up tired." Whether they represent purely intervertebral or or a type of costo-vertebral dysfunction is still moot. They all require a technique which applies flexion, sidebending toward the sore side, and rotation away. One of the most unfortunate mistakes of the first book was an illustration showing a much larger amount of sidebending than the ideal. I have been trying to talk students out of mimicking the illustration ever since publication. The ideal position is limited in the amount of sidebending.

If this limiting is not done, it is impossible to find the ideal position of mobility. I do this by having my patient seated at the table draping one shoulder over my knee and thigh (covered by a small pillow). Patient rotates his face toward the pillow and rests his head on it and leans on operator's thigh. Limitation of sidebending is provided by a pressure from the medial side of the operator's thigh against the side of the patient's chest. Now flexion can be enhanced by pressure on top of the shoulder of the affected side, from the operator's forearm. This technique is far superior to the one illustrated in the old book.

Especially for the anterior eighth thoracic, it is a transitional segment and may be more easily and effectively included with those just below than with those above it.

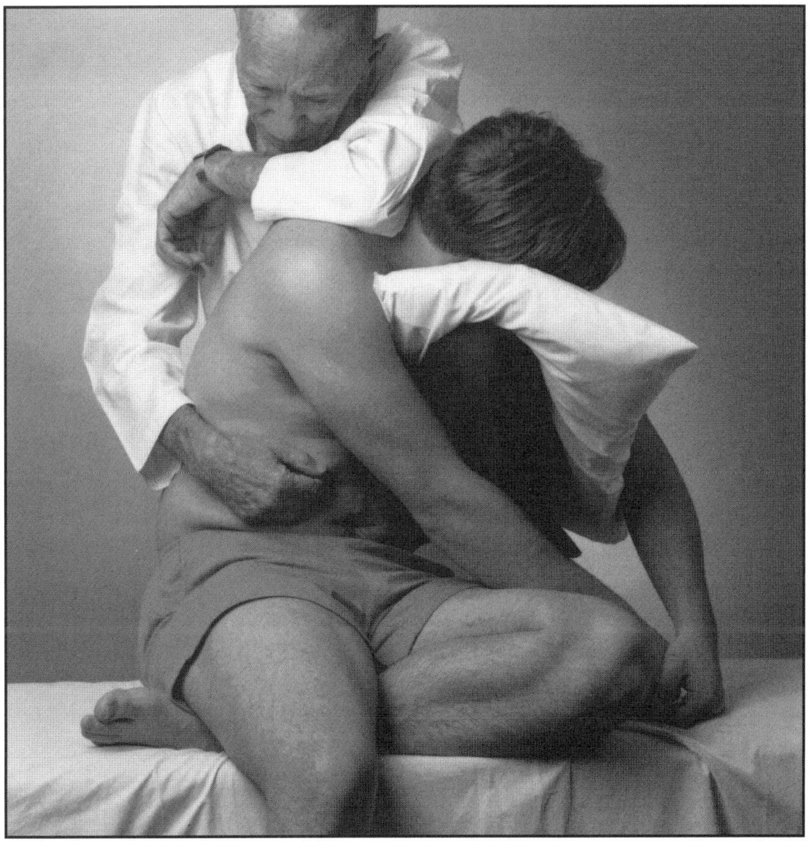

Anterior T9, T10, T11, T12, and L1—These are an important source of low back pain with inability to extend the spine. Fortunately they are relatively easy to relieve. Tenderpoints except for the T12 are located near the midline deep in the abdomen. That for the AT9 is about one centimeter above the umbilicus. The one for the tenth is one to two centimeters below the umbilicus and that for the eleventh about two inches below. The point for the T12 is found on the inner table of the ala of the ilium in the midaxillary line, approaching it from above. That for the AL1, included here because it is relieved like the others, by starting an inch medial to the anterior superior spine of the ilium, pressing deeply and laterally. All or any of them may be relieved with marked flexion and mild rotation of the legs toward the sore side.

These will be best treated with the use of a table that can have one end elevated. If you are limited to a flat top table, most of them can still be relieved with the patient lying supine with a large pillow doubled under his hips so as to allow the segments of the lower thoracic and upper lumbar spine room to flex. With minor variations one treatment will relieve any of them. Roll the knees and legs up about 135 degrees and pull the knees lightly toward the tender side, perhaps twenty degrees. Besides the slow return of the legs, the removal of the pillow must be done very slowly. To be effective, the treatment must stretch the segment indicated.

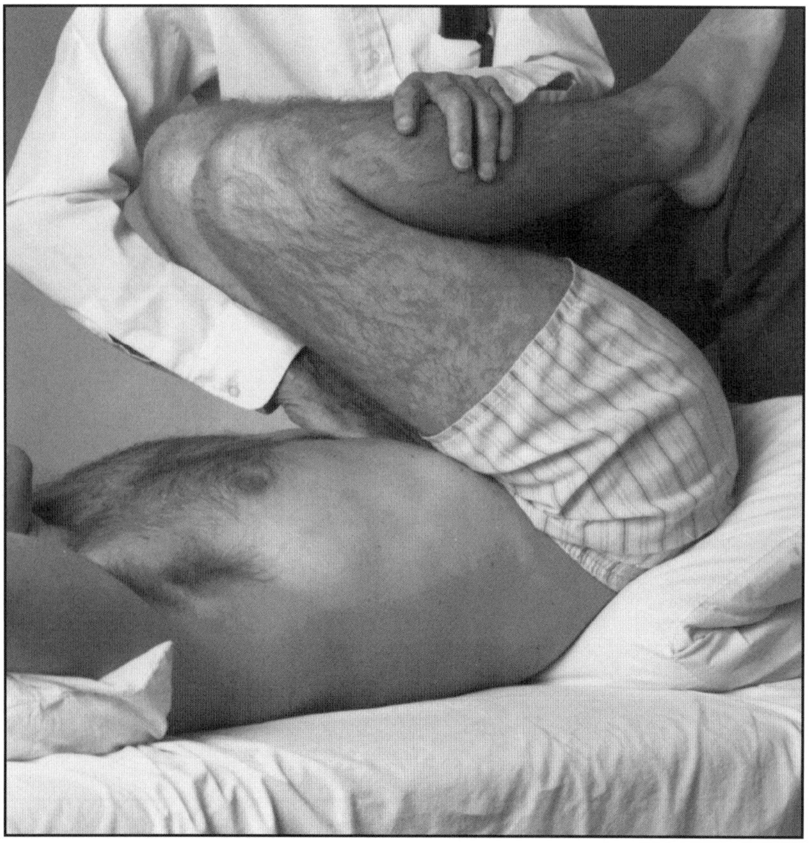

COSTO-VERTEBRAL JOINTS

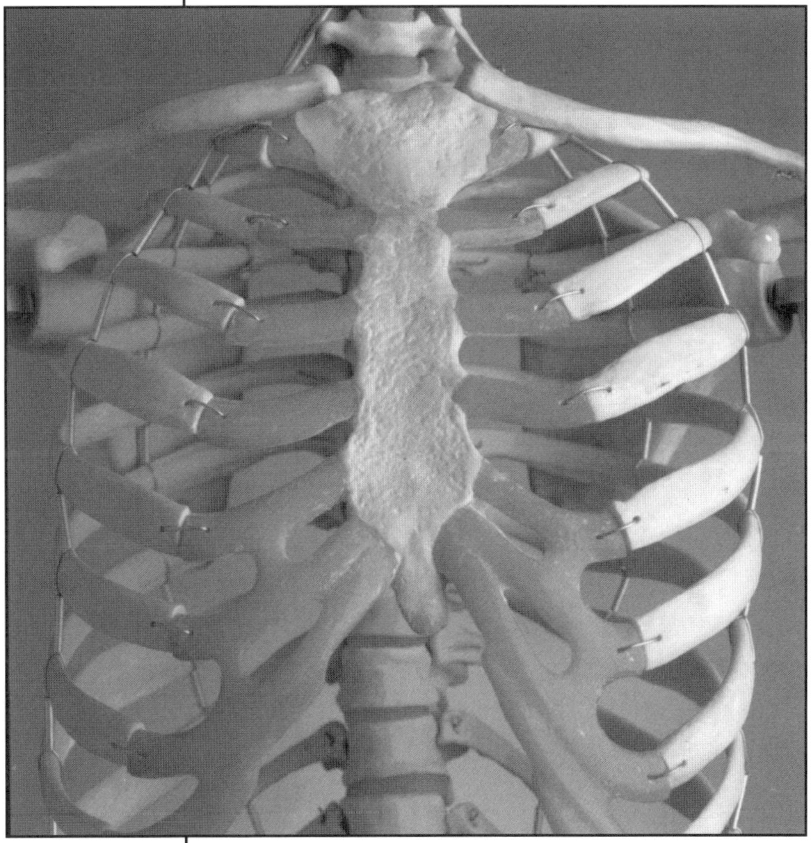

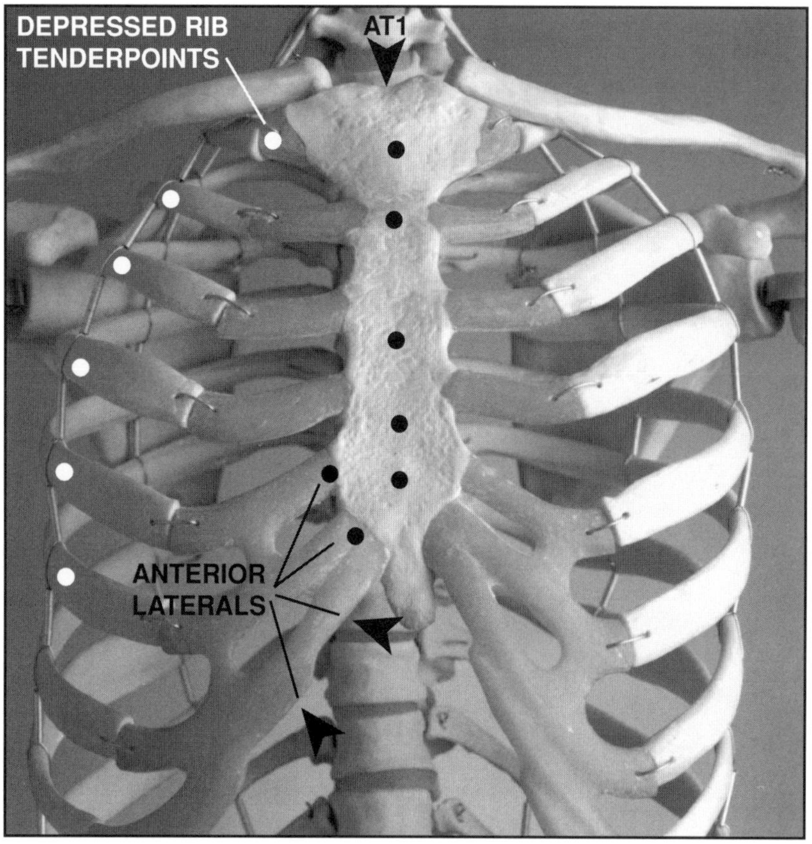

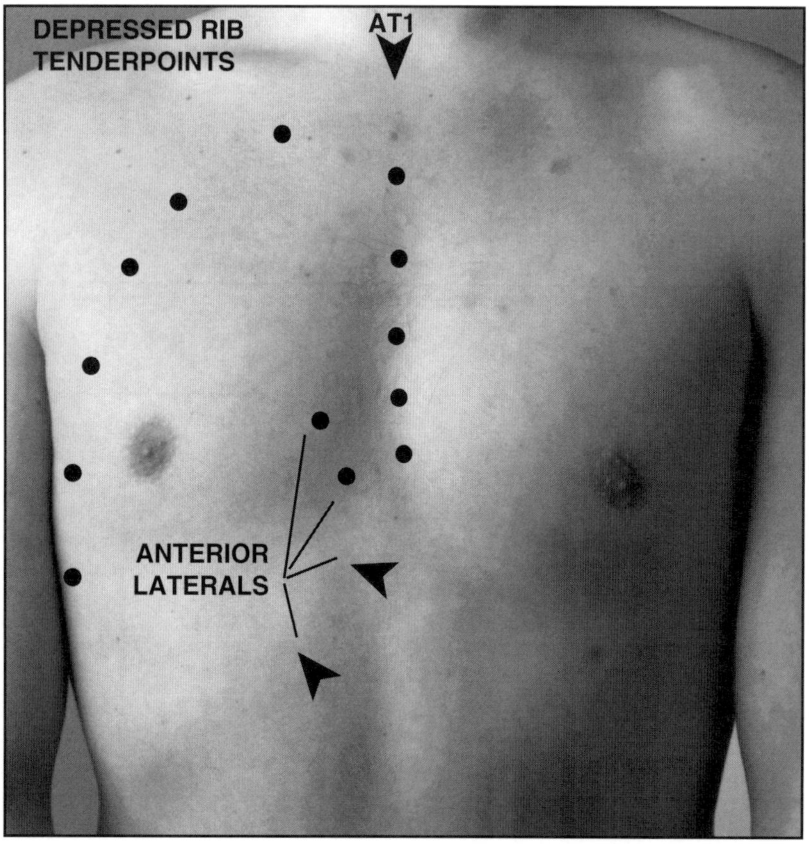

GENERAL

Most costo-vertebral joint dysfunctions occur with thoracic intervertebral dysfunctions. The ones we are most concerned with are the top five intervertebral segments and the top six ribs, with an occasional trouble on the eighth and tenth ribs. Since rib problems and the upper five thoracic intervertebral joint dysfunctions appear to be so strongly interdependant, I never fail to examine one without the other.

In the part of the book dealing with sequencing of treatments, we speak of treating the most painful first. Here is the exception. Most often the ribs are more painful than the intervertebral joints, but the intervertebral should be treated first because of the location of the rib heads (with the exception of the first rib) between two adjacent vertebrae. Without normal intervertebral relationships, it can prove frustrating trying to relieve the costo-vertebral joints.

Though the first book classified the interspace tenderpoints as rib problems, here we will classify them with lateral anterior 5, 6, 7, and 8 intervertebral joints, as the treatment is identical with that for these problems. Many improvements in the newer book over the older book have come from physicians who have not been entirely satisfied with the way I suggested they treat something, and have found a better way. Here is one offered by Murray Black, DO, who practices in Yakima, WA. I have used his method since he told me and have found it effective and easier than mine. Just one more evidence that there is much room for improvement. I am always grateful when a student of mine contributes something better. For anterior mid thoracic dysfunctions, Dr. Black treats his patients in the supine position, using traction of the arm and internal rotation (pronation) of the forearm with traction caudad and slightly anterior. I think his method may be better than mine.

Because of these changes of interpretation, we are left with just two types of rib problems, elevated ribs and depressed ribs. Before I learned to trust pain and comfort of the patient to tell me what the rib needed, I used to spend much unnecessary time trying to decide whether one rib was high or the other one was low. Since we believe that any asymmetry shows the body's inability to return to a symmetrical position, we call ribs which we relieve by pushing them down, depressed ribs, and any we relieve by elevating, elevated ribs. By pursuing this concept we have excellent success with ribs. We will discuss them from below up, because the treatments and tenderpoints form a pattern for ribs up to the second.

I had forgotten to ask Dr. Goering to demonstrate Dr. Black's techniques. My fault. These are my techniques.

DEPRESSED RIBS THIRD AND BELOW

Tenderpoints for these are found on the anterior axillary line. An easy way to locate this line is to search just beneath the outer edge of the pectoralis major muscle. Treatment is sidebending of the spinal area at that level toward the affected side and rotating toward it with a little flexion. For me this has been easily accomplished by having my patient rest his arm of the opposite side over my knee and thigh, padded by a pillow. Like the story for the lateral anterior mid and upper thoracics, the illustrations of the first book led most students to use too much sidebending. We do here as with the others push against the side of the chest with the side of the operator's thigh to limit the amount of sidebending. For operators not able to get a table low enough for them to do this with comfort, they find they can substitute their shoulders for their thighs. They sit beside the patient with a shoulder under his arm, close to the chest wall. This device may be used for elevated ribs too.

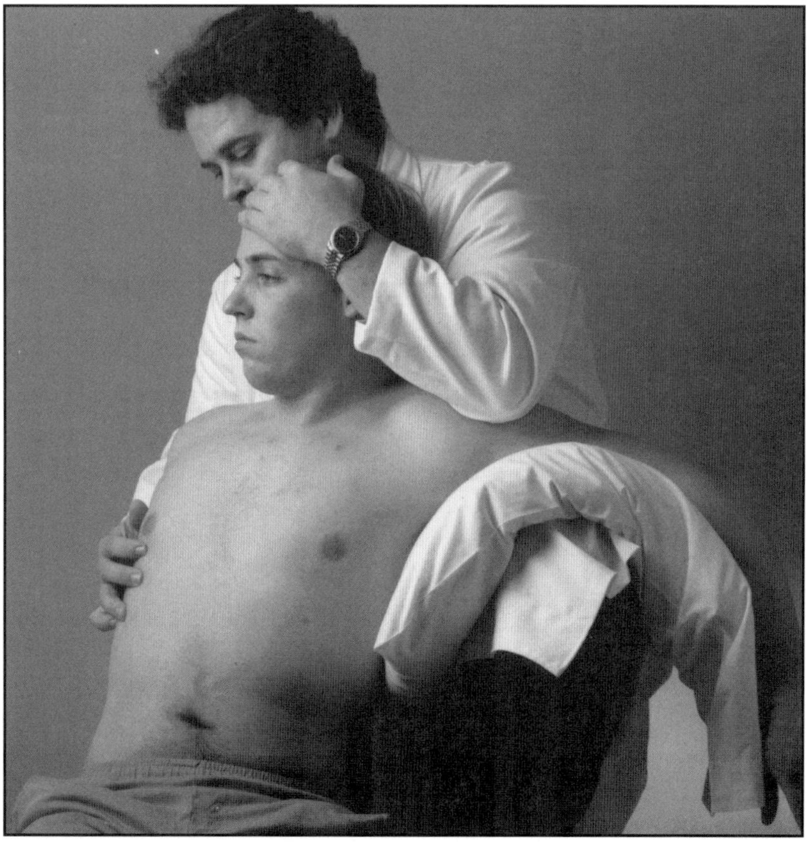

DEPRESSED
FIRST AND SECOND RIBS.

These are atypical both in location of tenderpoints and method of treatment. A depressed first rib has a point of tenderness just beneath the clavicle and just lateral to the margin of the sternum. The depressed second rib is tender one and one half inches below the middle of the clavicle.

Treatment is the same for both. The patient lies supine and the operator lifts the head and neck about forty degrees and rotates and sidebends toward the sore side about forty-five degrees. Like other depressed ribs, pain is usually in back of the shoulder although the tenderpoints are in front.

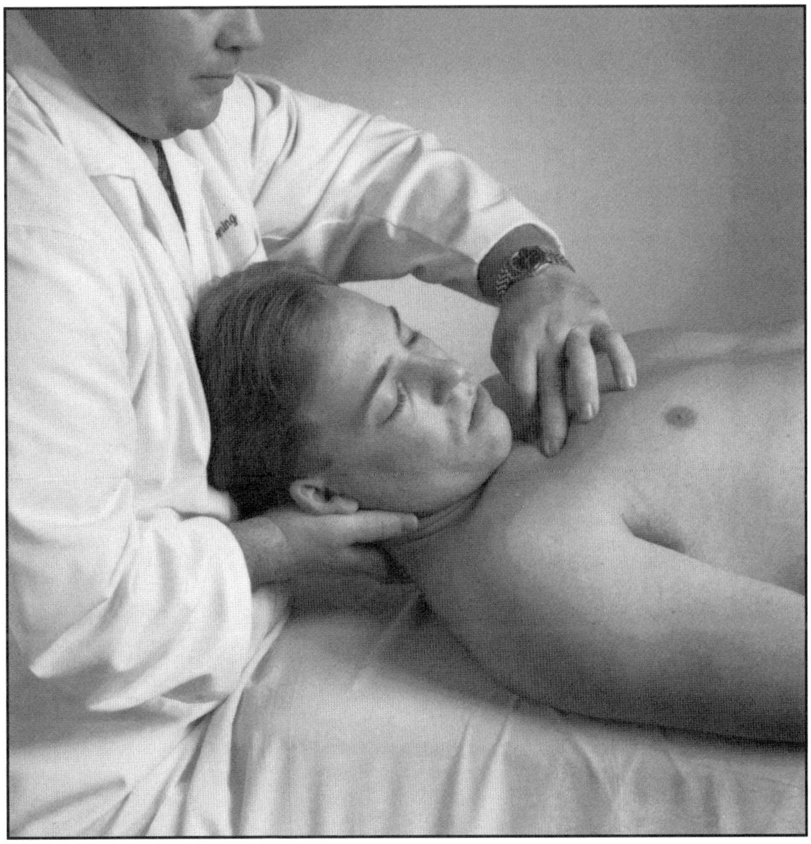

ELEVATED RIBS THIRD AND BELOW

(usually ribs 3, 4, 5, and 6)

Tenderpoints for these problems can be found on the ribs involved in two areas of the chest. The original book listed an area on the back of the thorax, on the angles of the ribs, about two and a half inches lateral to the midline (not an inch or less, which would indicate a lateral intervertebral problem). It will save considerable confusion if you adopt a rule of pulling the arm of the affected side across the front of the chest to move the scapula away from the rib angles you are probing. Besides being tender at these points, the affected rib usually will be less prominent posteriorly than normal in contrast to depressed ribs, which when probed at this area will usually be excessively prominent posteriorly. There is another area of tenderpoints almost as useful for elevated ribs right on the mid axillary line (not the anterior axillary line).

Regardless of which area you use to diagnose and monitor, treatment involves sidebending and rotating the joints involved away from the sore side with the same limitation of sidebending discussed above, because we will not find the position of mobility for the rib unless we do. Motion between ribs is often easy to feel when the position is ideal.

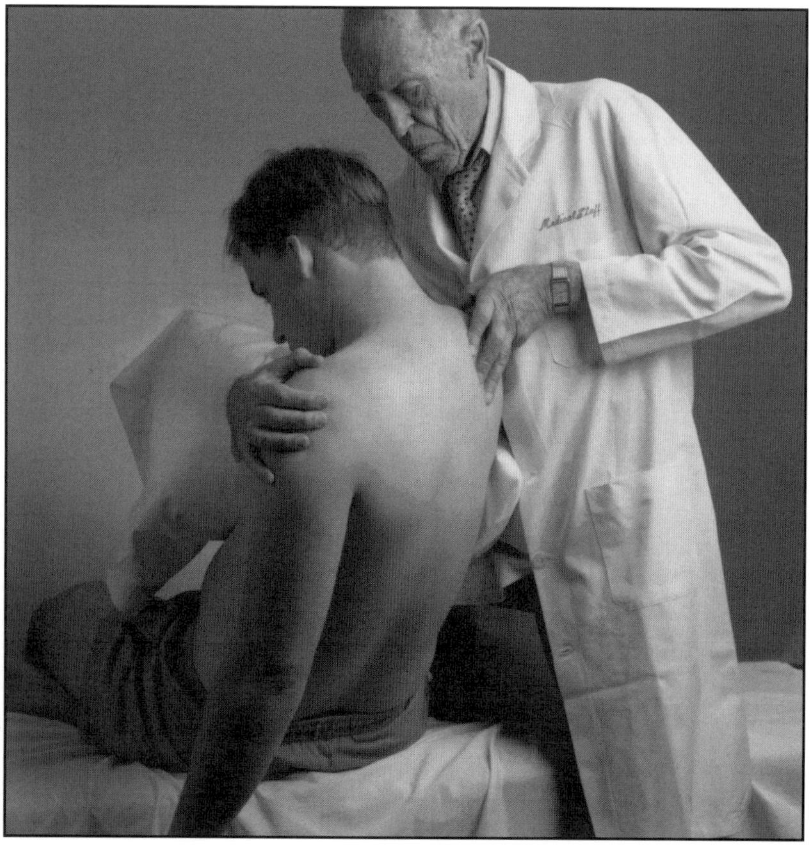

ELEVATED SECOND RIB

We discuss the second rib because it is different only in that its treatment needs a twisting and sidebending of the neck in addition to the rest of the treatment. The force on the shoulders alone doesn't affect ribs this high enough to release the dysfunction.

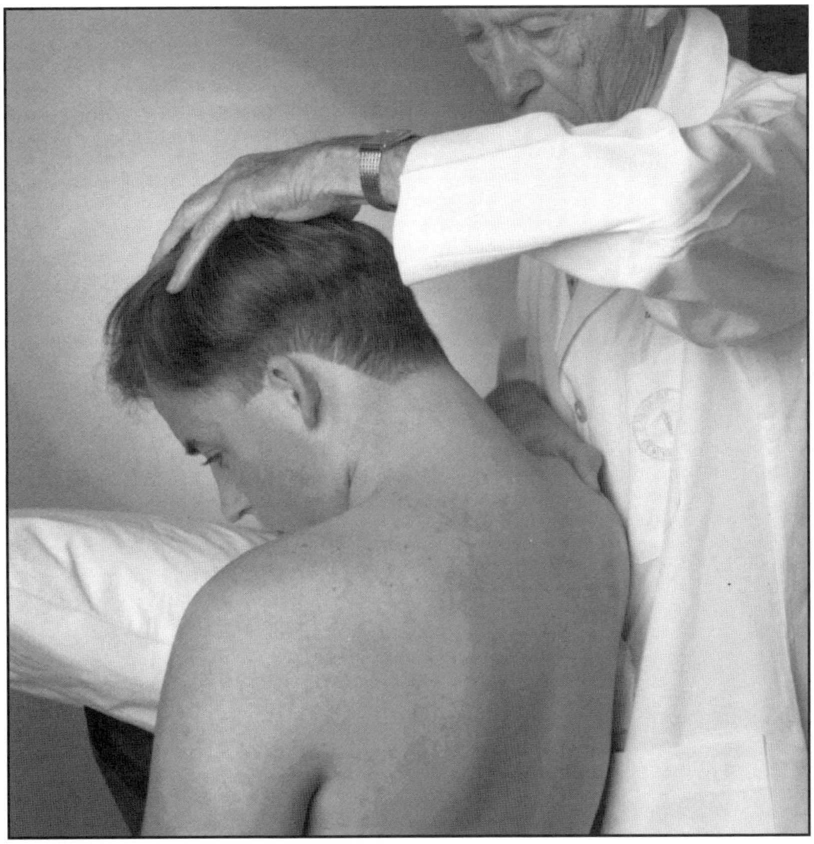

ELEVATED FIRST RIB

The elevated first rib is tender on it superior surface close to its attachment to the spine at the base of the neck. Probe down through the superficial muscles until you feel bone. Treatment is accomplished entirely with neck extension and this is very slight and with hardly any force. This treatment is much more effective than the brutal thrust I was taught and uses less than five percent of the force. Any rotation or sidebending to find the easily palpable position of mobility will confirm your success.

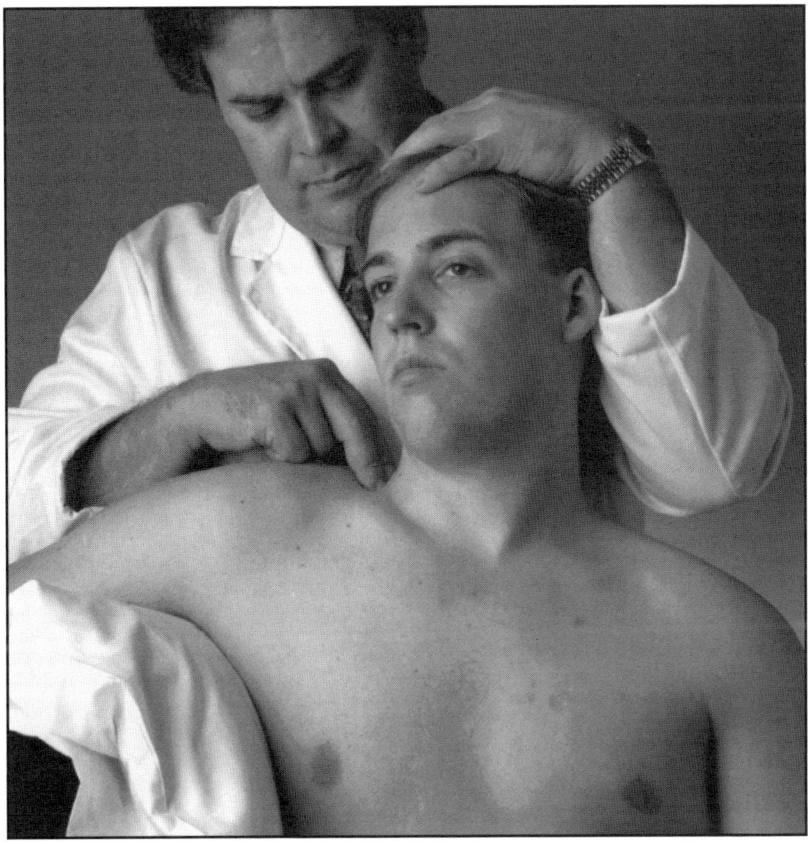

LUMBAR JOINTS

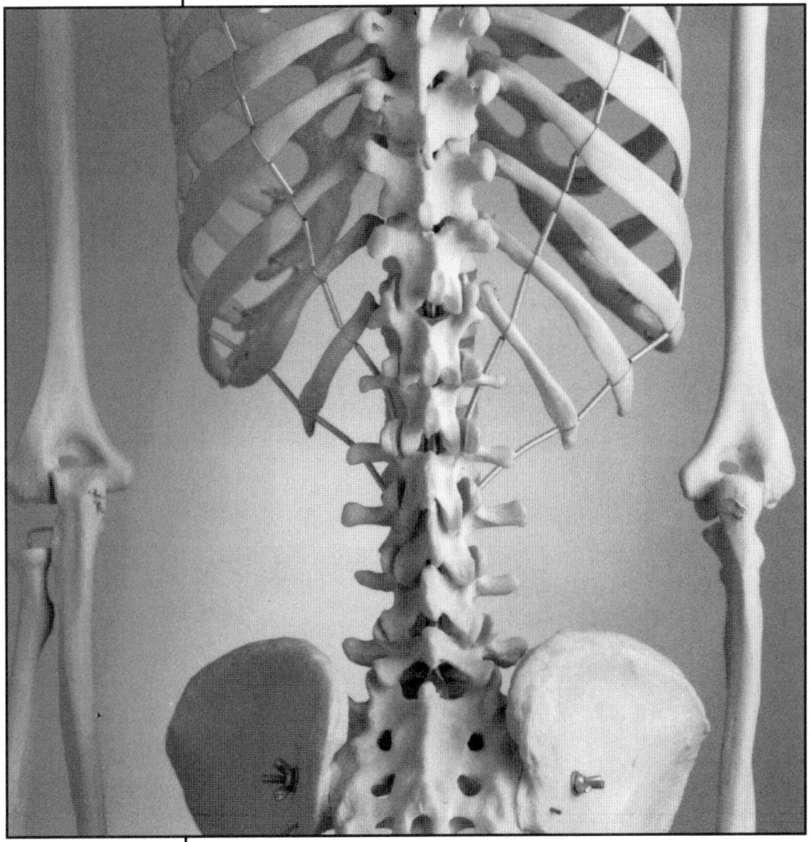

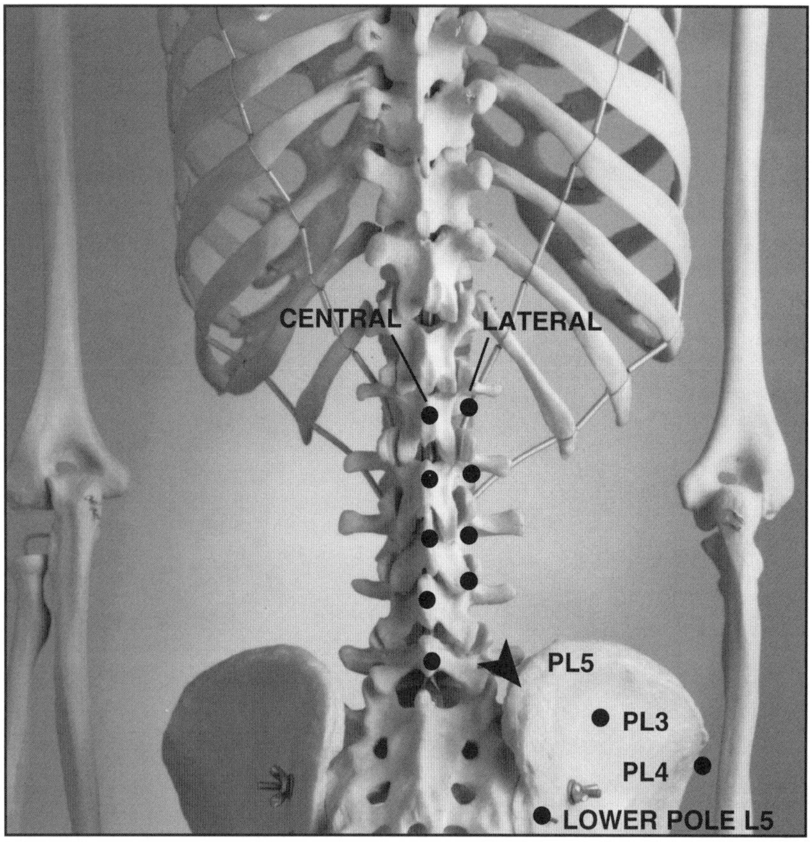

POSTERIOR LOWER THREE LUMBARS

Because of relative importance these will be discussed from below up. The common complaint of low back pain is often related to the lower three lumbar joints which are best diagnosed from discrete points on the posterior pelvis. An important landmark here is the posterior superior spine of the ilium which can be found high and about one and a half inches lateral to the midline. Its superio-medial edge is the place to look for dysfuncton of the L5.

Another landmark is the strong tensor fascia femoris on the side of the pelvis extending up from a third useful landmark, the greater trochanter of the femur. One centimeter behind the tensor halfway up between the trochanter and the crest of the ilium is the spot for the L4. When these are located, the point for the L3 will be found halfway between the points for L4 and L5.

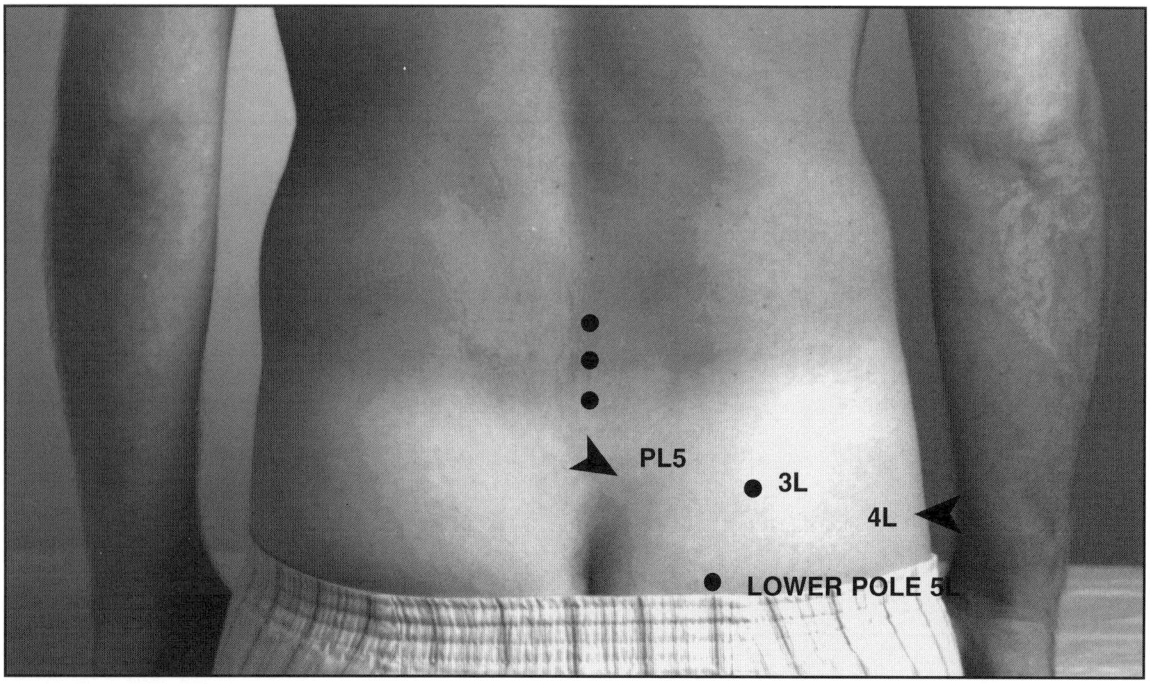

With small variations, one treatment will relieve all of these dysfunctions with extension of the leg of the painful side. The variations are in the degree of rotation and extension. A lifting force on a prone patient, applied just below the knee will permit the knee to reman straight while the femur and lower lumbar vertebrae are extended. I do it with my flexed knee. If a second lifting force is applied six inches above the knee, the effect on the low back will change from pure extension to less extension and more rotation. The first position will ease a L5 dysfunction. The second will relieve a L3 dysfunction. The L4 will be eased by a stretch halfway between the other two. The fifth lumbar and the fourth lumbar are more common than the third. The author puts a padded, flexed knee under the tibia and pulls with his hand to produce the variation, but operators of different stature using tables of different relative height adopt various other means producing these stretches.

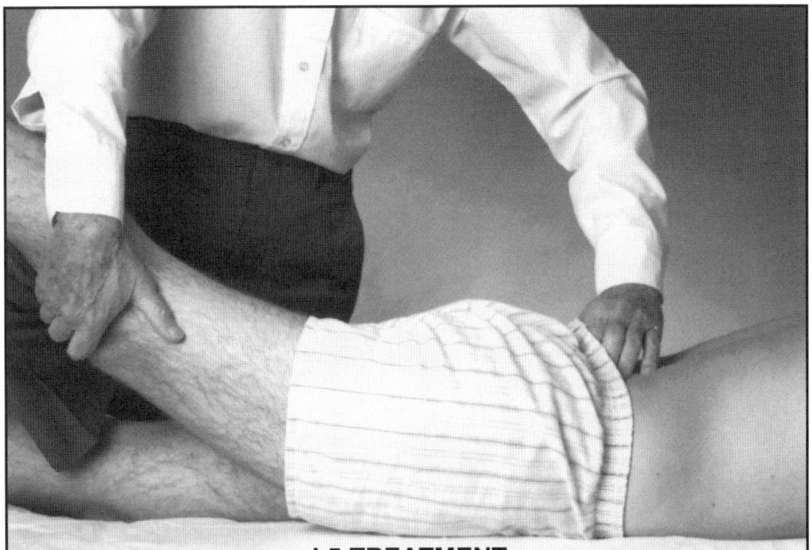

L5 TREATMENT

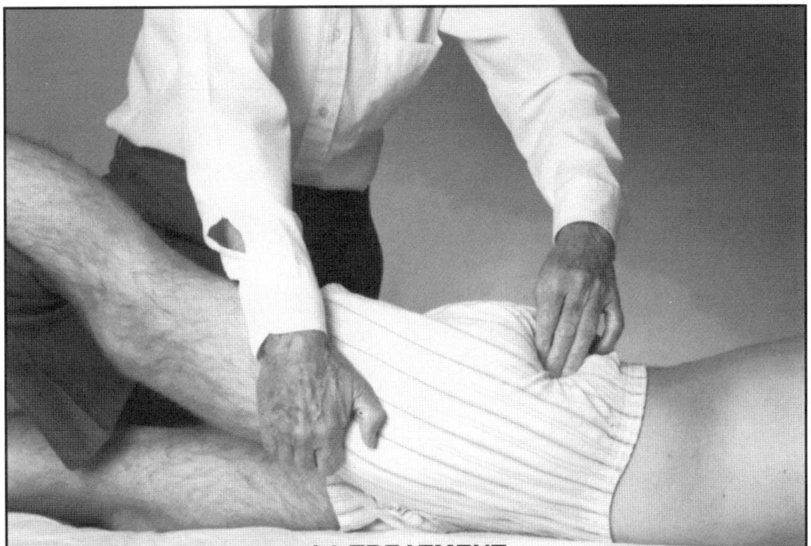

L3 TREATMENT

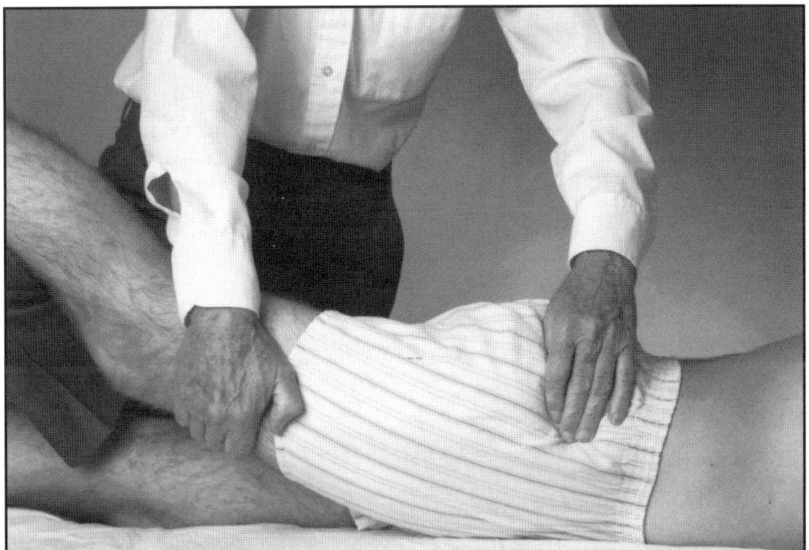

L4 TREATMENT

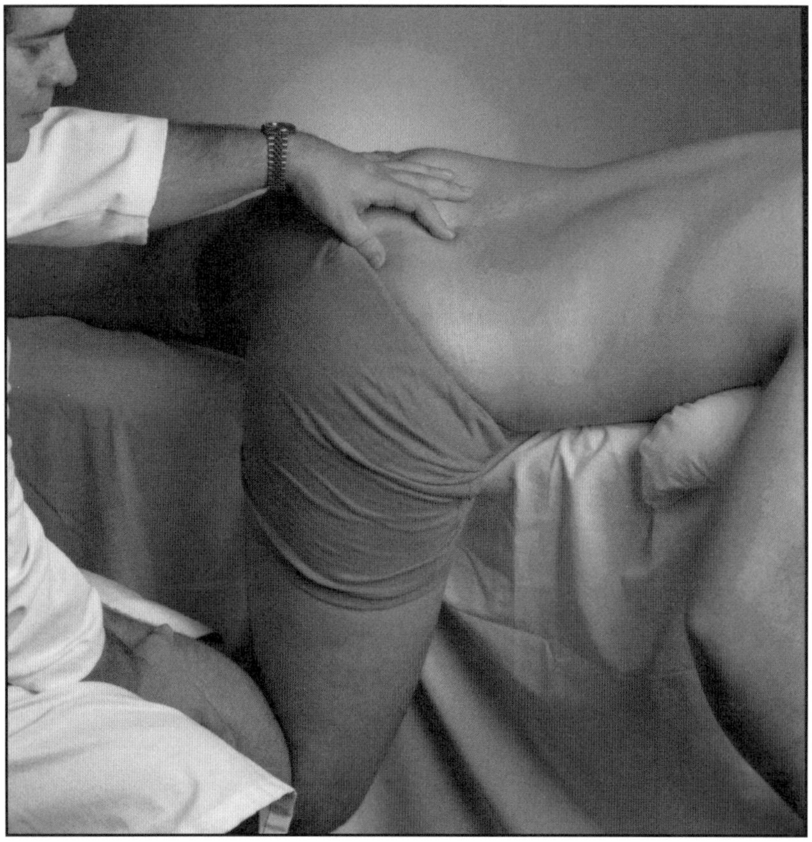

LOWER POLE FIFTH LUMBAR JOINT

There is another L5 tenderpoint with a different treatment. It is located an inch just below the posterior spine of the ilium. This treatment is accomplished with the prone patient's leg on the affected side hanging off the side of the table with the femur vertical and the knee pushed slightly under the edge of the table top. Usually this is done easily with the knee also flexed ninety degrees.

An alternate tenderpoint is on the upper surface of the top spinous process of the sacrum.

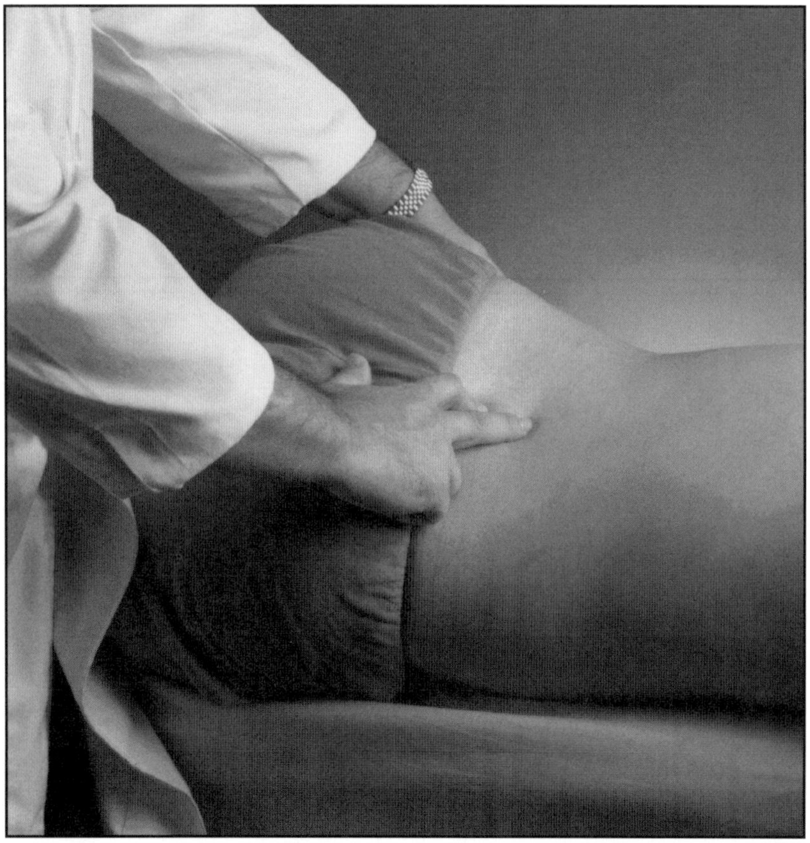

TREATMENT FOR TENDERPOINTS ON THE SPINOUS PROCESSES

As in the lower thoracic and first lumbar area there may be tenderpoints on the spinous processes of the lumbar vertebrae. These again, if tender, are diagnosed as to rotation by pinching of adjacent spinous processes and exaggerating any deformity found. At this level there is no need to have extension. Rotation is produced by grasping the anterior superior spine and rotating the pelvis about forty-five degrees. The second lumbar may be one of these.

ANTERIOR LOWER LUMBARS 2, 3, 4, AND 5

Tenderpoints for the L2, L3, and L4 are found on a small knob one and three fourths inches below and a little medial to the anterior superior spine of the ilium, the anterior inferior iliac spine. This is recessed deeper than the superior spine and takes some practice to learn to find it. It is easiest found with the patient supine with both knees up. This little knob must be learned because of these important tenderpoints.

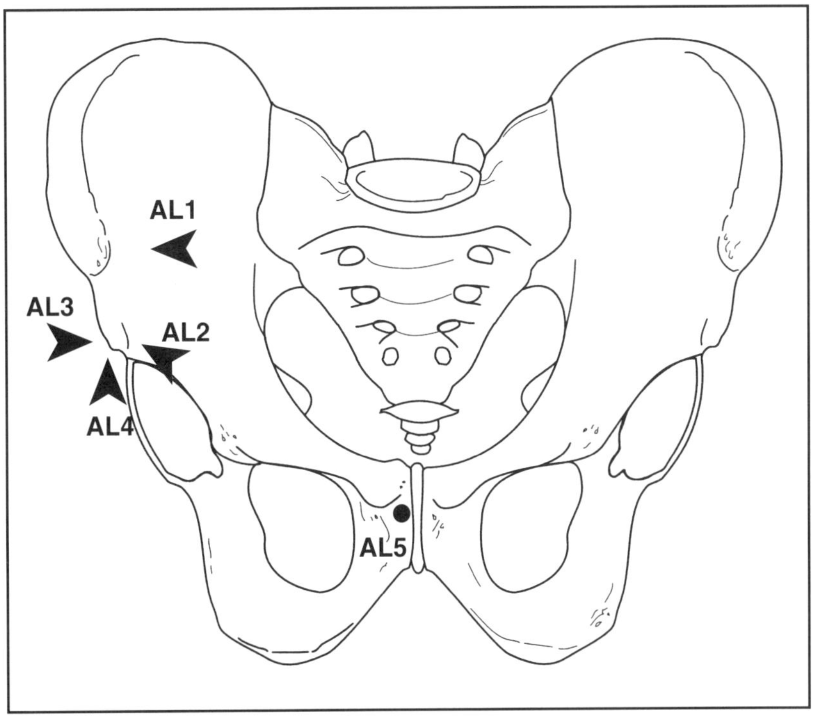

TREATMENT FOR ANTERIOR SECOND LUMBAR

The point for the important AL2 is on its underside of this little spine and a little medial. Treatment for this problem requires much rotation of the flexed femurs away from the tender side with about sixty degrees of rotation. This will often produce a strained feeling in back of the hip, which can be eliminated by a force of traction on the higher femur by pulling behind the flexed knee. If the patient is relaxed, his feet will fall to the side and produce a little sidebending away from the sore side. This is helpful.

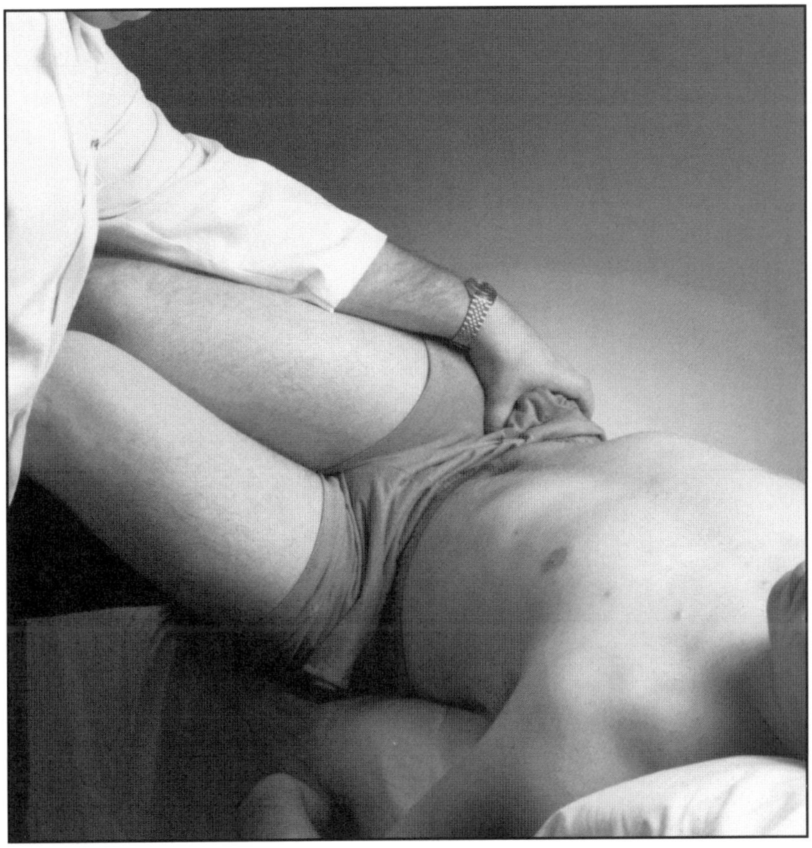

ABDOMINAL SECOND LUMBAR

There is another tenderpoint blamed on the second lumbar, because of its treatment position, which is like the last treatment position but with rotation reversed. The legs are rolled toward the affected side. Sidebending remains away so instead of supporting the knees in the roll and allowing the feet to hang down, the holding of the leg is low enough on the calf to produce a little lifting of the feet and sidebending away from the sore side. This tenderpoint is located in the abdominal wall two and a half inches lateral to the umbilicus and a half inch lower.

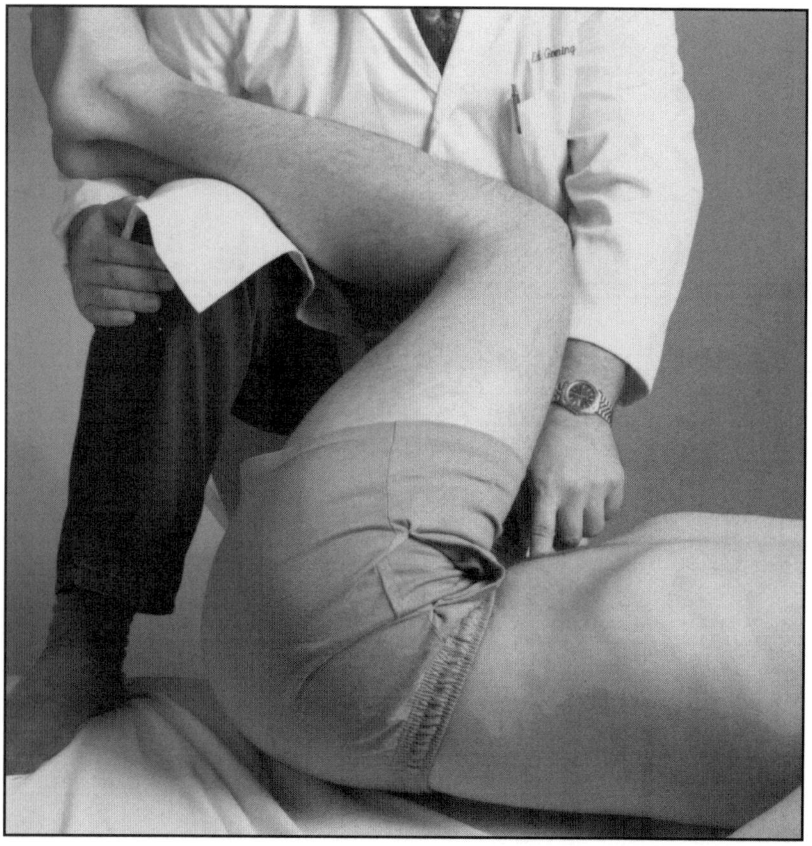

ANTERIOR THIRD AND FOURTH LUMBAR

Back to the anterior inferior iliac spine: tenderness against its lateral side indicates dysfunction of the third lumbar. Tenderness on its exact underside is interpreted as anterior fourth lumbar. These two are much less common and important than the second. They are both relieved with the knees straight above the pelvis and the feet pulled away from the painful side to produce in the lumbar spine a sidebending. For some reason beginning students seem to confuse rotation of the lumbar spine produced by pulling the knees laterally and this sidebending with the feet pulled laterally.

(Occasionally there is another tenderpoint on the superior medial side of this small knob, which we blame on the pelvis. It is relieved with further flcxion of the femur of the affected side.)

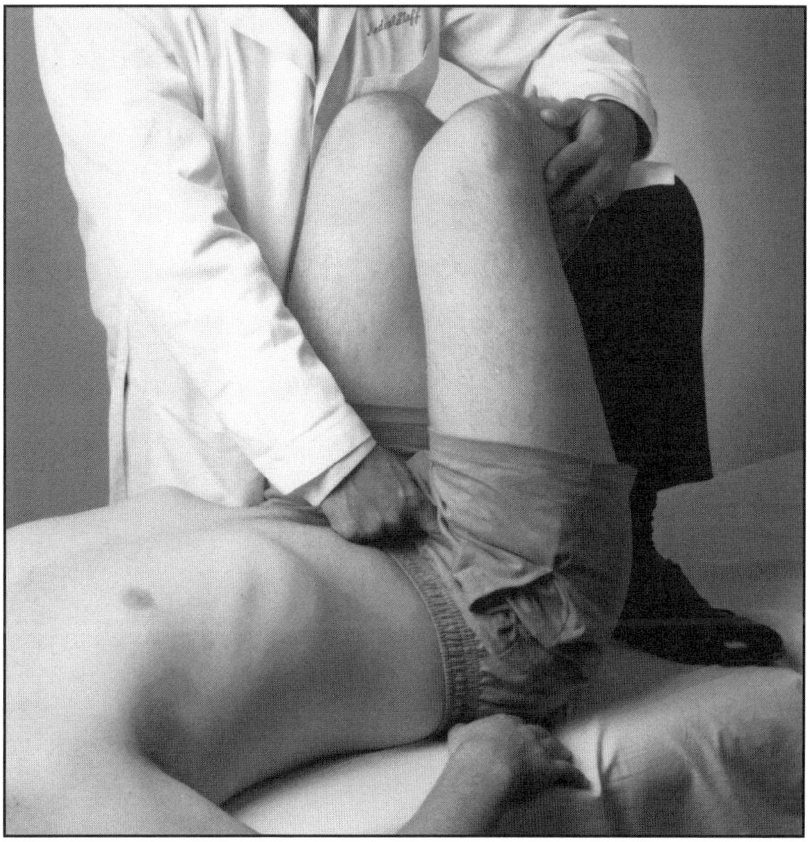

THE ANTERIOR FIFTH LUMBAR

This common dysfunction has its tenderpoint on the front of the pubic bone within a centimeter of the symphisis pubis. It is relieved on a flat table by increasing the flexion of both femurs to about 135 degrees and pulling the knees a little toward the side of pain and tenderness.

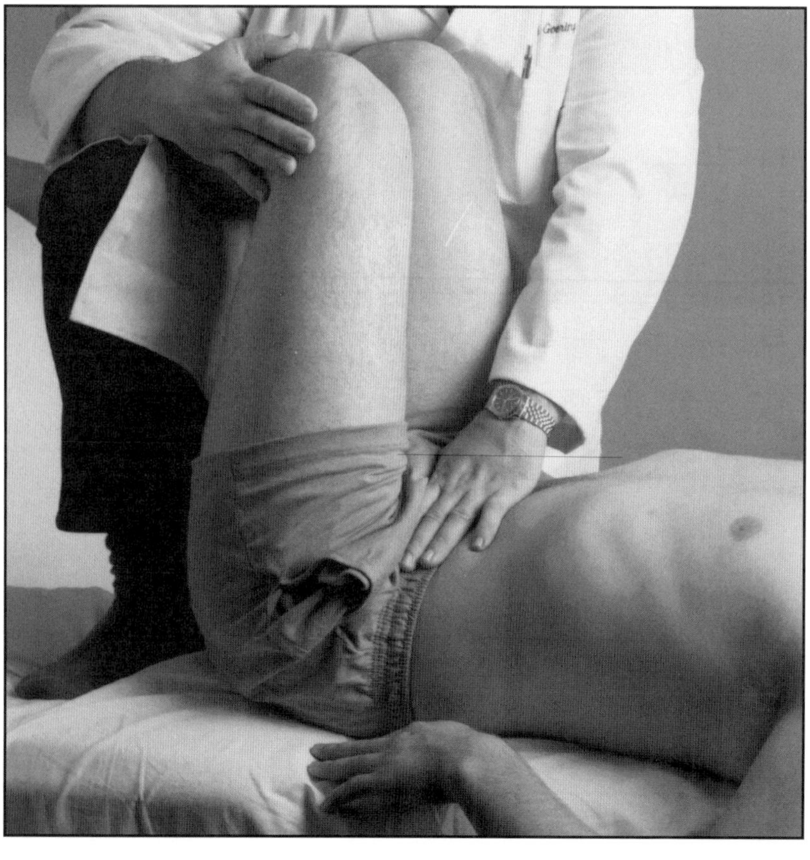

THE PELVIS

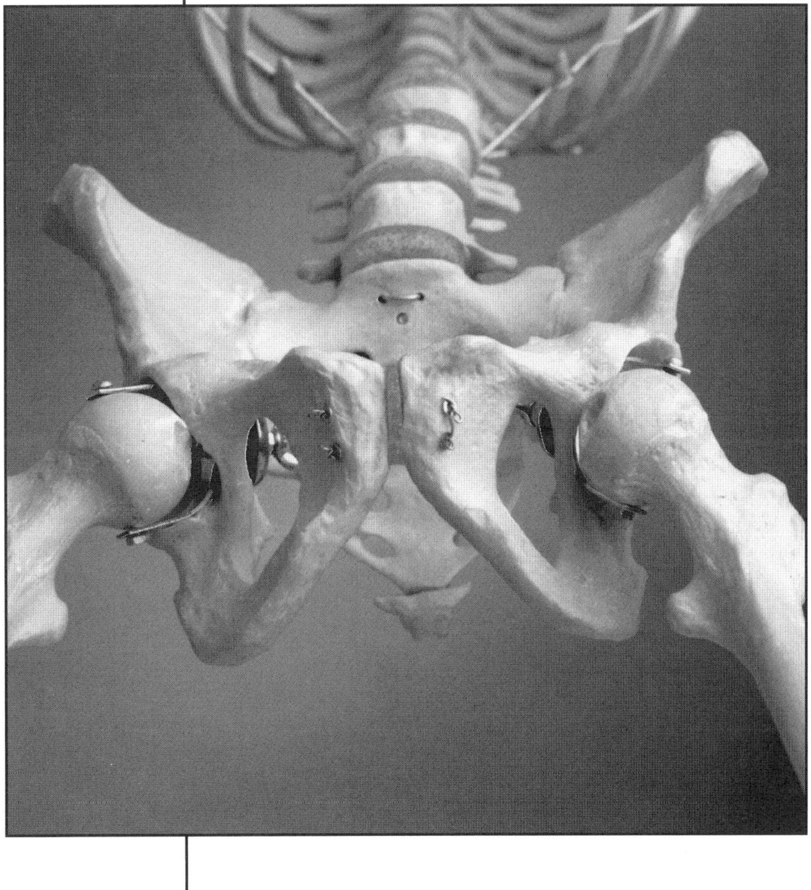

GENERAL

The pelvis is different from the torso especially in the fact that we do things that move one side of the the body in relation to the other side, rather than move the entire spine in some direction. In the beginning we thought only of sacro-iliac disorders, probably because our concept of this disorder as a joint subluxation at that time made it hard for us to imagine such a disorder affecting a joint still capable of a hundred and eighty degrees of motion as is the case in the enarthrosis of the femoral joint.

With the change in concept from subluxation to dysfunction of proprioceptor reflexes, it became reasonable to believe in an enarthrosis capable of developing false strain reflexes that would persist. It is well we did, because we were often at a loss to explain several pains related to things in the pelvis. Now after years of finding many more types of dysfunctions in the pelvic area of the body I am, if anything, less certain of the parts of the pelvis involved in many of the dysfunctions painful there and often radiating into the thighs.

This may appear to be very discouraging, but I have rationalized that what we believed to be true before was less true than we thought. At least we can now think we have one answer to a cause of degeneration of the head of the femur as well as that of lumbar intervertebral discs.

One thing remains fairly clear. In dysfunctions we believe to be related to the femoral joint, pain is especially influenced by the position of the femur. One position of the femur will aggravate the pain; another will ease it. For example, "It only hurts when I sit."

The same is true in the shoulder enarthrosis. Pain is much more related to the position of the arm than pain arising from a dysfunction just from an intervertebral joint in the thorax. If we still present these as sacro-iliac or femoral joint

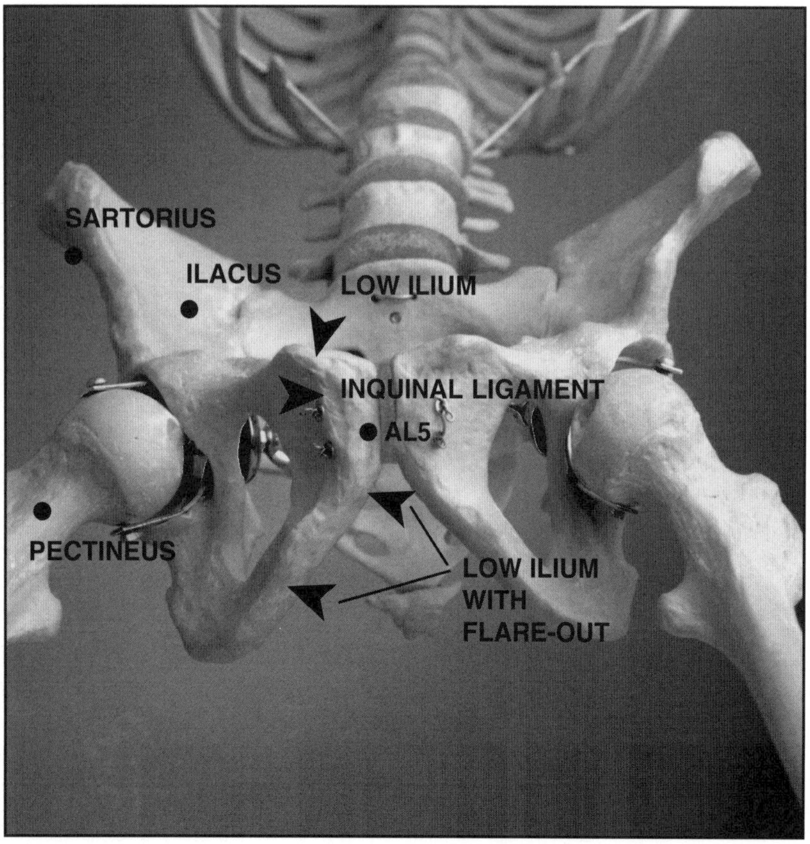

dysfunctions, it is partly based on these observations.

Since we are so dedicated (for diagnosis and for treatment) to reliance on location of a tenderpoint as evidence of a dysfunction and its marked and immediate decrease in tenderness when our position is ideal, we can from a practical standpoint proceed, knowing that the body's responses to our efforts will keep us on the straight and narrow path.

Because the posterior pelvis is so heavily covered with muscle and fat, we are especially dependent on the use of landmarks to enable us to locate tenderpoints. The most obvious one of these is the posterior superior iliac spine (PSIS). We also use the greater trochanter of the femur and the tensor fascia femoris (formerly tensor fascia lata), a strong and discrete muscle on the mid axillary line, and the posterior surface of the sacrum itself. For landmarks in front we use the lateral ramus of the pubic bone, a point on its superior surface close to the symphisis pubis and in the perineum on its descending ramus.

DYSFUNCTIONS OF SACRO-ILIAC JOINTS

These are described according to the abnormal position of the posterior border of the ilium in relation to that side of the sacrum. For those more accustomed to speak of an anterior or posterior sacrum, our high ilium would relate to a posterior. We think more of a rotation between the bones, over a transverse axis than a front to back, shearing type of strain.

HIGH ILIUM

The tenderpoint for this is found by pressing against the lateral side of the posterior superior spine of the ilium, starting out about an inch from it. Treatment can be accomplished on a prone patient by holding the leg just below the knee and lifting it to produce extension (forward rotation) of the ilium on the sacrum. Fine tuning for finding the ideal position is done by slight abduction or adduction of the femur.

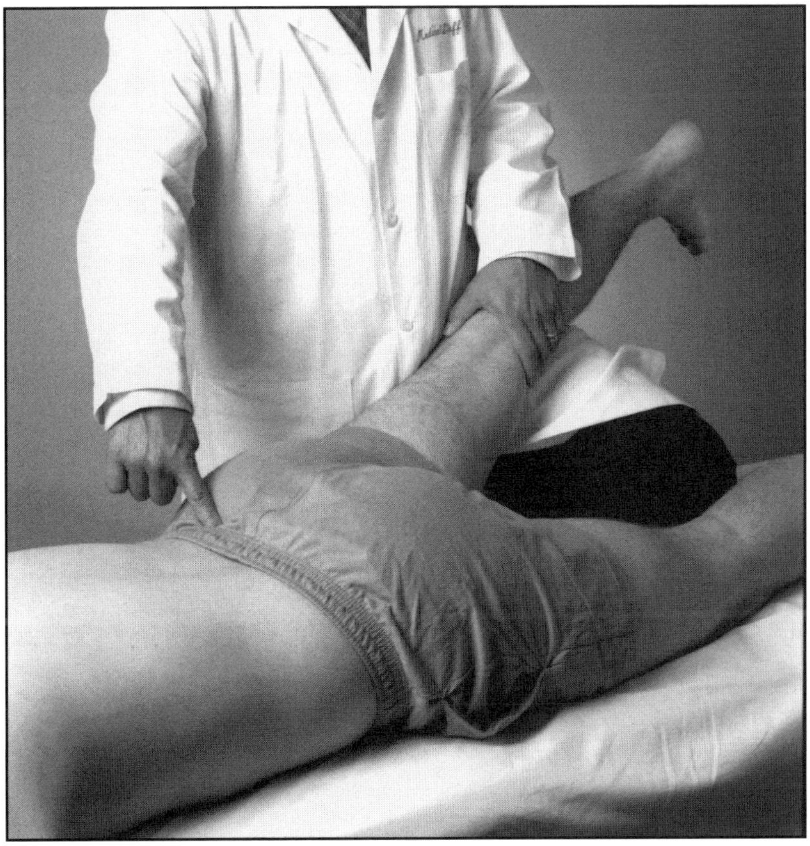

HIGH ILIUM WITH FLARE-OUT (HIFO)

Flare-out here refers to an apparent gapping of the upper (cephalad) part of the sacro-iliac joint with a relative compression of the lower part. We use it in combination with high and low ilium descriptions. We also do things that produce a flare-in of the sacro-iliac joint, among other things.

The tenderpoint for the HIFO is found one and three fourths inches below and one fourth inch medial to the lower edge of the PSIS; not ten centimeters as reported in the first book. (The only way I can guess that I managed to make that mistake in the first book was that I transposed from inches to centimeters and then did it again. 1 3/4" = 4 cm. 4" = 10 cm. It has served to mislead students ever since.) It is one and three fourth inches or four centimeters. Treatment is easily accomplished on a prone patient by extending the femur of the affected side, holding the leg just below the knee and pulling it back behind the other leg. After trying and failing for about two years to relieve coccigodynia by moving the coccyx on the sacrum, I began to hear from patients that this HIFO treatment had stopped their coccyx pain and tenderness. This has a high success rating. It must be valid.

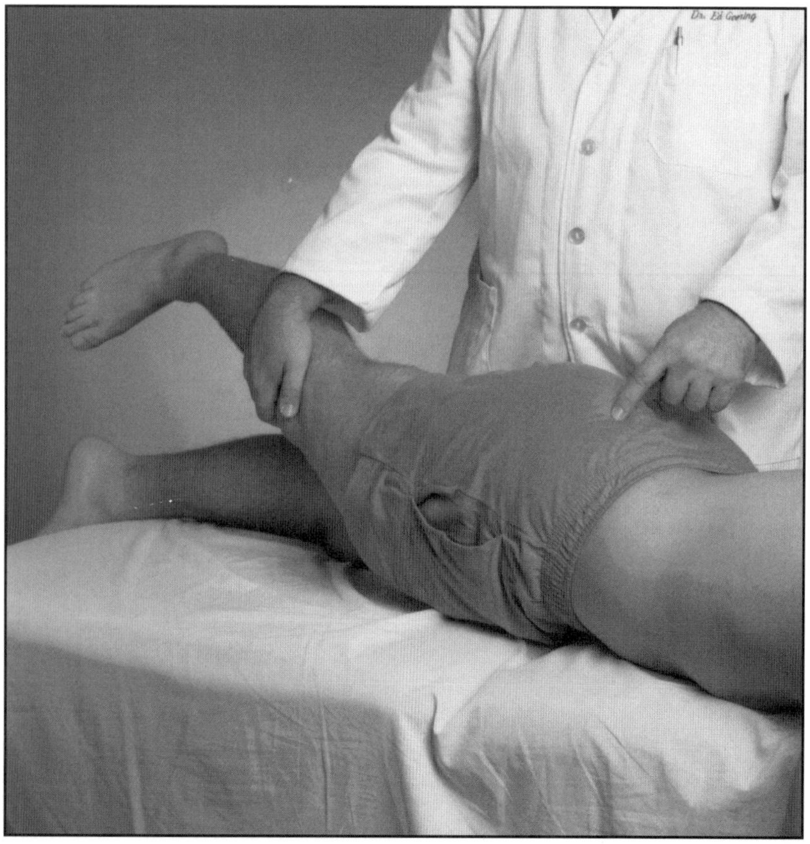

LOW ILIUM

This is named for what I think happens posteriorally to the ilium in relation to the sacrum in effective treatment. Patient lies supine with knees up. The tenderpoint is on the superior (not anterior) surface of the lateral ramus of the pubic bone, out about one and a half inches from the midline. Treatment, with the patient in the supine position, is marked flexion of the femur on the affected side. Pain most often is in back or side of the hip or thigh.

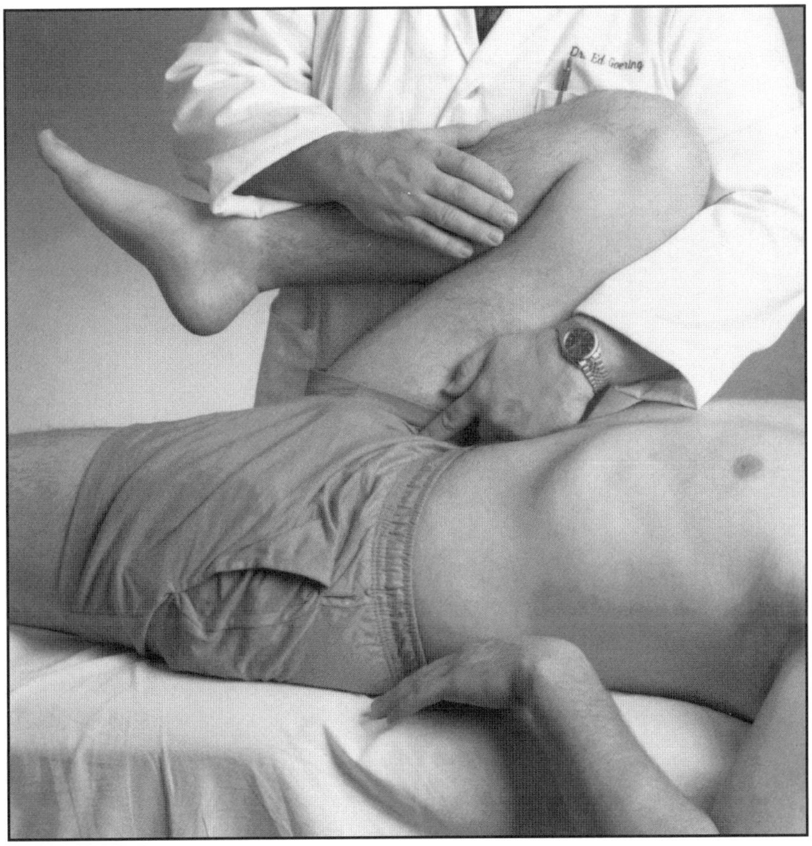

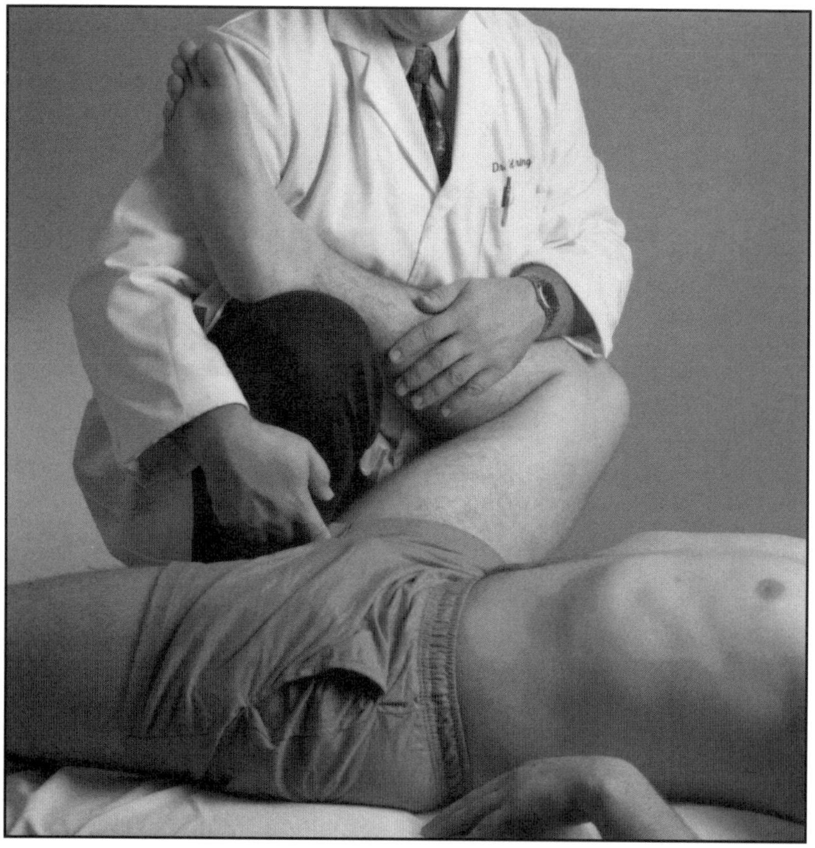

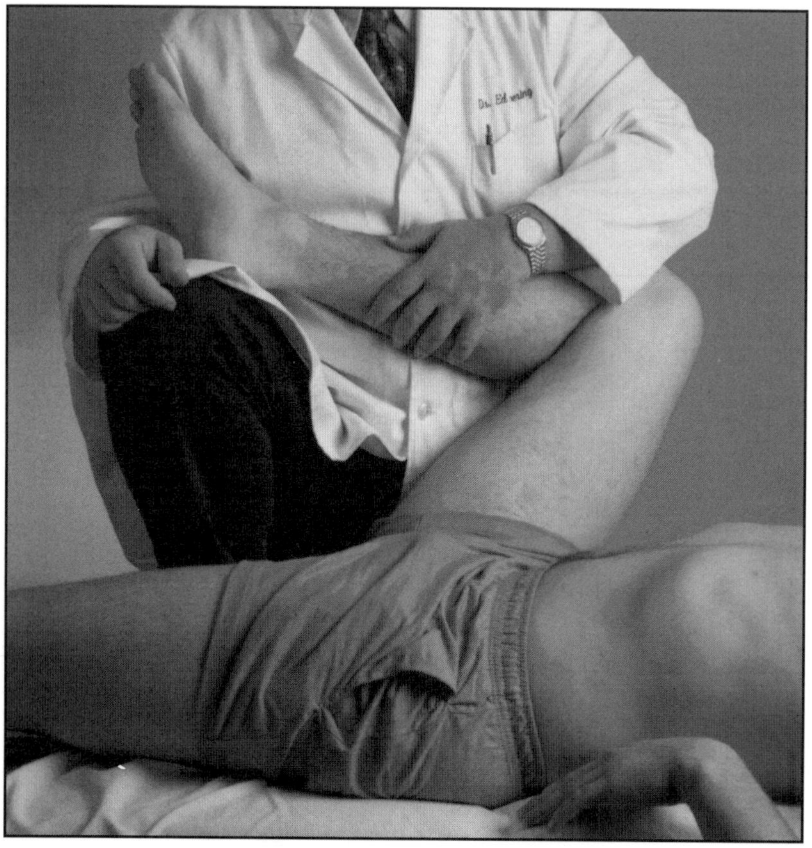

LOW ILIUM WITH FLARE-OUT

The tenderpoint for this dysfunction is in the perineum on the medio-inferior side of the descending ramus of the pubic bone. Because of its proximity to the vulva, it is wise to explain why a search will be made in a painless area for the cause of a pain in the buttock. Also since the tenderpoint is on a bone to the side of the vulva, it will be less threatening to a female patient for your search to start by pressing on the ischial tuberosity and moving up toward the symphisis pubis about an inch and a half, all the time pressing against the bone of the ischium or pubic bone. This is a common and important dysfunction. Treatment has much femur flexion but also the femur is markedly abducted and the foot kept near the midline to produce abduction and external rotation of the femur in addition to flexion.

There is a second, less common, tenderpoint much nearer the symphisis pubis, but still on the medio-inferior edge of the pubic bone. The external rotation of the femur is about the same as the former one, but the abduction is about one third as much.

FIDGETY LEG SYNDROME

I am indebted for this one to an English physician. who was practicing in Calgary, Alberta, Canada, Douglas Longden. Since he was especially impressed with the peculiar history in patients with this dysfunction, I have adhered to his name for it. He observed that these patients told how they couldn't keep from fidgeting their leg, constantly trying to discover a position of comfort. The position he found for them was extending the leg of the affected side off the edge of the table in hyperextension. He found a tenderpoint on the superior surface of the pubic bone very near the symphisis.

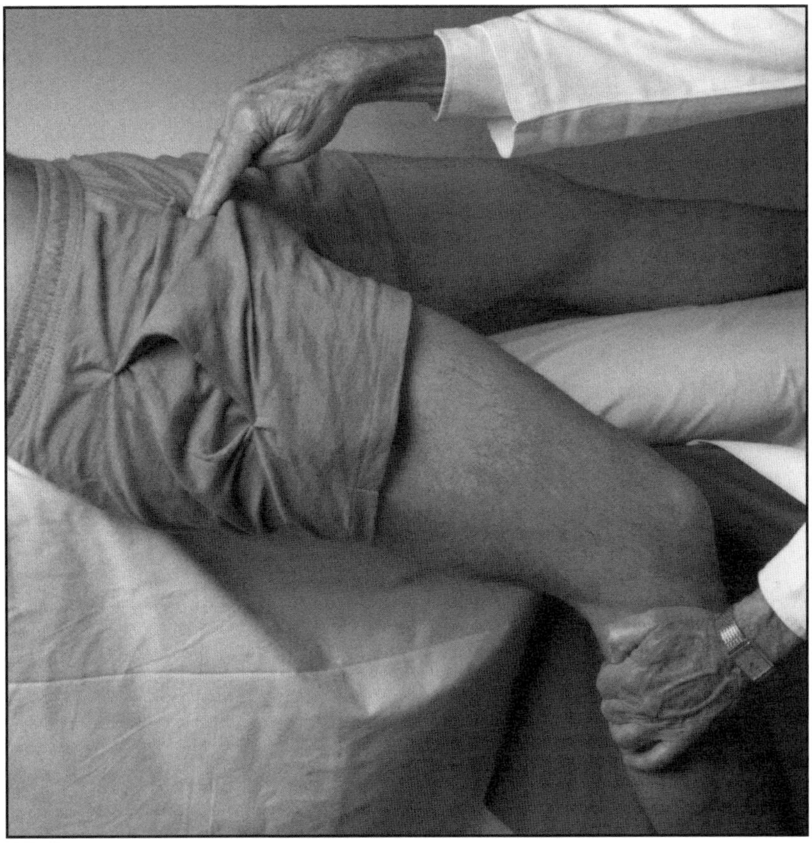

FLARE-IN SACRO-ILIAC

(Formerly called Mid Pole)

The tenderpoint for this relatively uncommon problem is at about the middle of the gluteus maximus muscle, down about four inches below the lower edge of the PSIS and slightly lateral. It is relieved on the prone patient by holding the leg in abduction.

Early in my practice, long before I had learned of proprioceptor reflex dysfunctions, I used to treat a patient who suffered severe dysmenorrhea. She had a sore spot in her buttock and came to me faithfully every period for several visits to have me press on her tender spots hard enough to hurt her severely, because it partially eased her cramps. Years later I realized that this sacro-iliac tenderpoint was her point for dysmenorrhea. By this time I had established myself as a manipulator for back pains and was seldom consulted for dysmenorrhea, but whenever I found one of these on a young woman I asked whether she suffered cramps. Successful treatment of this dysfunction often did decrease severity of cramps by the second period after treatment.

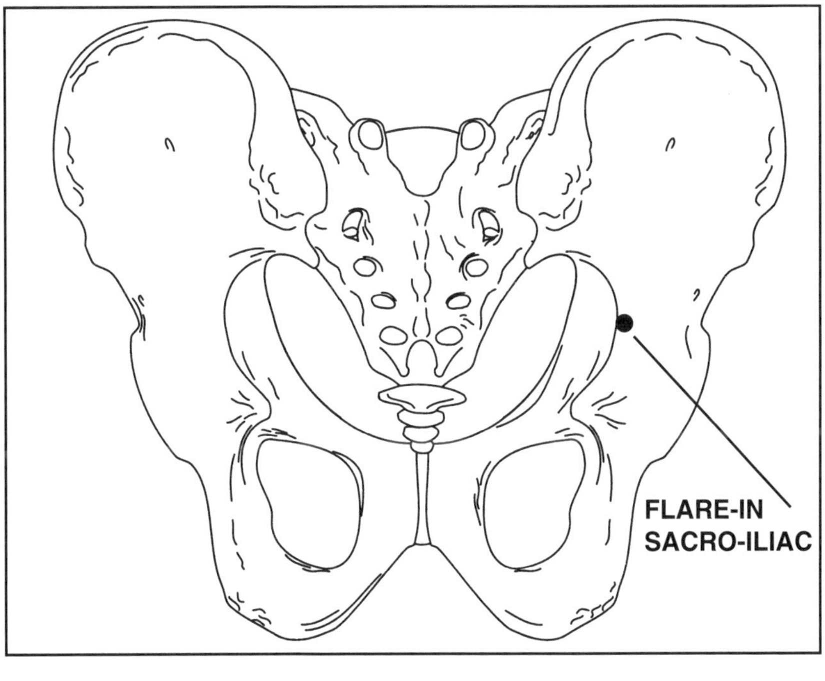

WORK OF MAURICE ANTHONY RAMIREZ, DO, PH.D.

(Maurice Anthony Ramirez; Jerry Haman, DO; Leonard Worth, DO. "Low back pain: Diagnosis by six newly discovered sacral tenderpoints and treatment with counterstrain technique." *Journal of the American Osteopathic Association,* July, 1989. Vol. 89, No. 7, Pg. 905+.)

Many of the later things I have learned have been discovered and perfected by other physicians using Strain-Counterstrain methods. One such was a paper Ramirez published in the *Journal of the American Osteopathic Association* on finding and treating dysfunctions by locating tenderpoints on the back of the sacrum. Unfortunately for me personally, his paper appeared after I had closed my office to devote my remaining energies to teaching, so I haven't had enough practice to learn his techniques perfectly. I found several things I could do using his tenderpoints and techniques. I don't offer my version of his work as thorough as his, but it had seemed that he found a spot to press heavily on the back of the sacrum as far away from the point of tenderness as he could. By doing this I was able to ease sacro-iliac dysfunctions in ways I had not known of before. Too often for my comfort I found some of his points after I thought I had given an adequate treatment for sacro-iliacs. There is a lot yet to be learned before counterstrain is perfected.

To keep this simple and practical, I search for the tenderpoints; when one is found, I press on the sacrum as far away from the tenderpoint as possible.

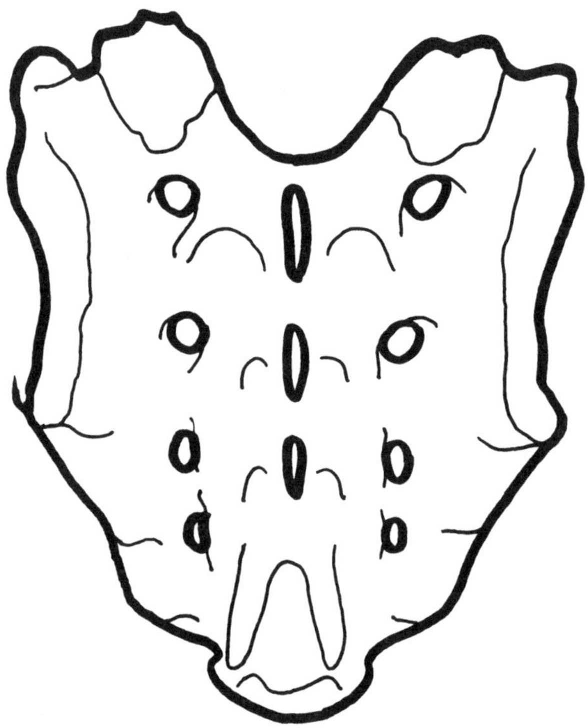

Sacrum

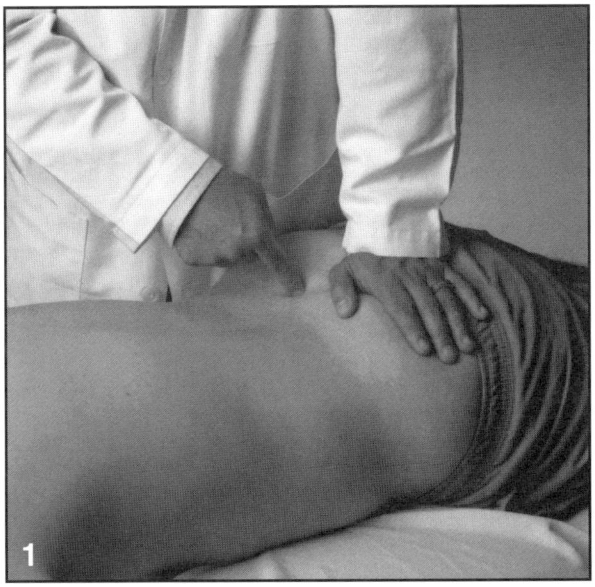
1

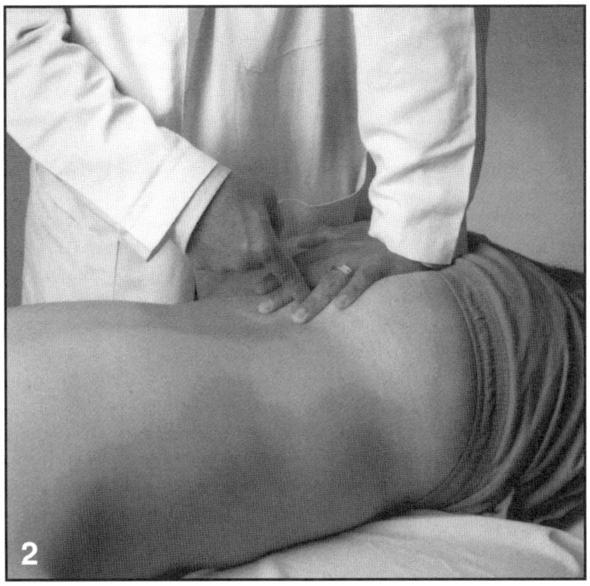
2

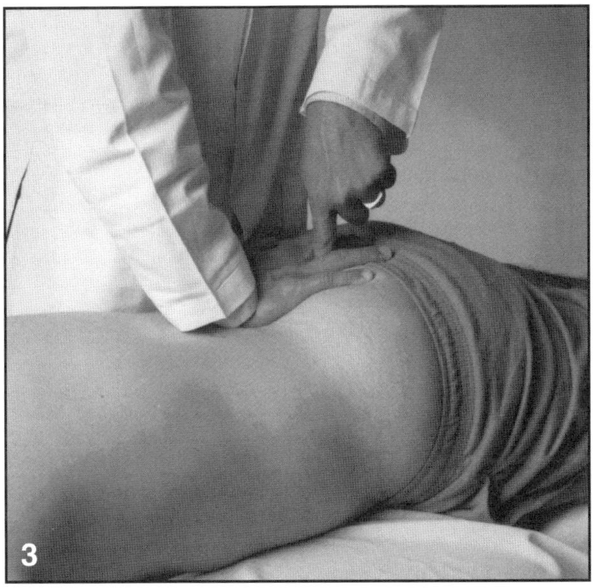
3

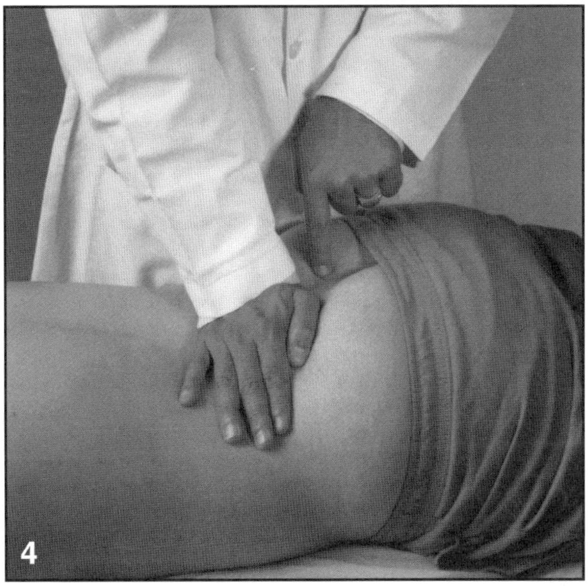
4

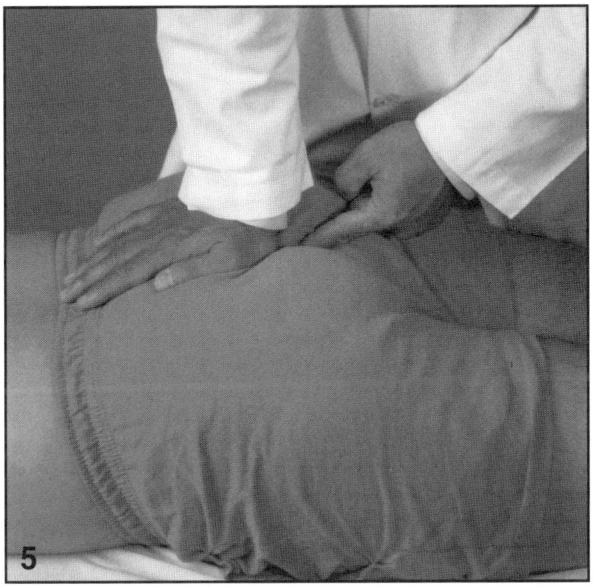
5

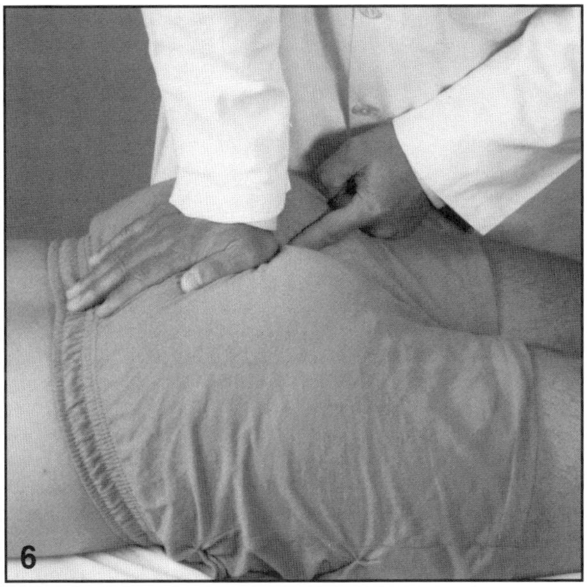
6

Dysfunction in Muscles Moving the Femur

As I learned more and more about the pelvis, I became more uncertain of what to blame for each pain and stiffness. The most certain difference is that pains from muscles that move the femur are more position oriented.

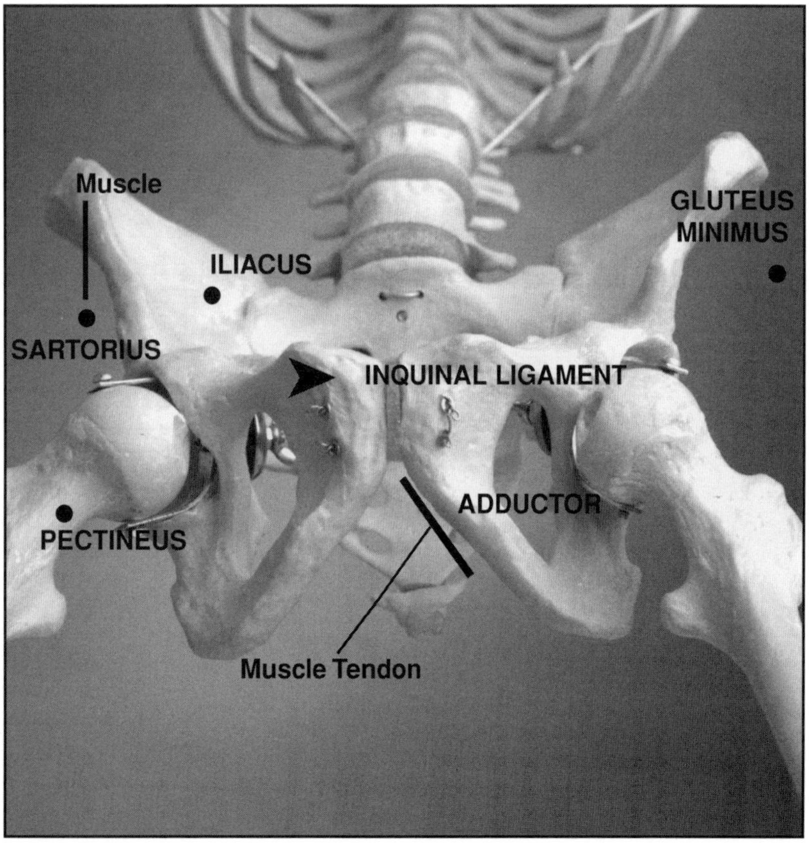

ANTERIOR

ILIACUS

This is a good one to start with because it seems, among other things, to be the most likely culprit for recurring low ilium and low Ilium flare-out dysfunctions. Tenderness is deep in the fossa of the ala of the ilium, about two inches medial and slightly below the anterior superior iliac spine. Treatment is bilateral, even when the tenderness is unilateral, which is usually the case. Knees are raised and widely separated on the supine patient, but the feet are crossed. Any time there is a knee complaint, put that leg's foot on top. This treatment produces flexion, marked external rotation, and abduction of the femoral joint. Whenever you have a patient with a sacro-iliac problem that keeps recurring, be sure to check for this dysfunction. It is also very common even when there are no sacro-iliac dysfunctions.

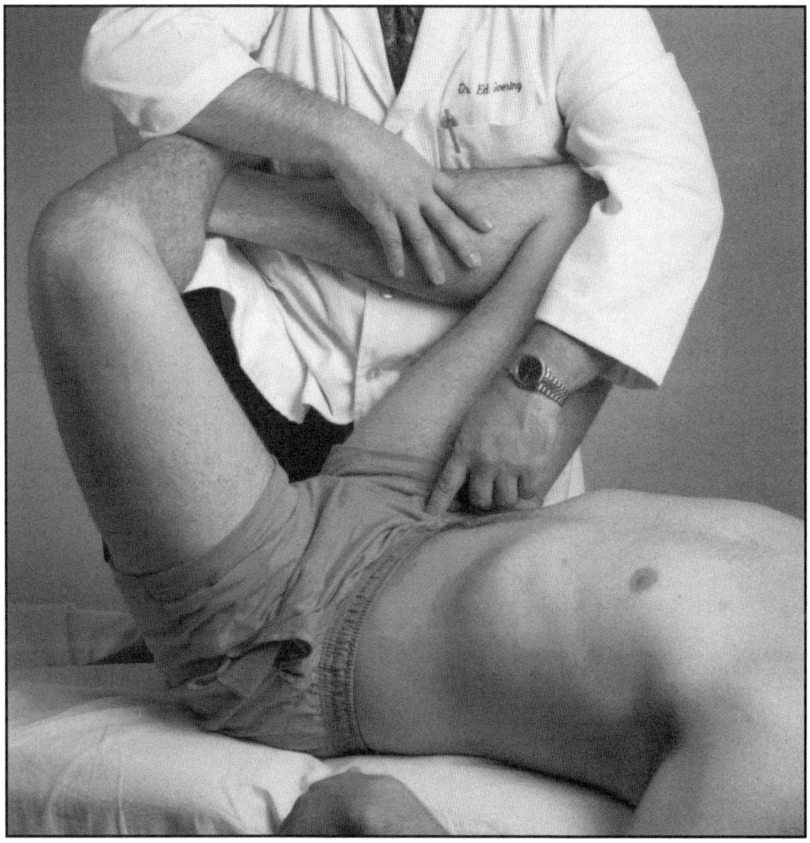

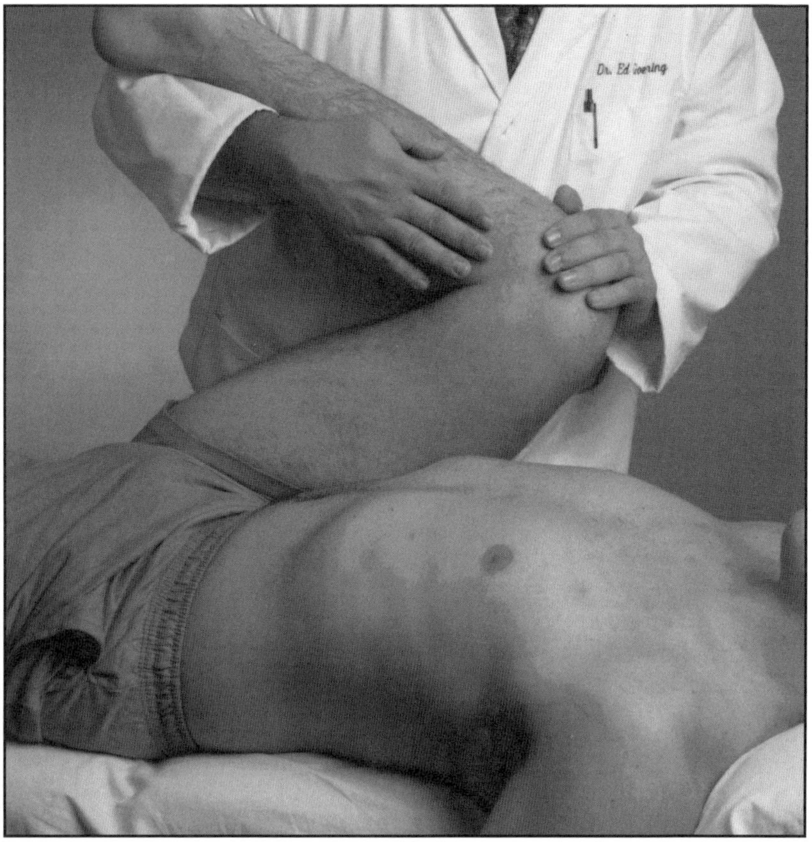

SARTORIUS

(Called anterior trochanter in the first book, because I found the first tenderpoints for hip socket problems and I tried to relate everything to tenderness around the greater trochanter of the femur.)

Tenderpoint is about an inch caudad to the anterior superior spine of the ilium, on the tendon of origin of the sartorius muscle. When it is markedly shortened, by flexion of the the femur, it will recover nicely.

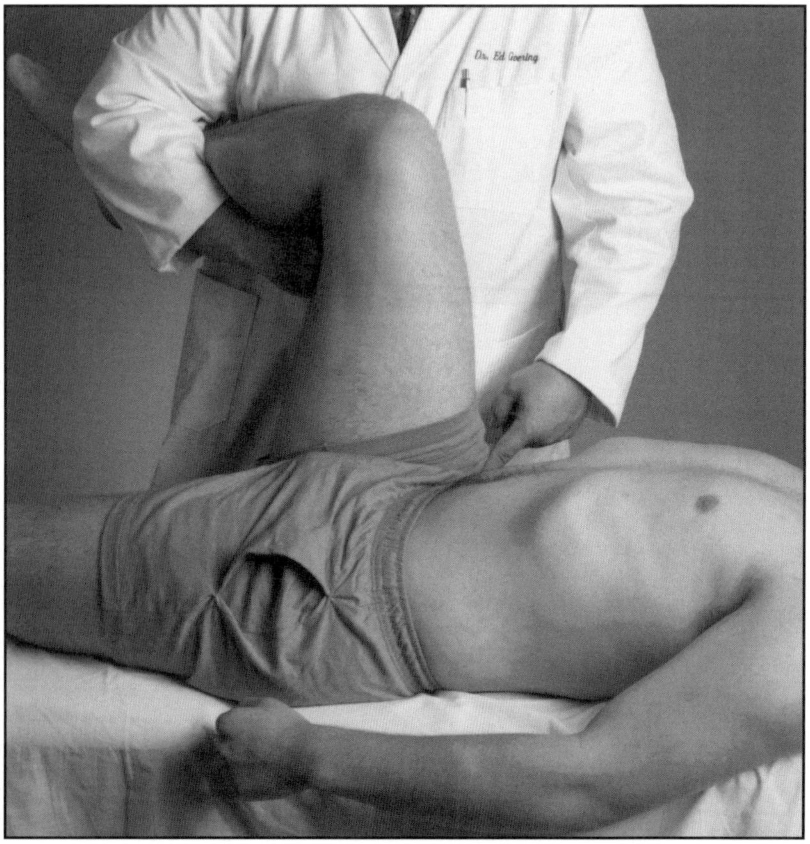

GLUTEUS MINIMUS

This is not found behind as I had thought at first, but about two and a half inches down and out from the anterior superior spine of the ilium. This and the gluteus medius are common causes for pain on the lateral part of the pelvis, after a long drive in a car in a sitting position. The weight is carried on the ischial tuberosities and the greater trochanters of the femurs hang down in an external rotation strain.

A fairly marked femur flexion with slight abduction and internal rotation of the femur, produced by pulling the foot more lateral than the knee, will stop these.

INGUINAL LIGAMENT

So-called, not because I suspect involvement of the ligament, but because the tenderpoint is found on the side of the front part of the pubic bone. It is a difficult thing to find until you probe close to the medial attachment of the inguinal ligament, which here serves as a landmark. Most of us can find an inguinal ligament. It is eased by ninety degree flexion of the femurs of the supine patient and a crossing of the knees. The knee of the affected side is crossed under that of the well side. Internal rotation of the femur is produced by mildly pulling the ankle laterally. Fine tuning here is done by small amounts of moving the knees laterally.

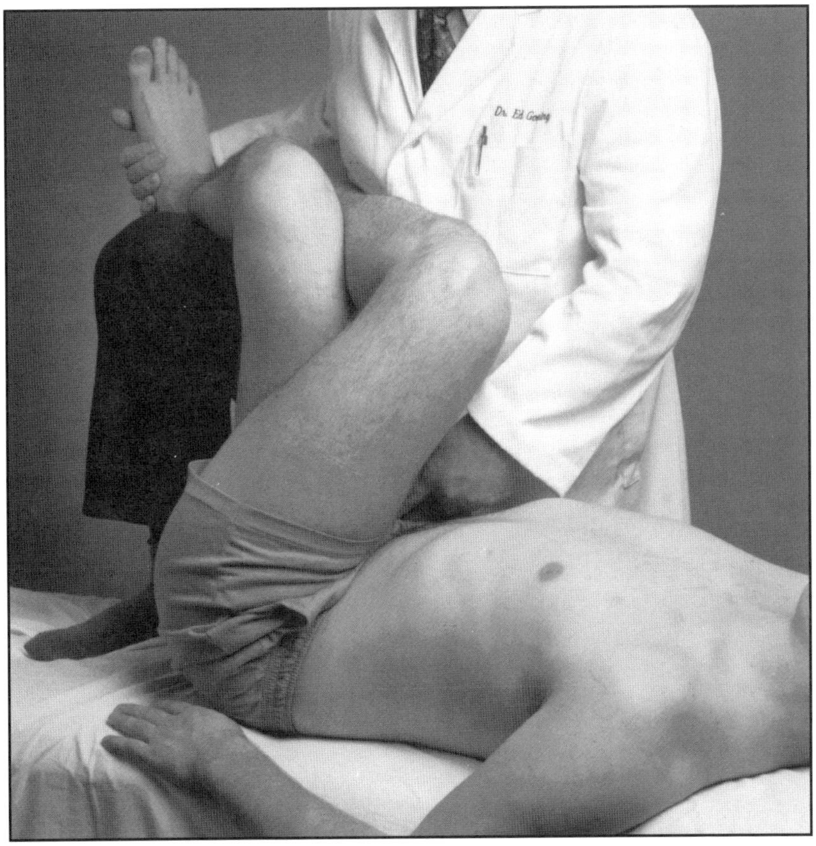

ADDUCTORS

These often occur along with inguinal ligaments so when I find one I look for the other. Tenderpoints are found high in the adductors, close to the the attachment to the pubic bone. As you might expect, they are relieved by adduction, with the thigh either slightly flexed or extended depending on what part of the adductors you find.

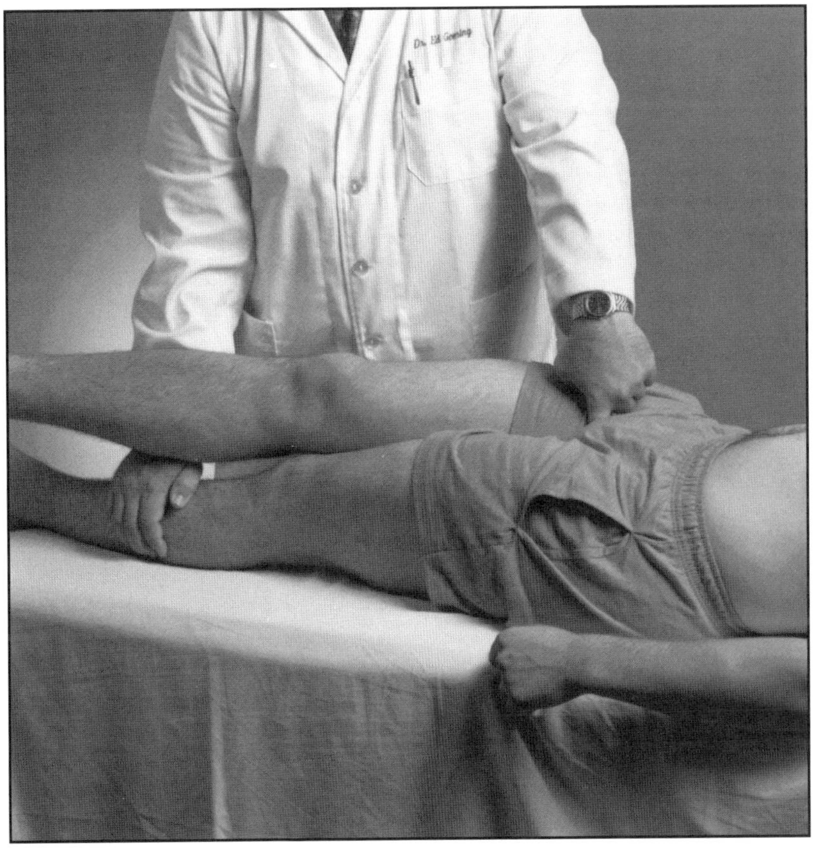

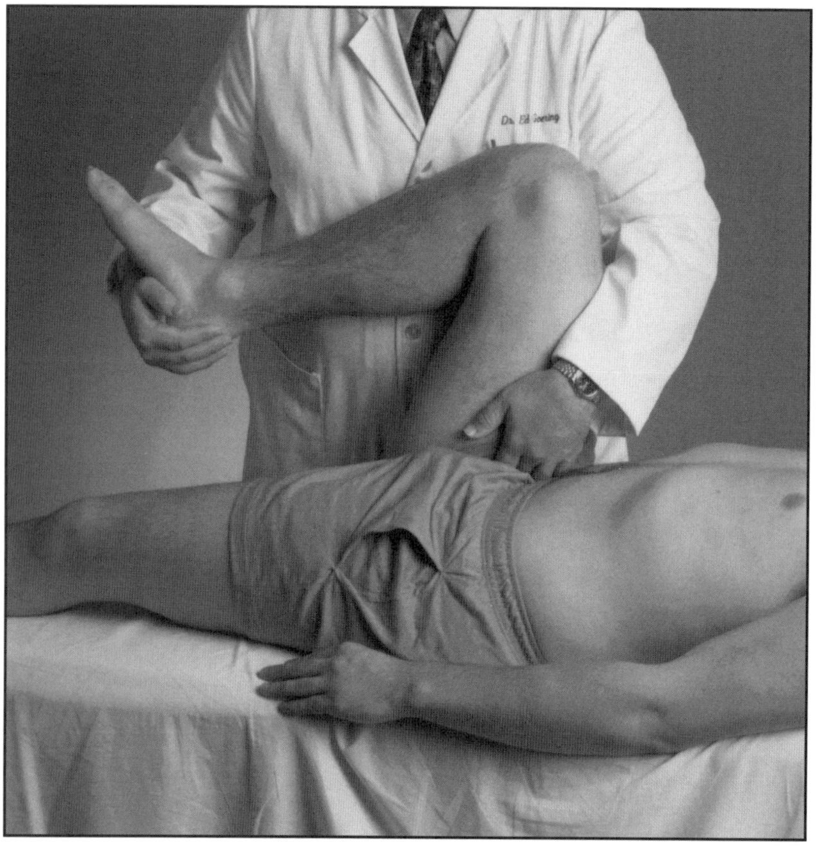

PECTINEUS

This is the name of a tenderpoint as deep in the groin as it is possible to probe. It is best done with patient supine and knees drawn up. All I am really certain of is that there is a tenderpoint here that is common. It will be relieved with marked flexion of the thigh. It seems to be close to the anterior margin of the acetabulum. I don't even have an idea what muscle or muscles are involved, but it eases some pelvic pains.

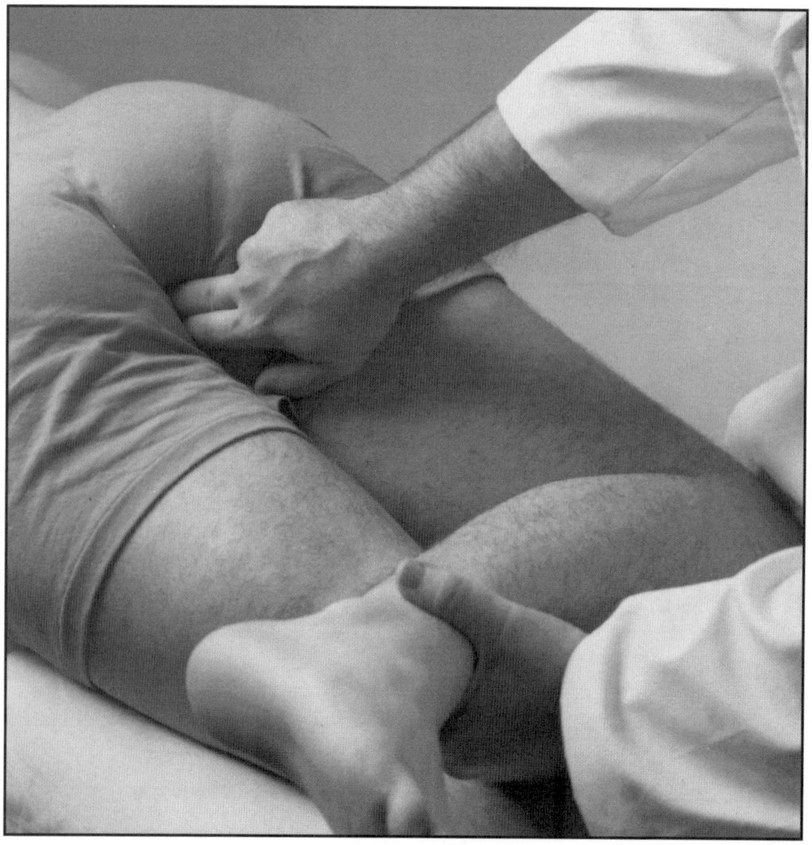

OBTURATOR

The tenderpoint named for the internal obturator muscle is found on the medial aspect of the pelvis minor. The obturator muscle takes its origin from within the pelvis minor and extends through the lesser sciatic foramen and inserts on the medial aspect of the greater trochanter of the femur. Enervated by L5 and S1, it may be irritated by L-S somatic dysfunction, as well as acetabular inflammation. Correction of this tenderpoint requires a prone patient with external rotation of the thigh as shown in the picture.

POSTERIOR

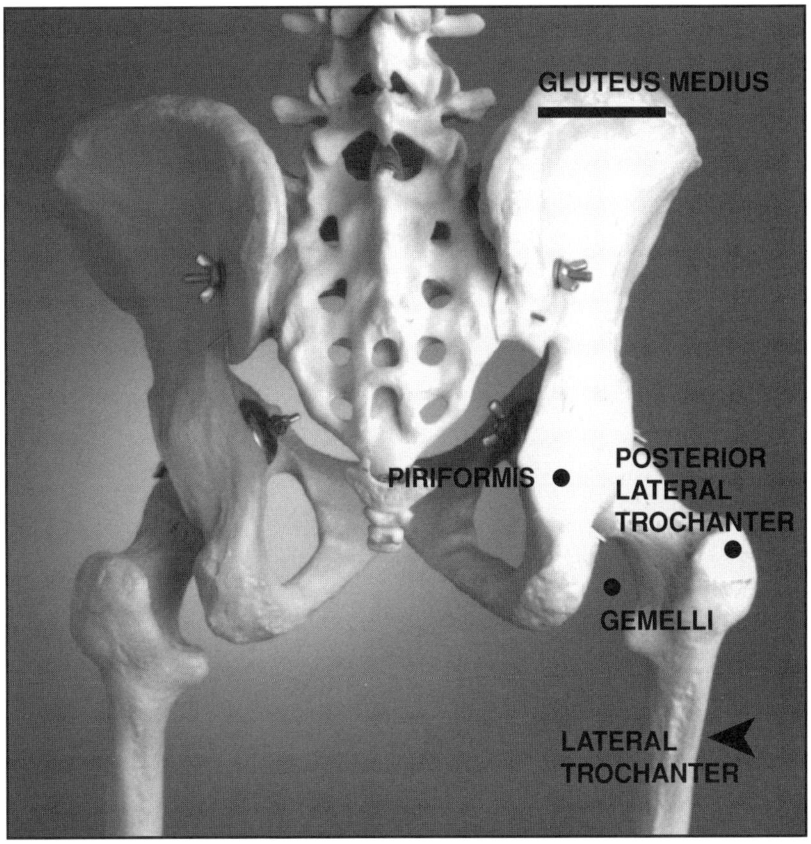

GLUTEUS MEDIUS

This is a common trouble that has its tenderpoint behind the tensor fascia femoris about two inches down from the rim of the ala of the ilium. It is occasionally found further back. It is relieved by extension and internal rotation of the femur with a little abduction. One patient told me after this was successfully treated on him that it had freed him from his impotence. Too short a series from me but a surprised urologist I know says that it has worked for some of his patients.

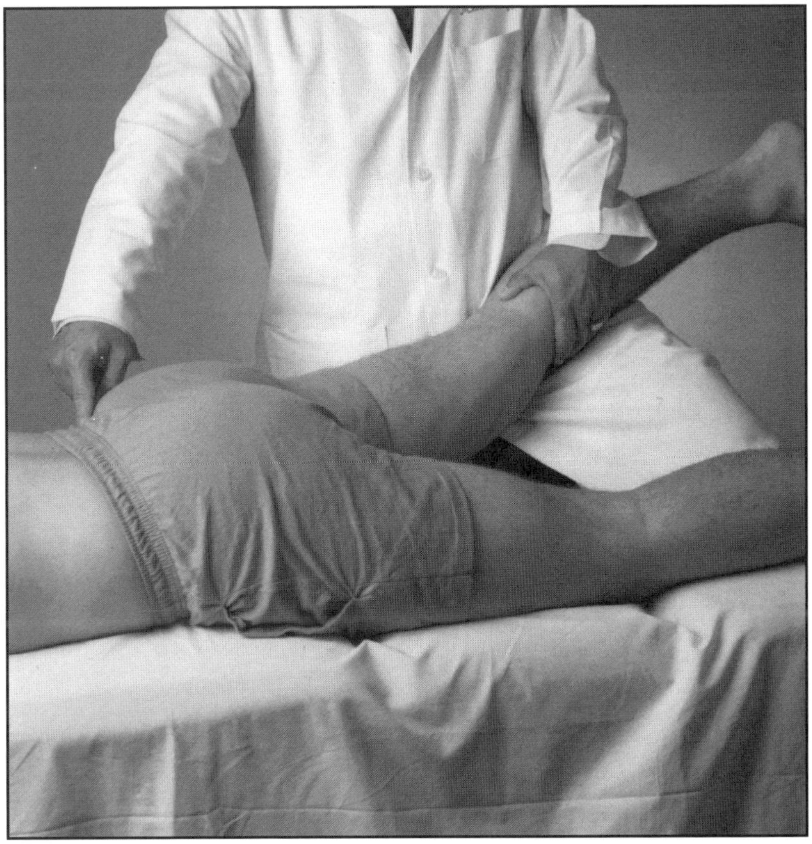

PIRIFORMIS

Many manipulators blame this poor muscle for most of the sciatic pains around the hip. It is common, but not universal. If the probing is done starting at the upper posterior corner of the greater trochanter where the tendon runs, and proceeding along the muscle moving medially and a little superior for a muscle not much wider than an inch, you are likely to be on the piriformis. Treatment is accomplished on a prone patient with hanging the knee off the edge of the table flexing about 135 degrees and strongly abducting the femur. This will often also ease a tenderpoint on the posterior lateral trochanter itself. If not, it can be relieved with the leg straight but markedly externally rotated by placing the doctor's knee under the front of the thigh high enough to produce marked external rotation of the femur.

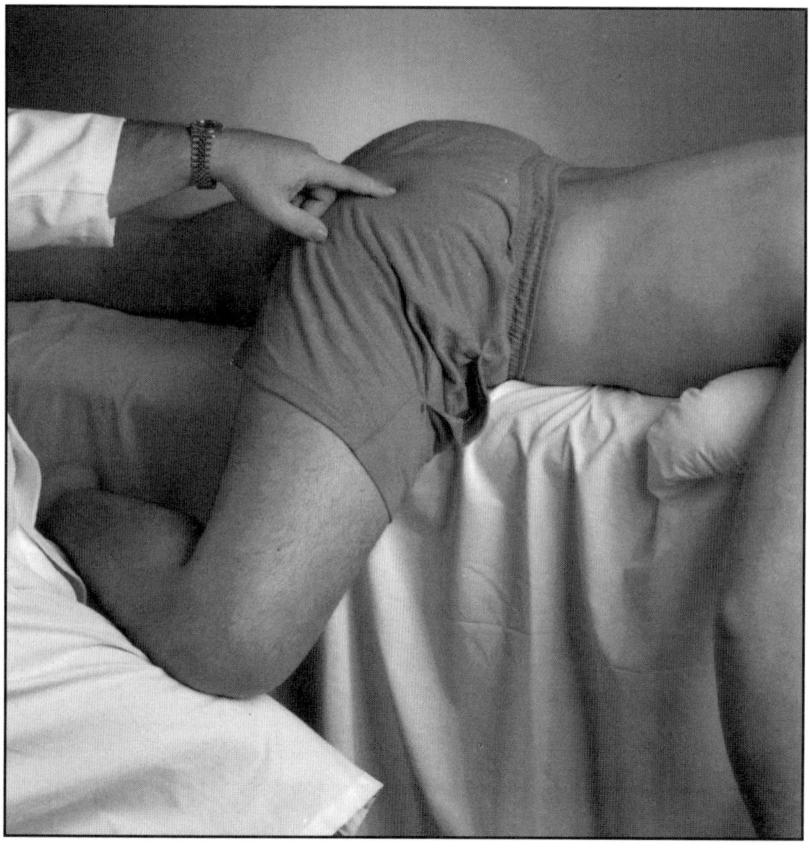

LATERAL TROCHANTER

This seemingly obvious dysfunction has a tenderpoint on the lateral surface of the top of the greater trochanter and another, more tender, on the lateral surface of the shaft of the femur five inches down from the trochanter. It has given me much trouble when I used the technique of abducting the femur until tenderness eased. Apparently it eased very well, but the dysfunction was usually back again at the time of the next visit. Better results were obtained after I found, on most of them, tenderpoints in the adductors and using adductor techniques for further treatment.

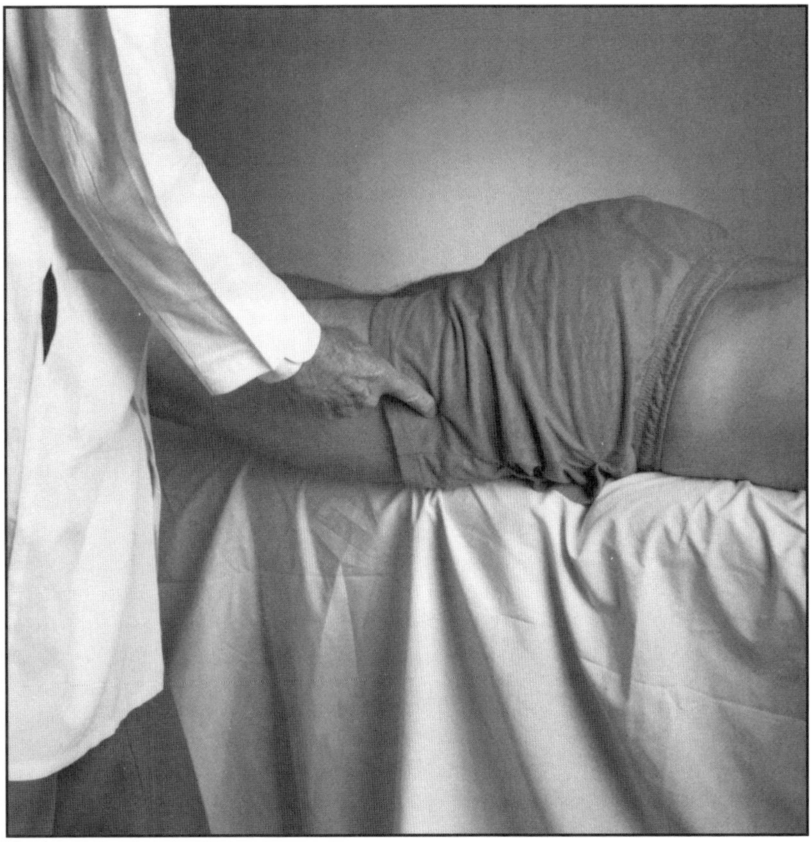

GEMELLI

These are the site of a tenderpoint behind and medial to the greater trochanter (before called posterior medial trochanter). This patient complains of pain at the fold of the buttock. Relief is obtained by extension adduction and external rotation. An easy method for me is to have the patient prone and pull the ankle and knee back and across behind the other leg, pinning the ankle under my elbow.

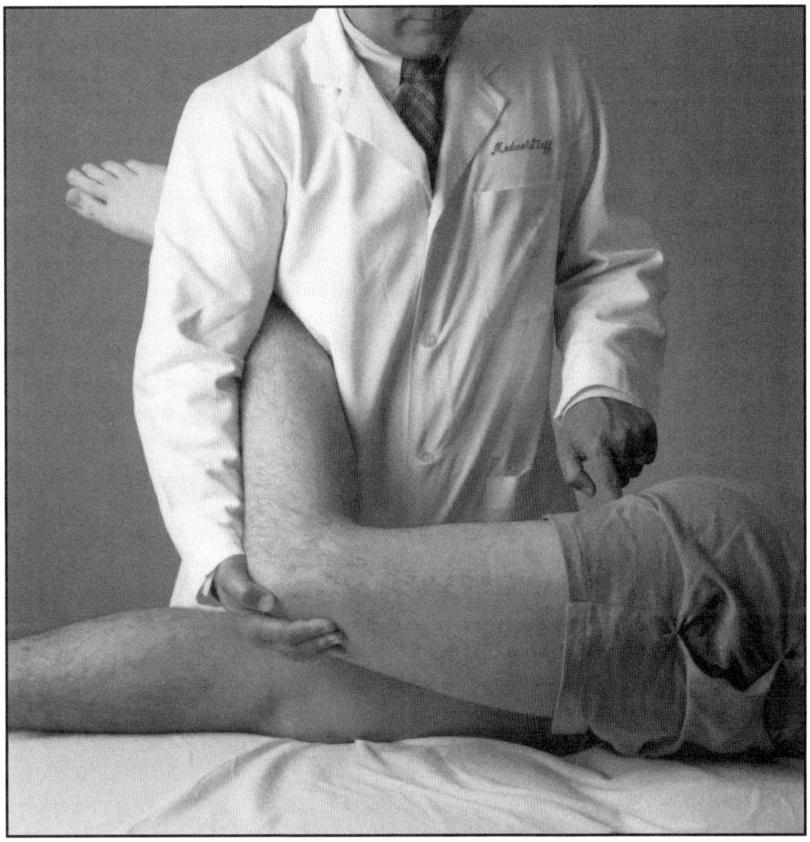

KNEES

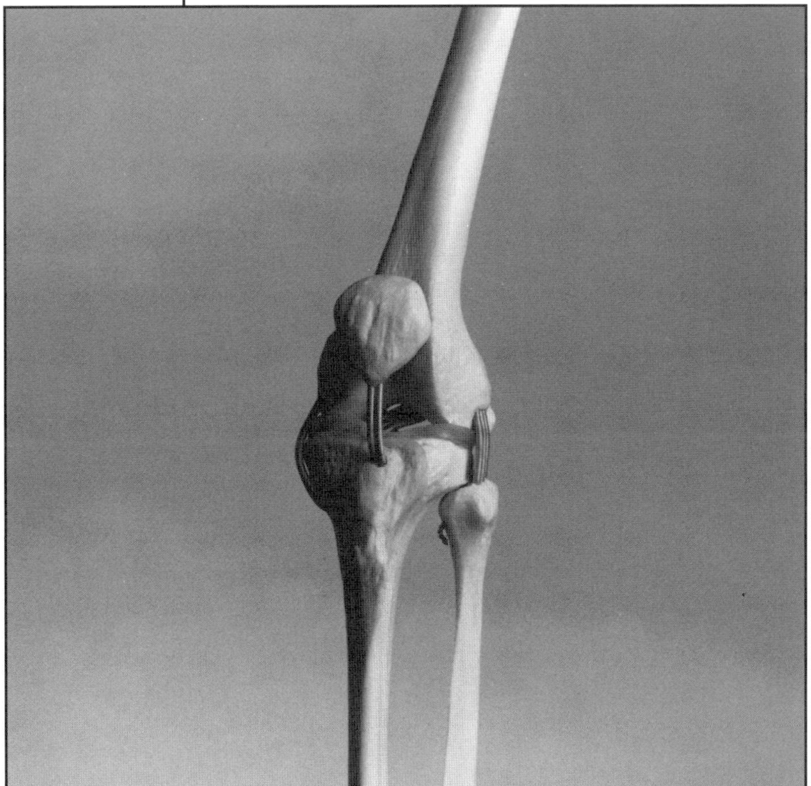

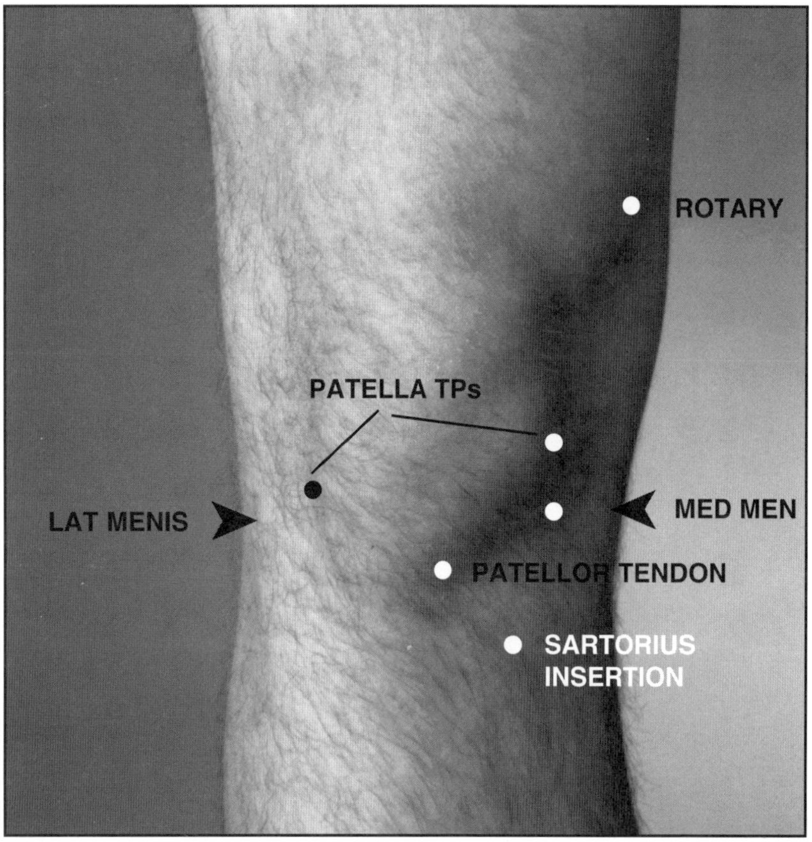

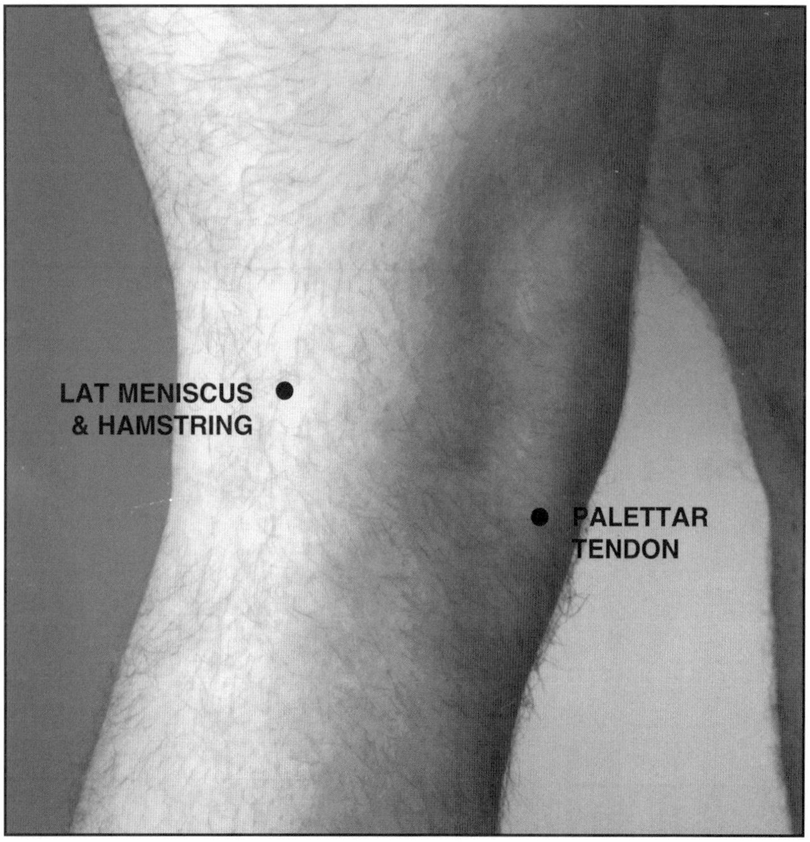

GENERAL

Arms and legs may have dysfunctions just related to the joint involved, but they may have a local problem complicated by some other, less obvious problem, from an area more proximal. In the case of the knee it seems that the fifth lumbar joint is often present and should be checked, especially the anterior fifth lumbar.

The knee is different in another way. Two of its problems seem to have their origins in the cruciate ligaments. Here we have two shearing type strains between the femur and tibia that cannot be explained by muscle strains, because no muscles do what these cruciate ligaments do.

The knee is a far more complicated joint than previously thought. Besides its obvious hinge actions, there are rotary actions betweeen the femur and the tibia and fairly marked changes in the lineup of two bones in a saggital view, so that the knees in extension also develop considerable abduction. With the exception of the popliteus muscle, these actions seem to result from forces due to the structure and direction of powerful ligaments.

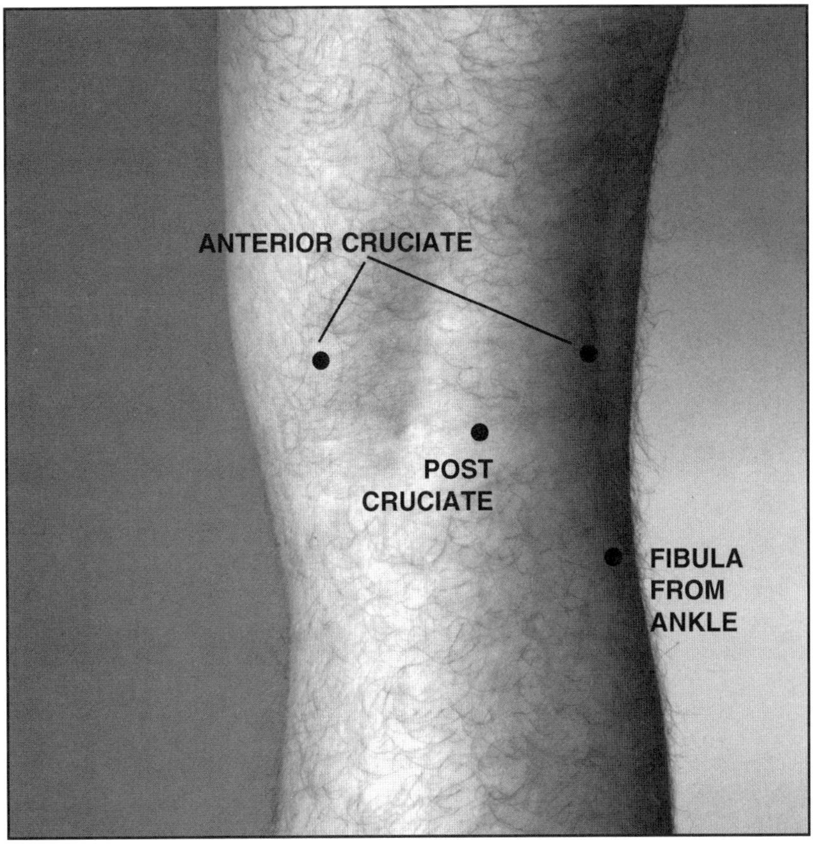
ANTERIOR CRUCIATE
POST
CRUCIATE
FIBULA
FROM
ANKLE

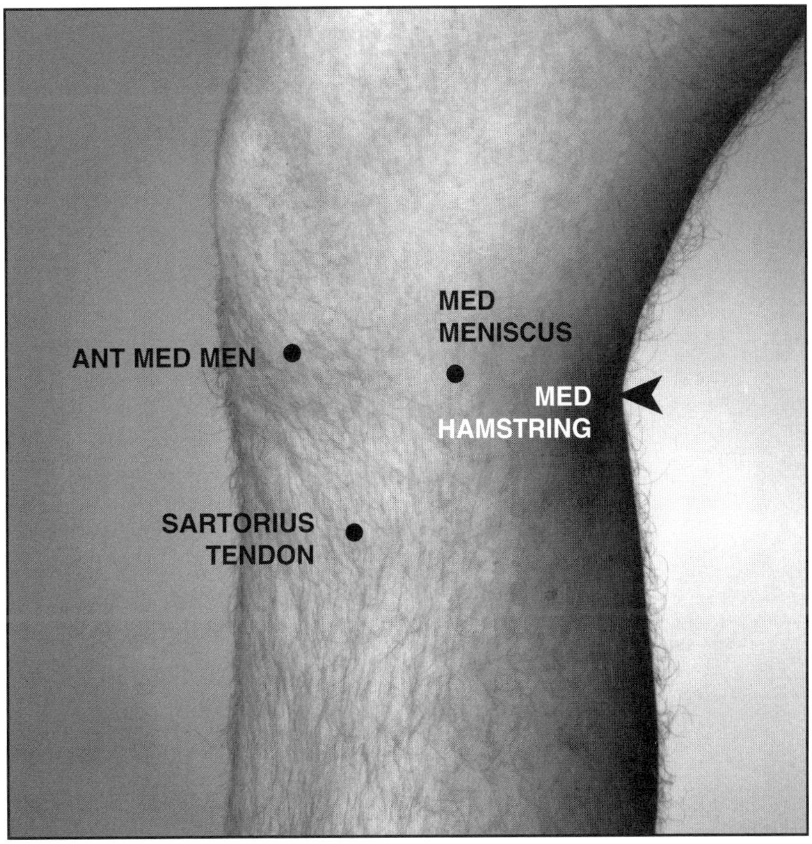
MED
MENISCUS
ANT MED MEN
MED
HAMSTRING
SARTORIUS
TENDON

POSTERIOR CRUCIATE LIGAMENT

In the mid-1990s there developed a great lot of reported sports injuries to the anterior cruciate ligament, but my personal experience in treating knees is that the posterior ligament suffers many more strains than the anterior. My opinion is based on the fact that I relieve more knees by forcing the tibia forward in relation to the end of the femur than the opposite. These ligaments are named for the site of attachment on the tibia. Thus a posterior cruciate ligament's principal attachments are the back of the tibia and front of the femur. My supine patient has this ligament shortened by my placing a rolled up towel on the table beneath his tibial head and use heavy force to push the femur end backward. This apparently shortens the posterior cruciate ligament enough to stop the false strain reflex in it. The tenderpoint for this problem is close to the middle of the popliteal space. Because this treatment uses no levers, more force is necessary.

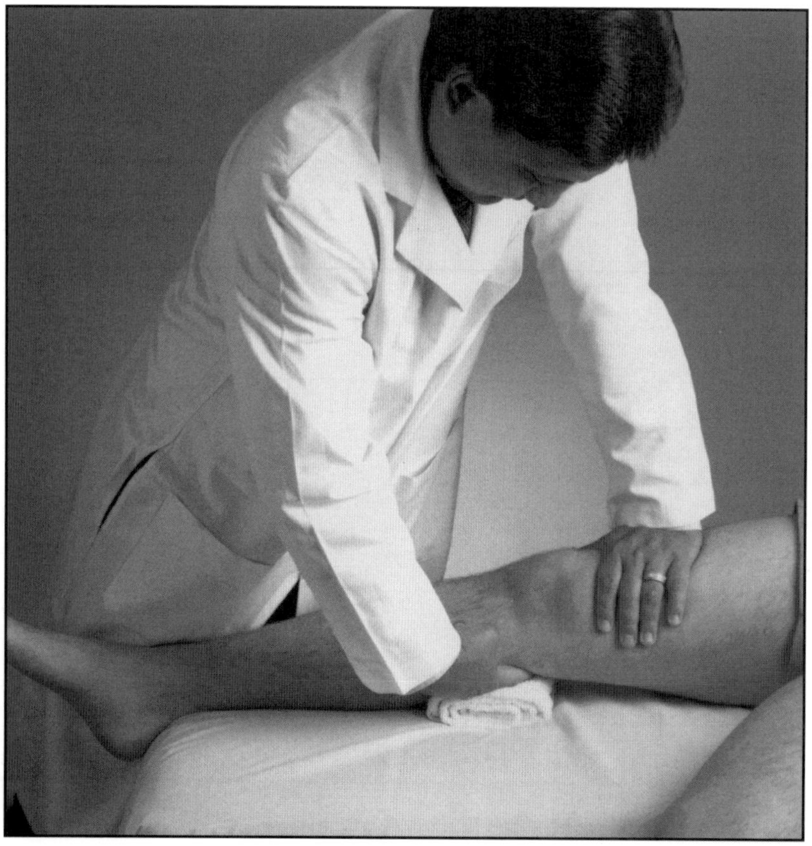

ANTERIOR CRUCIATE LIGAMENT

I need to treat this one much more rarely than the other. Tenderpoints are in the hamstring muscle tendons at the level of the widest part of of the popliteal space, possibly an inch and a half higher than one I name medial hamstring for another common knee strain, which is nearer the attachment of the hamstring tendon. Here the placement of the towel is under the end of the femur and the tibia is forced backward with heavy pressure. Several alarmed readers have questioned me about the amount of force I use on these (as much as forty pounds), but I point out that this treatment is unique in that it doesn't make use of any lever and so is much less powerful than we would first imagine.

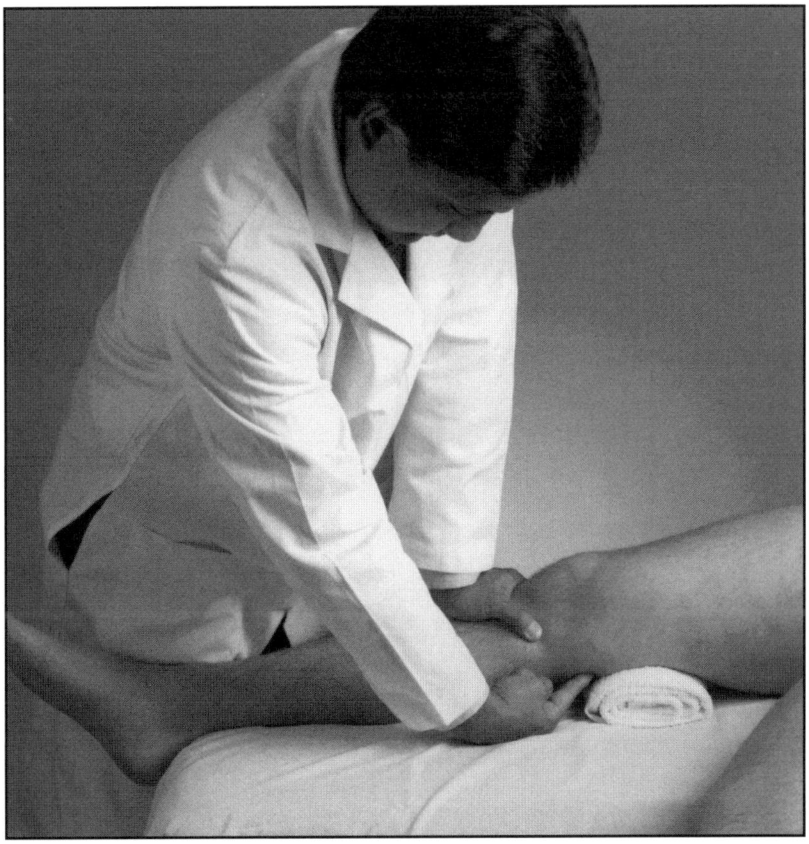

MEDIAL MENISCUS

(Semilunar cartilage)

This very common knee dysfunction has me at odds with orthodox concepts of knee injury. Orthopedic surgeons often speak of this problem as laceration of the internal lateral ligament. Because my tenderpoint is much more evident at the site of the perimeter of the medial meniscus, I still call it by that name. It can be felt at the level of the lower edge of the patella. It is most common on the inner line of the leg. Treatment is usually with my patient supine with his leg below the knee hanging down with about sixty degrees of flexion. Force applied is almost all internal rotation of the flexed tibia with slight adduction so that the ankle might be under the edge of the table. For this reason I suspect the popliteus muscle to be involved, as this rotation would shorten it.

Again I must warn against using much force of adduction, because the knee has scant ability to resist the powerful force possible, because of the long lever. Rotation doesn't present nearly so much lever force.

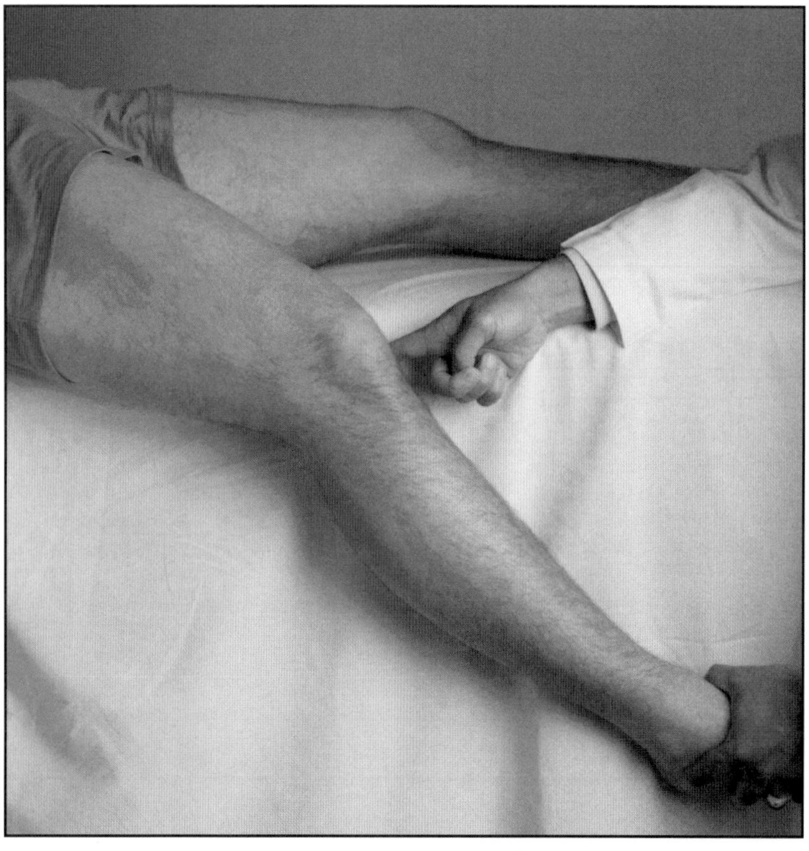

MEDIAL HAMSTRING

Medial hamstring is another very common and important knee dysfunction. The tenderpoint is located close to the attachment of the medial hamstring tendon, either in front of or behind it. Treatment easiest for me is with the patient in the supine position, knee flexed to about forty-five degrees, leg adducted and externally rotated with the force applied almost all rotation.

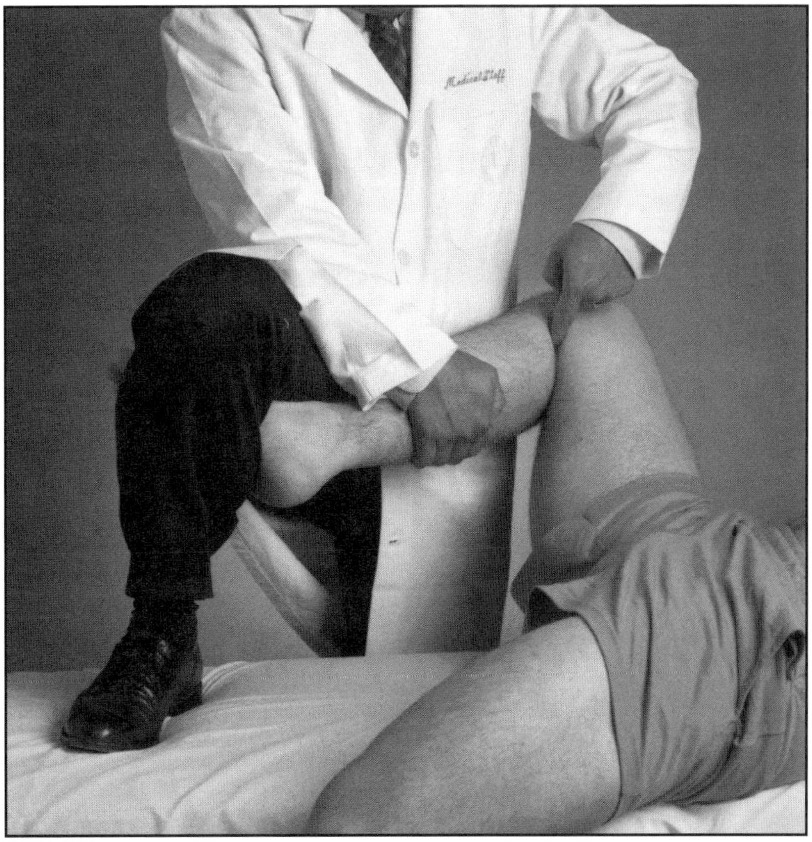

LATERAL MENISCUS OR HAMSTRING

The tenderpoint for this less common knee dysfunction is over the lateral meniscus or near the lateral hamstring. In either case this treatment is not consistent. It may be like that for the medial meniscus or it may have a little abduction rather than adduction or the rotation may be reversed. Treatment after you have fumbled your way through it is effective.

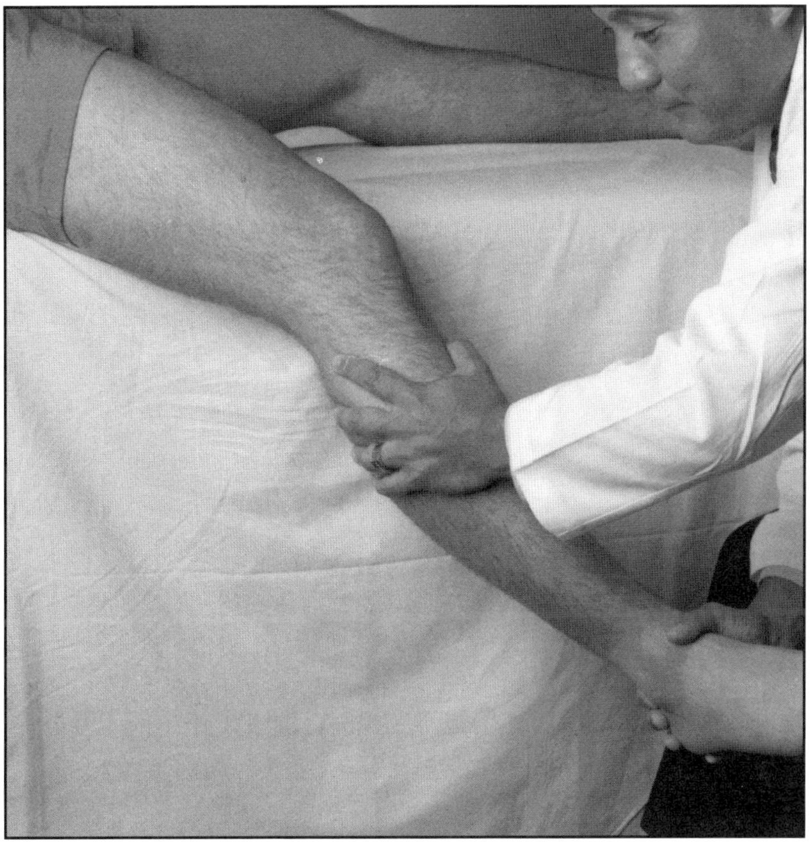

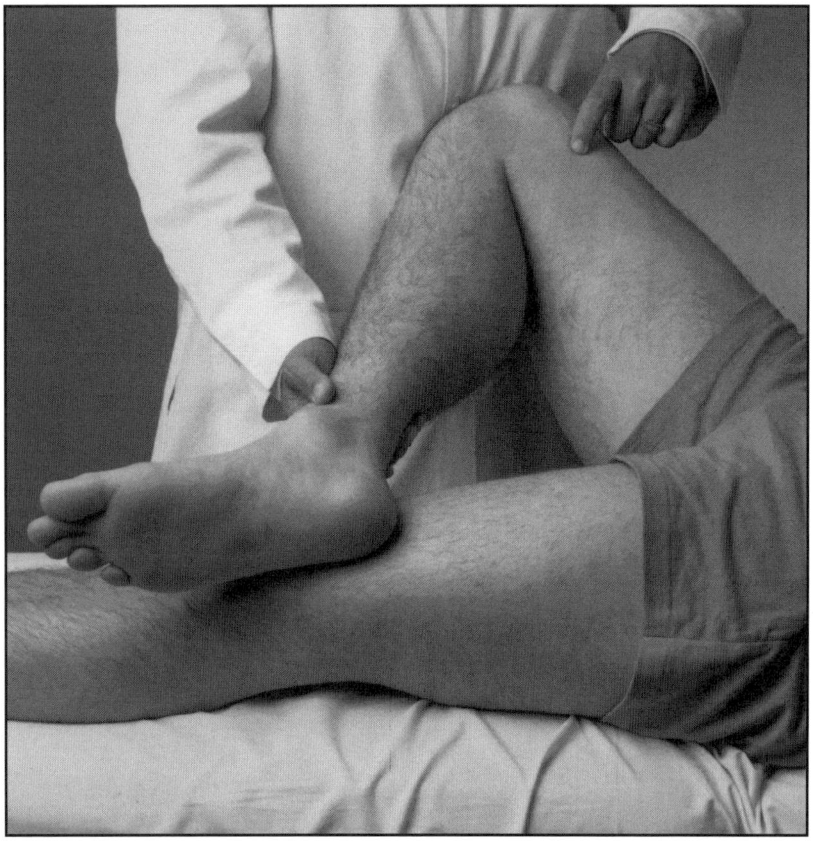

ROTATED KNEE

Rotated knee is another new dysfunction, although not all that uncommon. The tenderpoint is on the medial side of the knee, about an inch above the medial condyle. Treatment is ninety degrees of flexion and ninety degrees of rotation of the flexed leg on the femur. As the cause for this is so apparent, it is assumed to be crossing one ankle over the opposite knee while sitting. I recommend that when they catch themselves in this position, they ease back out slowly, supporting the leg with the hands.

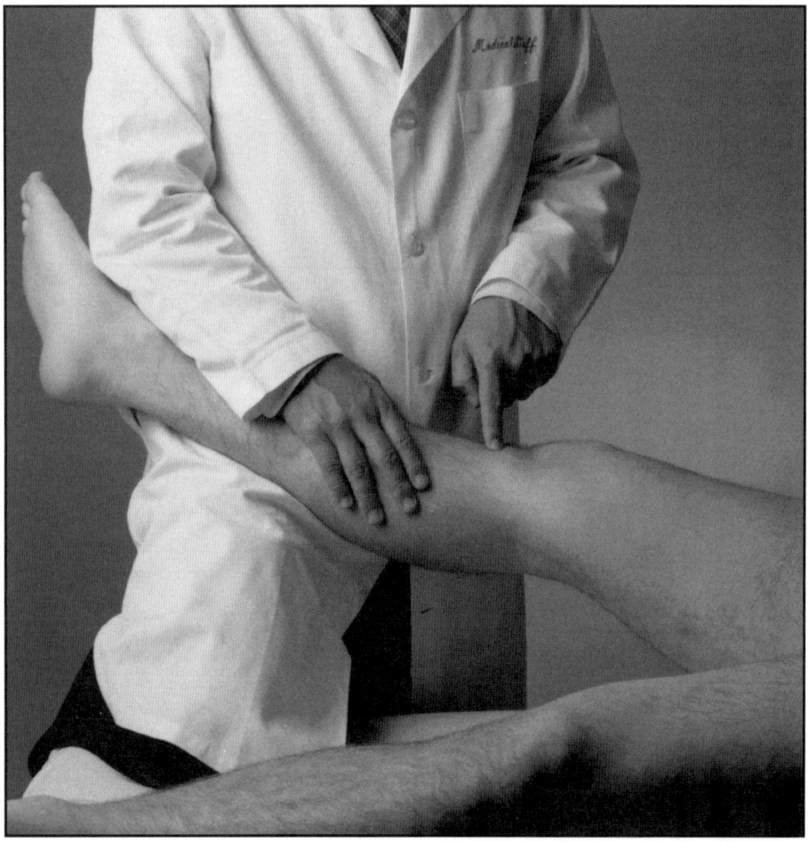

KNEE EXTENDERS

There are three main ones of this type with tenderpoints close together but distinct. The complaint is pain on hyper flexion like a squat and any strain of extension. The first tenderpoint is on the patellar ligament (actually an extension of the tendon of the rectus). Another near it is over the front of the medial meniscus. The third is on the front medial surface of the tibia in an area aparently free of muscle action. It can be thought that the aponeurosis of the sartorius could be the affected muscle. All are eased by hyperextension, the first two probably with a little internal rotation and the latter with a little external rotation.

PATELLAR TENDON WITH KNEE EXTENDERS

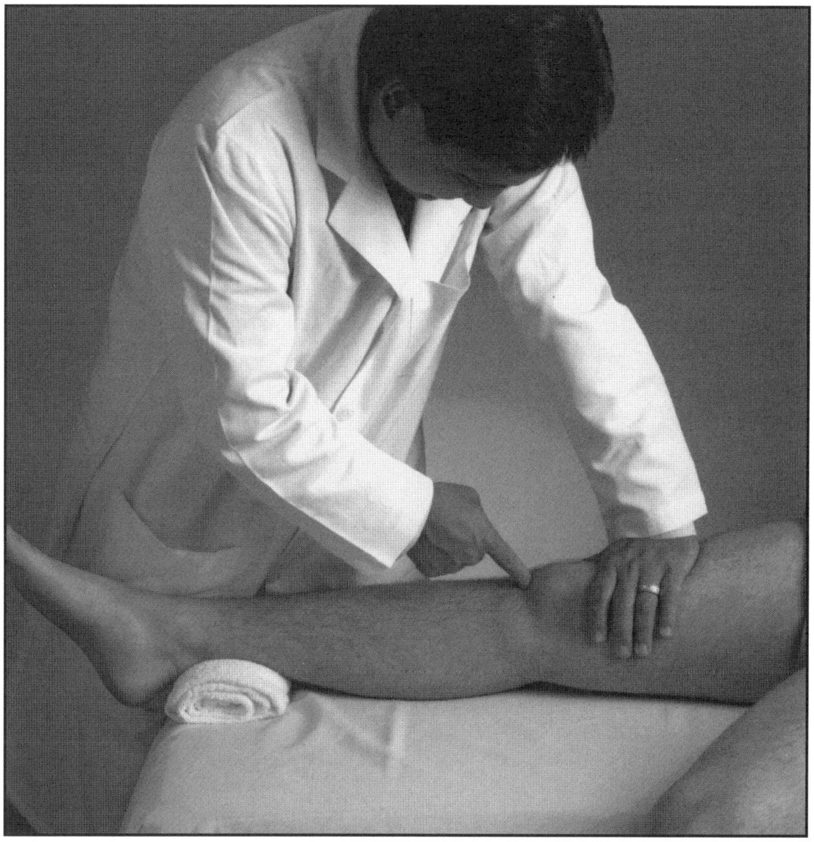

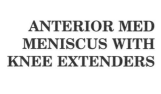

ANTERIOR MED MENISCUS WITH KNEE EXTENDERS

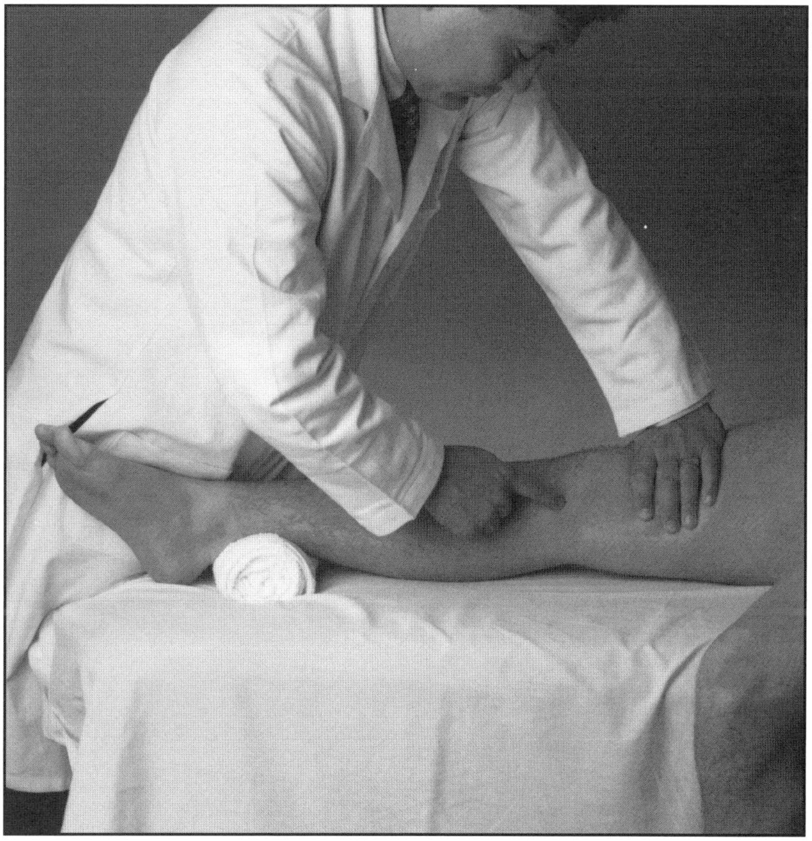

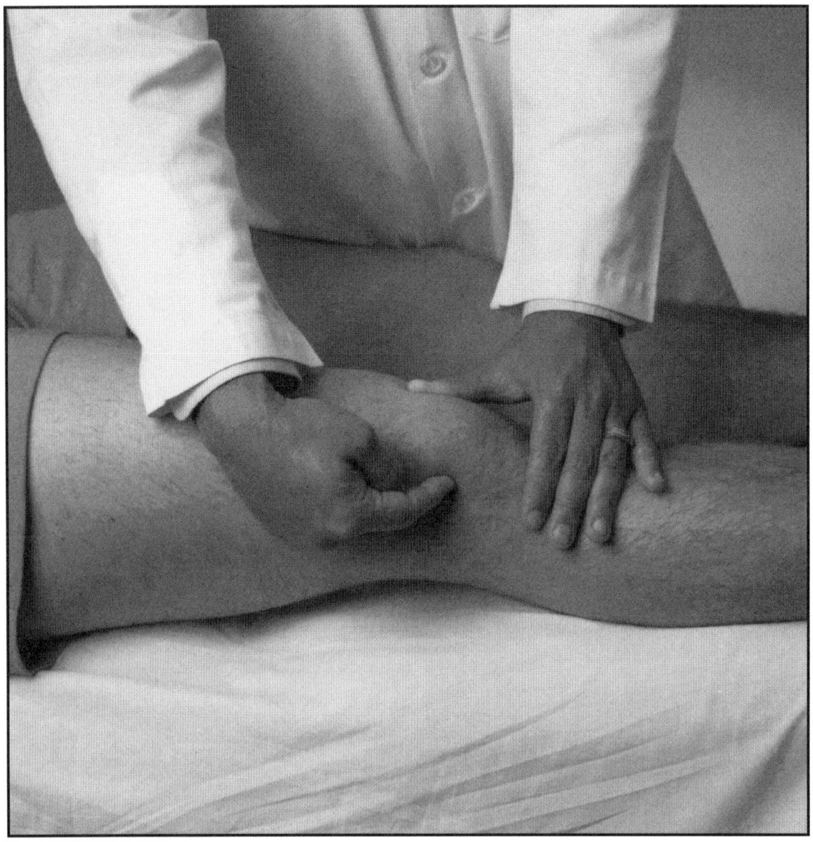

PATELLA

This one usually has a pain above the knee one and a half inches. Tenderpoints are on the perimeter of the patella. Treatment (surprisingly gentle for such a powerful structure) is pressure of a few ounces over the part of the perimeter of the patella that is opposite the tenderpoint.

UPPER TIBIO-FIBULAR PAIN

Although pain from this area would sometimes lead us to include this as a knee strain, successful treatment is almost always by stretches of the ankle. We will discus it with ankles.

ANKLES AND FEET

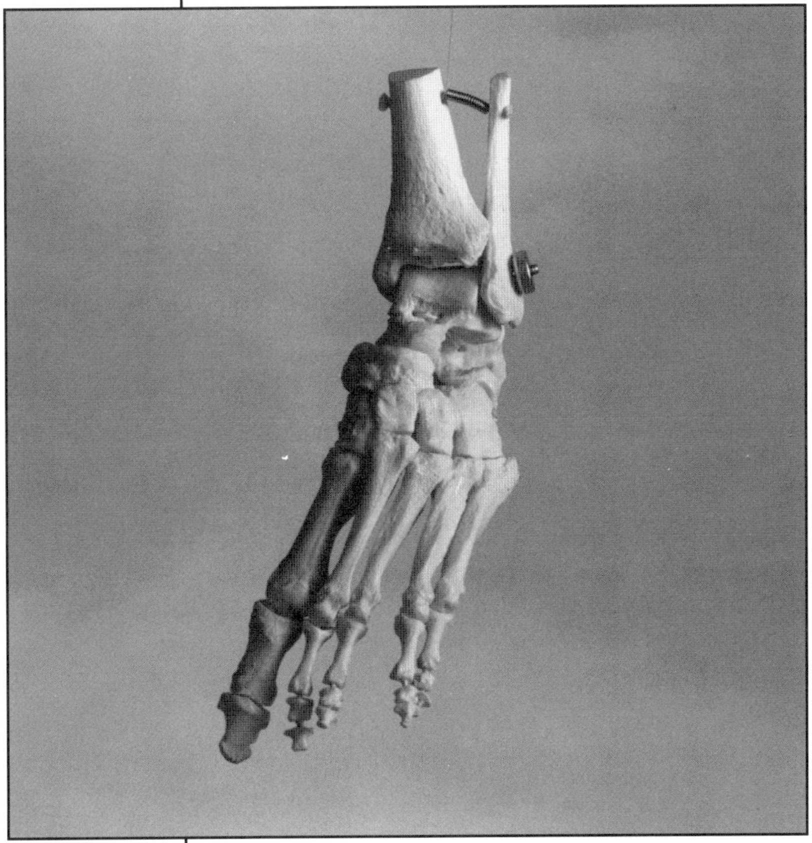

GENERAL

Feet are for many people the site of their greatest misery. Here is another part of the body that can be eased by comfortable stretches. Sixty years ago manipulators of feet were taught to use a direct force to overcome the resistance of the foot. The only thing wrong with this idea was that the foot and ankle are several times stronger than hands, and most operators found that effective foot treatment was likely to give them hand injuries. Maybe that was the reason that podiatrists like orthopoedic surgeons are dedicated mostly to surgery and take little interest in relieving foot pain by manipulation.

Again the salvation came by doing what felt good to the patient. If an operator does this, the foot doesn't resist, and he doesn't have to overpower it. My first paper on foot treatment was titled, "Foot Treatment Without Hand Trauma." The powerful foot still needs strong forces in many of its treatments, but they now are within the ability of most operators.

The right stretches will start the cure for ninety percent of painful feet, and the foot submits to any good feeling.

Chronic ankle irritations from old sprained ankles are a common yet not suspected source of trouble in the foot. All foot treatment should begin with a comprehensive check of the ankle. Almost every ankle sprain leaves a permanent dysfunction. Without proper treatment it will persist and be vulnerable for life. The patient does not complain of his continuous ankle sprain, just that he has a "weak ankle" or "a trick ankle."

Among other troubles in recovery, a sore foot is one of the hardest injured areas to rest between treatment. Except for the lateral ankle they are relieved the easiest for me with the patient prone. Because the plantar surface of the foot is so tough, tenderpoints on the plantar surface may require more forceful probing. Some of these have very tough tissue.

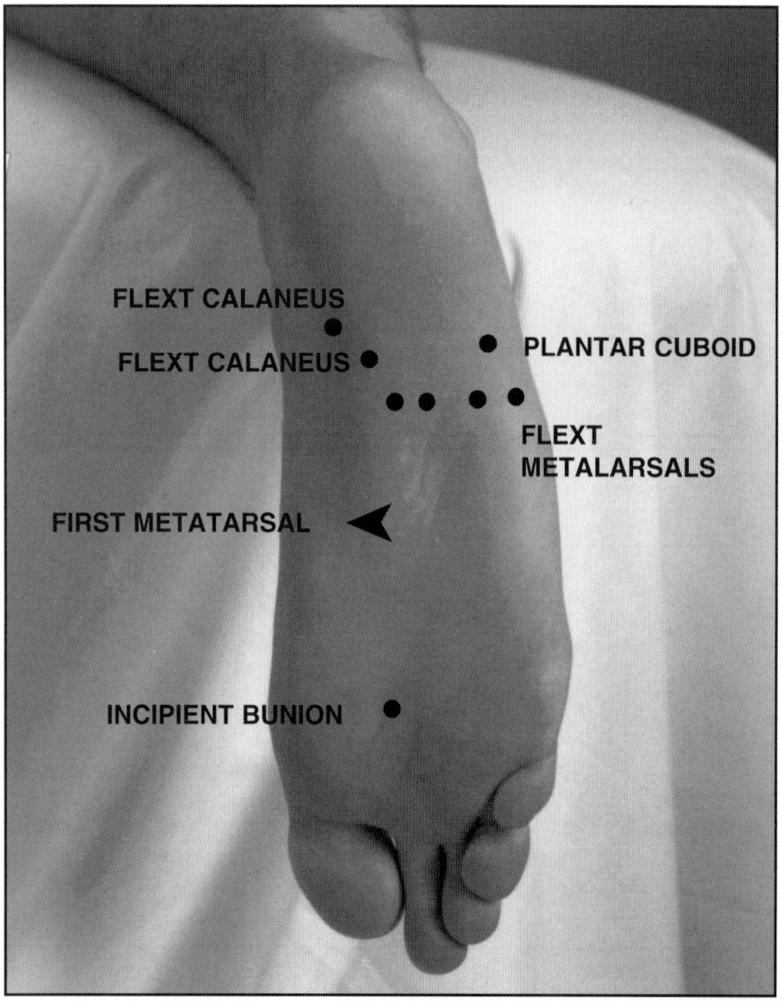

Since there are several directions a foot and ankle may be stretched and some difference in different author's descriptions, directions here are used as follows:

Extension ankle—Front of foot pulled away from knee;

Flexion ankle—Front of foot pushed toward knee;

Eversion—Foot rolls out to the side over an anterior-posterior axis;

Inversion—Foot rolls in over the same axis;

External rotation—Front of the foot turns out over a vertical axis;

Internal Rotation—Front of foot turns in over a vertical axis;

Plantar Flexion—Flexes the foot over its sole; and

Dorsiflexion—Front of foot pushed toward knee.

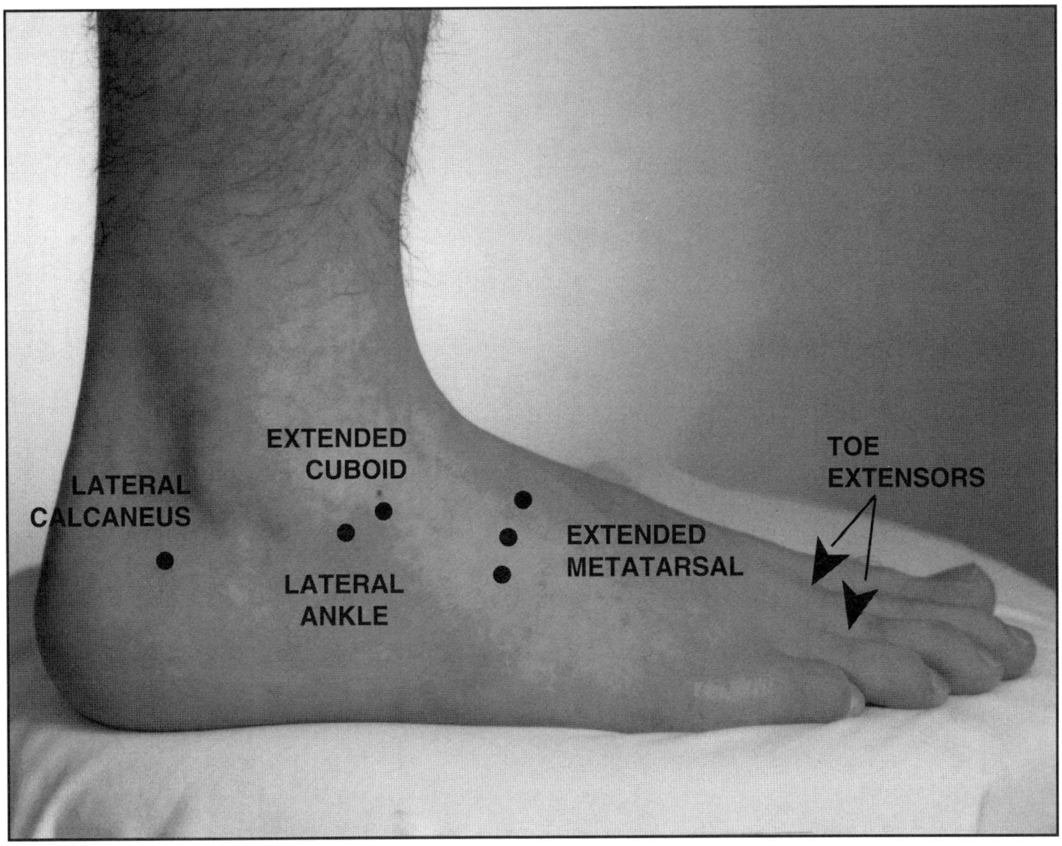
EXTENDED
CUBOID
LATERAL
CALCANEUS
TOE
EXTENSORS
EXTENDED
METATARSAL
LATERAL
ANKLE

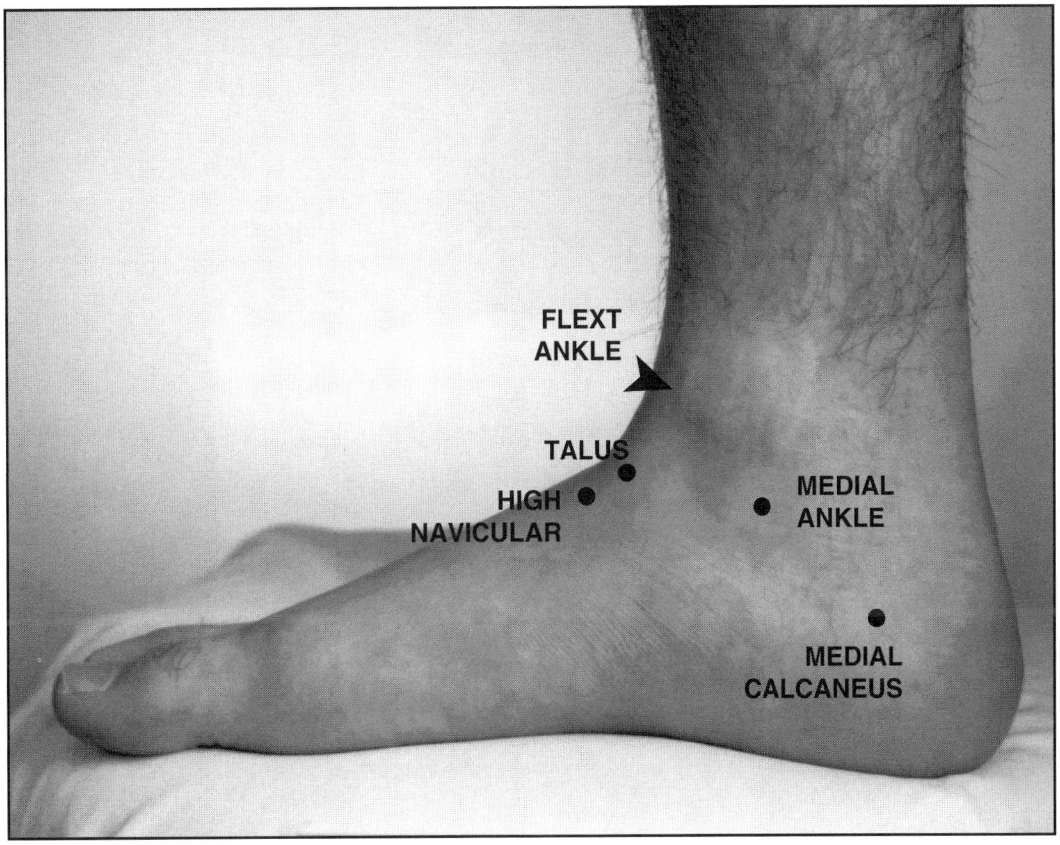
FLEXT
ANKLE
TALUS
HIGH
NAVICULAR
MEDIAL
ANKLE
MEDIAL
CALCANEUS

EXTENSION ANKLE

This very common dysfunction when severe can cause an apparent foot drop. The patient has strength to push off his foot walking but not enough to lift the foot when it leaves the floor. He scuffs his shoe and is especially prone to stumbling on any rough ground. He has a characteristic gait, lifting the knee extra high and flopping the foot upward. Milder cases just have a relative weakness of this type. The best tenderpoint is on one head of the gastrocnemius, usually the medial one. Treatment takes powerful extension of the ankle most easily provided by operator's thigh as he stands with one foot on the table. The foot is raised and the front of the ankle is laid over the fold where the operator's thigh meets his groin. Hands are used to hold the foot in his groin, which supplies the traction force for a powerful extension. Pressure is kept high on the instep to avoid straining metatarsals. Careless treatment here can damage weak tarso-metatarsal joints.

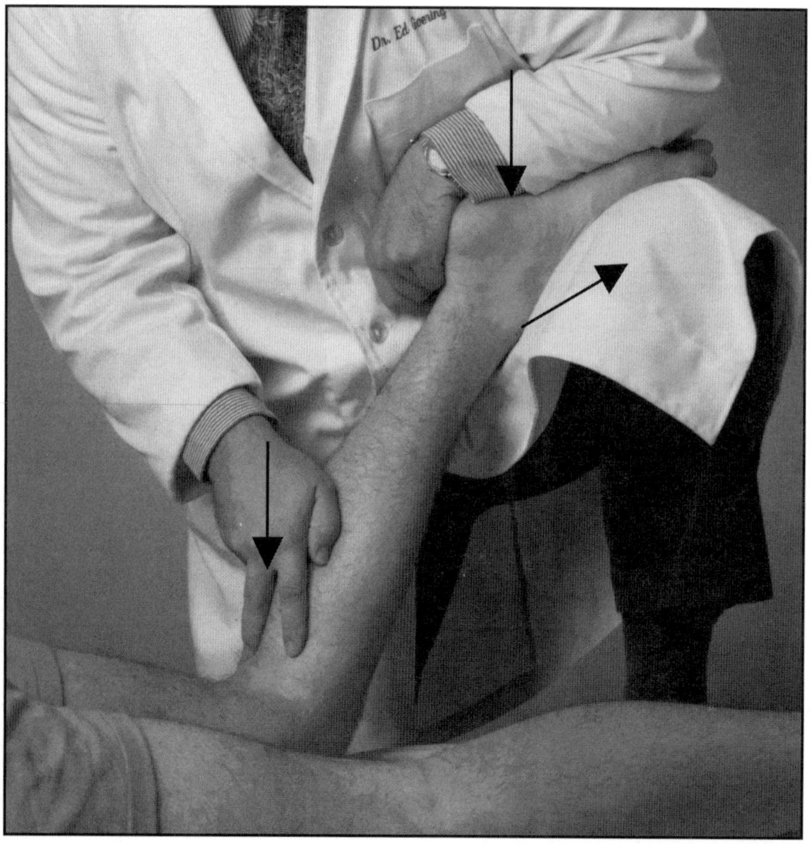

FLEXION ANKLE

This is the reverse of the force above. Tenderpoint is high in the front of the ankle in a depression just medial to the big extensor tendon. Exert force under the ball of the foot (can be reinforced by operator's chest). Fine tune with slight rotation.

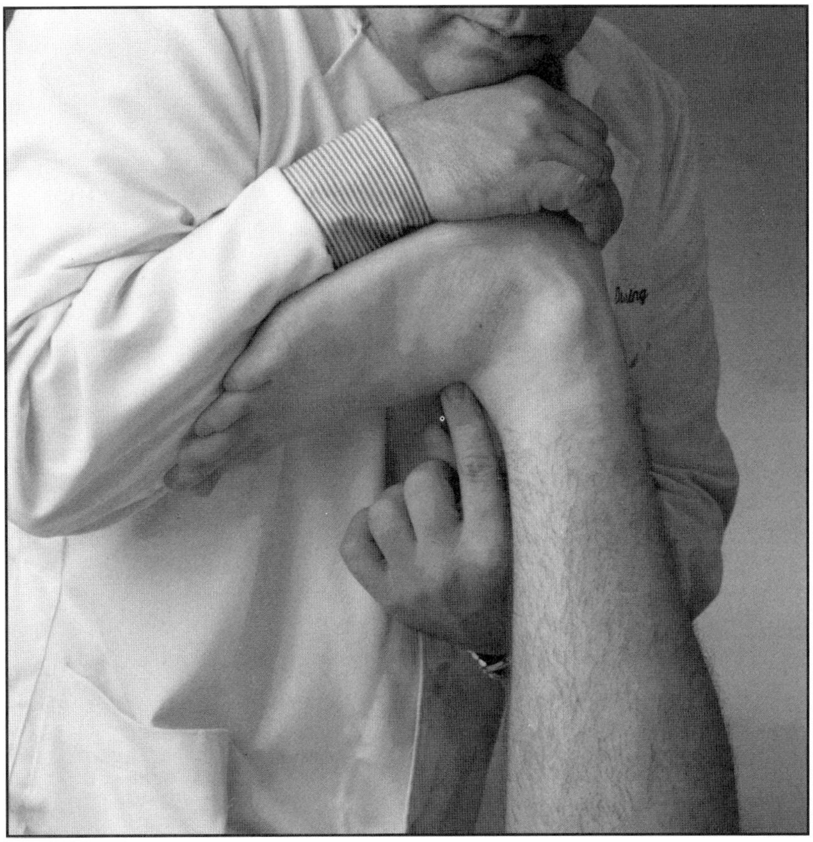

TALUS OR ASTRAGALUS

This is found in another depression high on medial side of the foot located in a little depressed area two centimeters forward from the medial malleolus. There is a little corner of the talus bone that is palpable in the bottom of this depression. Treatment is inversion and internal rotation of the foot. Fine tuning is done with flexion or extension. It may also have a tenderpoint on the medial border of the gastrocnemius.

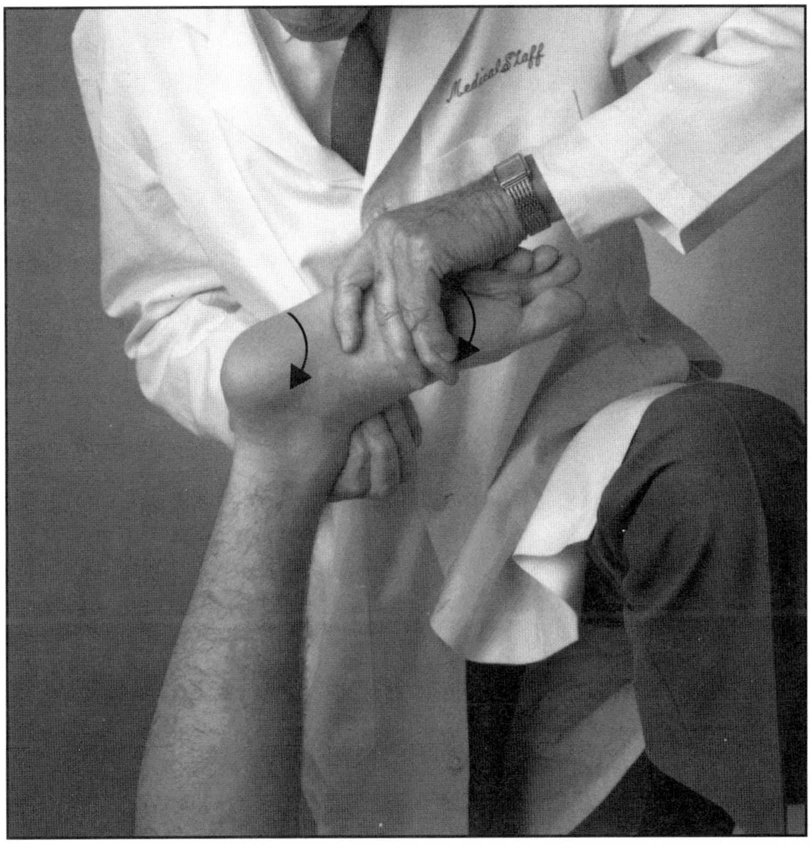

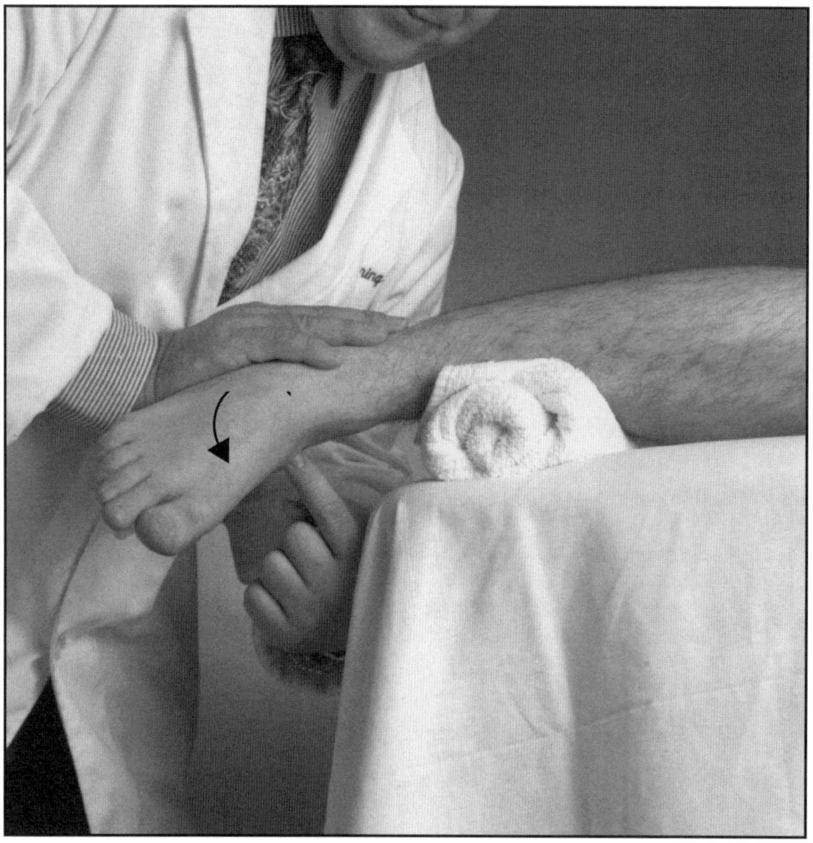

MEDIAL ANKLE

The tenderpoint is in a small arc below the medial malleolus. Treatment is mostly inversion of the foot without so much internal rotation as the talus.

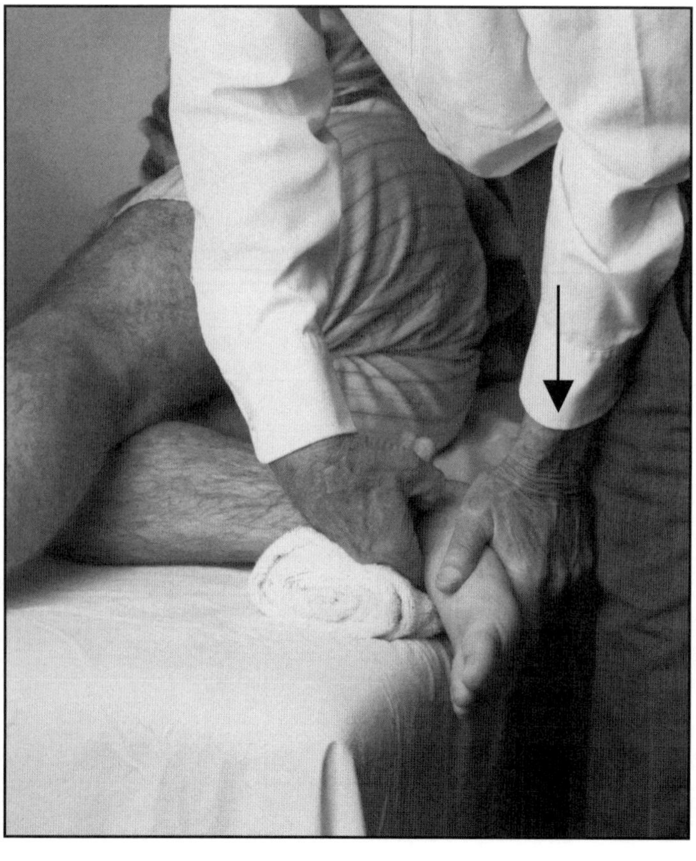

LATERAL ANKLE

This is another important and common ankle dysfunction. The tenderpoint is found in a depression three centimeters forward and a little below the lateral malleolus. As this trouble requires much force to relieve it, it is done with patient lying on the affected side, with knee bent and foot over the edge of the table with a rolled up towel under the ankle to protect the fibula. Force, up to forty pounds on a strong man, is applied three centimeters below the medial malleolus causing eversion of the whole foot. It is applied with the heel of the operator's hand. This can be a long ninety seconds for the operator unless he supports his elbow in his abdomen. While the treatment is in progress the point can be monitored by a finger of the other hand. There is also a mild external rotation. An alternate tenderpoint may be formed on the top of the fibula, but this is an ankle problem.

PLANTAR NAVICULAR

There is a tenderpoint beneath the navicular bone close to the cuboid. The physician wraps his index finger around the navicular bone. He reinforces the index with the third finger and with the thumb of the other hand to have enough power to stretch the navicular into inversion.

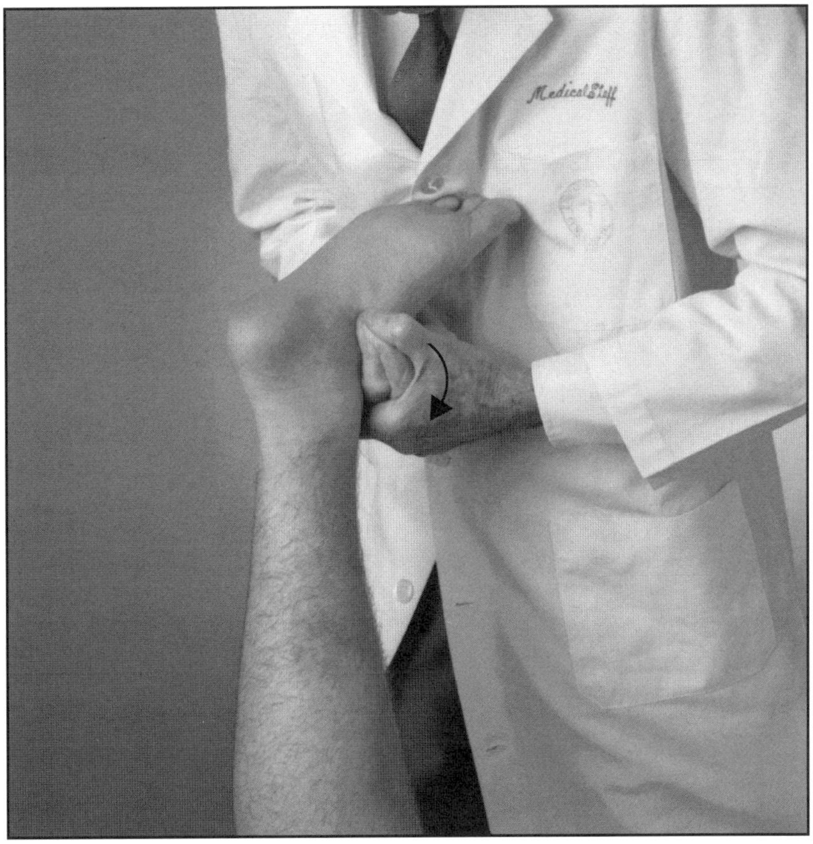

HIGH NAVICULAR

This tenderpoint was commonly found with flexed metatarsals and proved to be a valuable addition to their treatment. It is located high on the medial side of the bone. Treatment is much easier than that for the other navicular dysfunction. The operator puts his foot on the table and presses his knee against the lateral side of the foot. It can hurt the foot if placed wrong, so it is well to ask whether his knee hurts the foot. The foot is bent sideways over the knee by pulling the front of the foot and the heel laterally bending the foot laterally over a vertical axis. Not much force is needed.

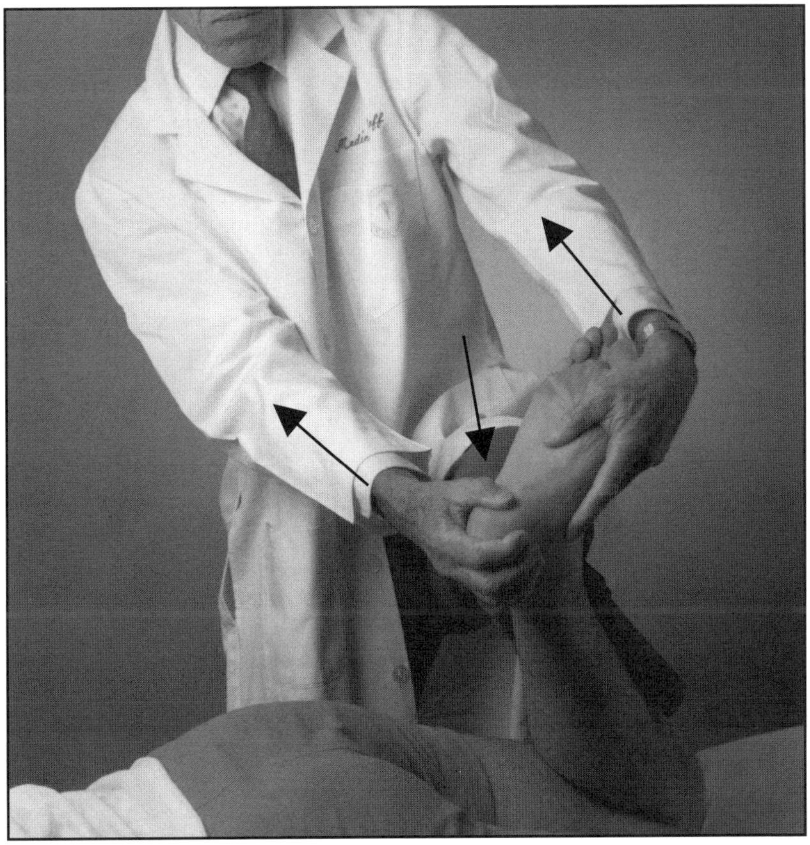

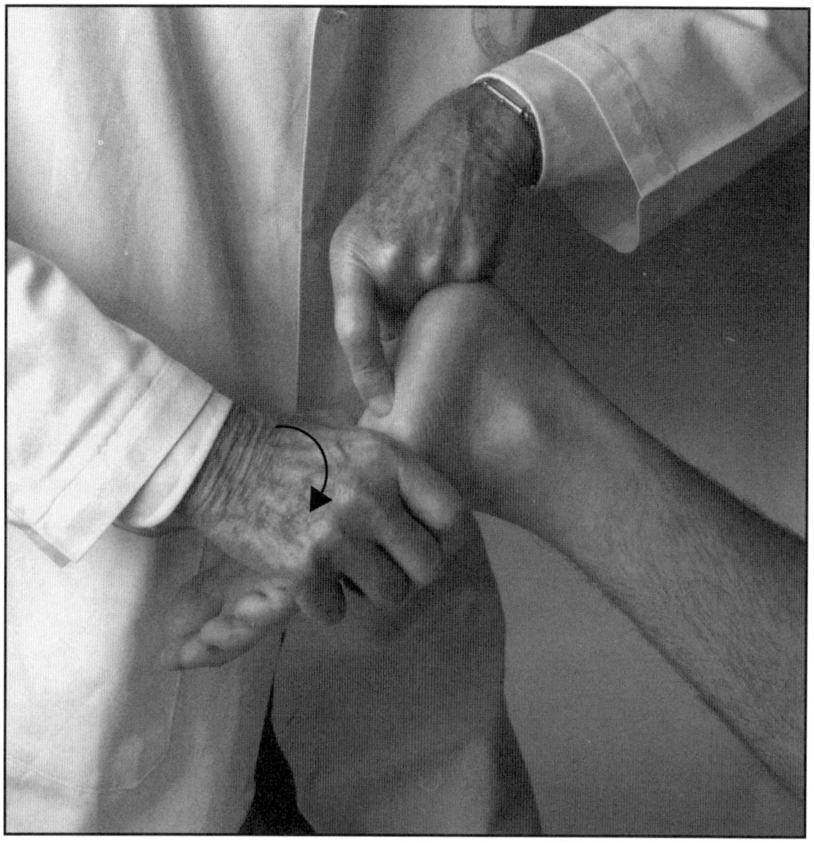

PLANTAR CUBOID

The tenderpoint on this uncommon dysfunction is on the tuberosity of the cuboid bone. This tubercle may be felt about three fourths of an inch back and medially from the base of the fifth metatarsal bone. It needs eversion which can be accomplished by pressure on the planter surface of the base of the fifth metatarsal bone. I do this most easily by pressing with the distal end of my second metacarpal bone, just behind the index finger. It needs a fairly strong force to produce enough eversion. This and the plantar navicular are the main troubles that I associate with flat feet. In spite of common belief that flat feet are the cause of pain, most sore feet have too high an arch.

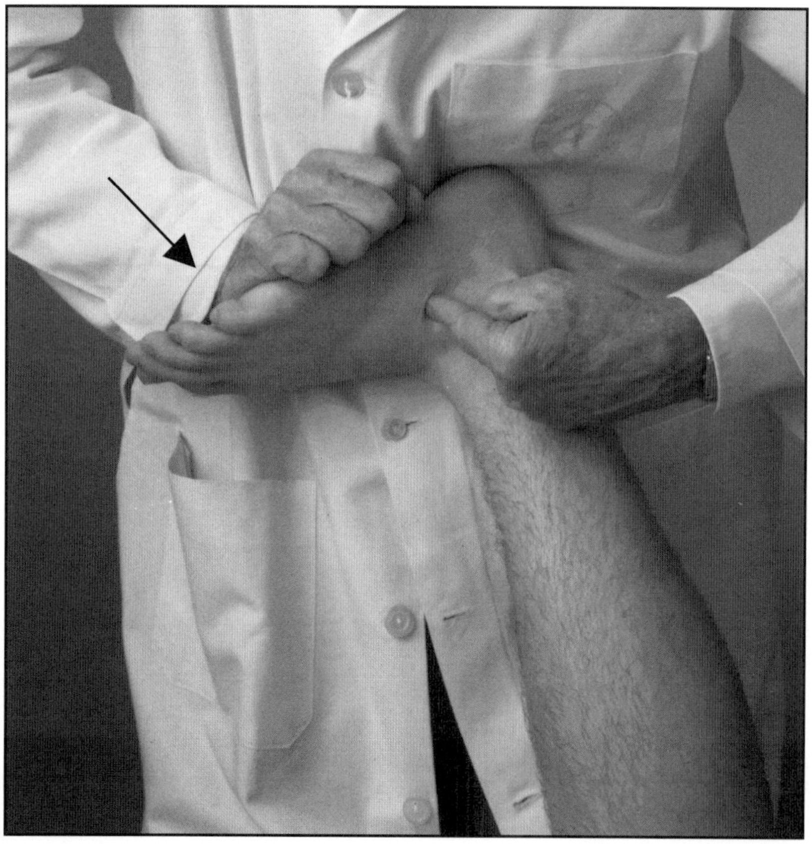

EXTENDED CUBOID

The tenderpoint for this is no more than one centimeter forward from the tenderpoint for the lateral ankle. Relief comes with a strong dorsiflexion of the lateral half of the foot.

THE CALCANEUS

This is involved in three common dysfunctions. Its treatment most often involves its relationship with the front of the foot rather than with the astragalus.

1. Flexed Calcaneus

The common term often applied to this problem is plantar fasciitis, because it is one of the principal causes of plantar pain. The tenderpoint is near the front end of the calcaneus in the medial part of the bottom of the foot. At the time of the publication of the first issue of this book the technique offered for treatment of this powerful area was difficult and not very effective. I found that I could avoid most of the difficulty by combining calcaneal treatment with extension ankle care (see Extension Ankle). Instead of just pushing the ankle into the fold of the operator's groin, the heel is pushed toward the front of the foot and the front of the foot is plantar flexed. This way effective treatment requires only moderate force.

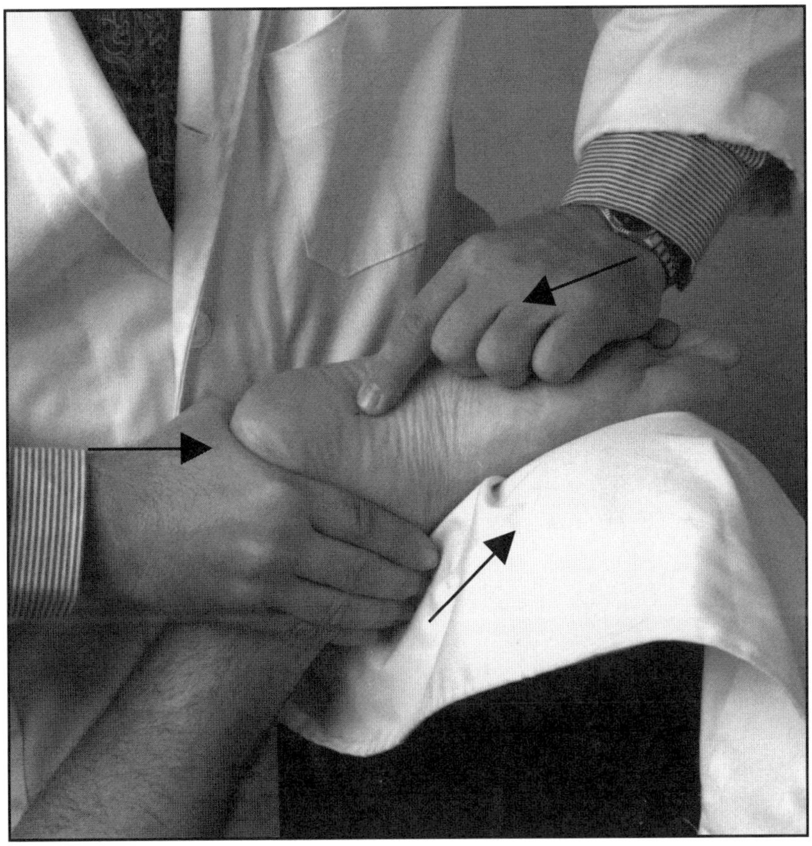

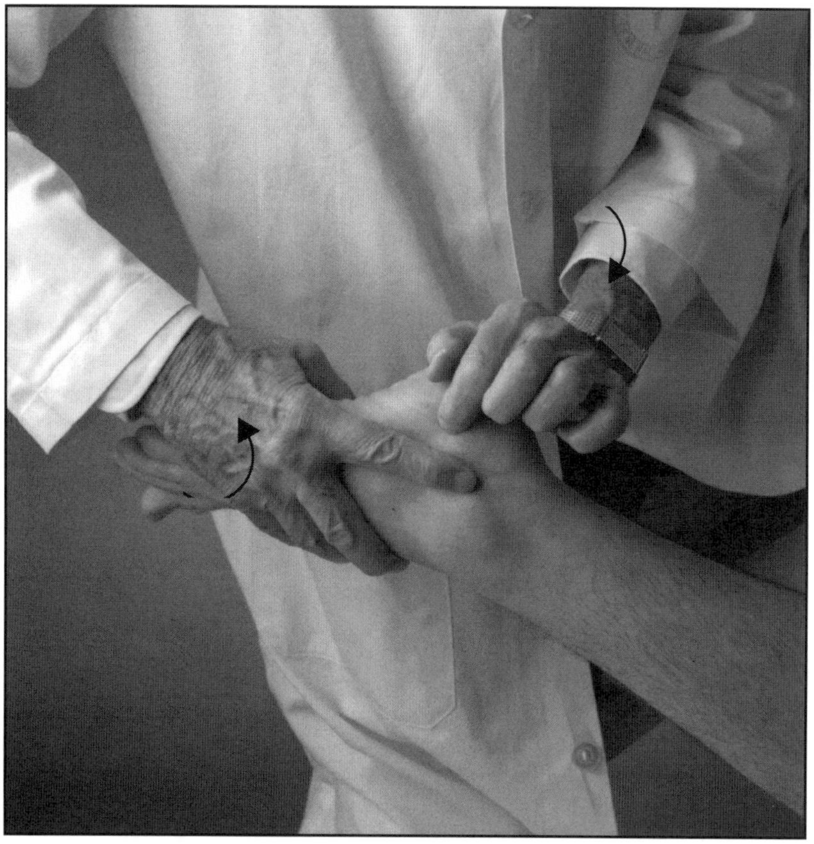

2. Lateral Calcaneus

There is a tenderpoint on the lateral side of the calcaneus about an inch down and back from the lateral malleolus. Treatment is a torsion stretch with the heel rolled out and the front of the foot rotated in into eversion. This is a source of calcaneal spurs.

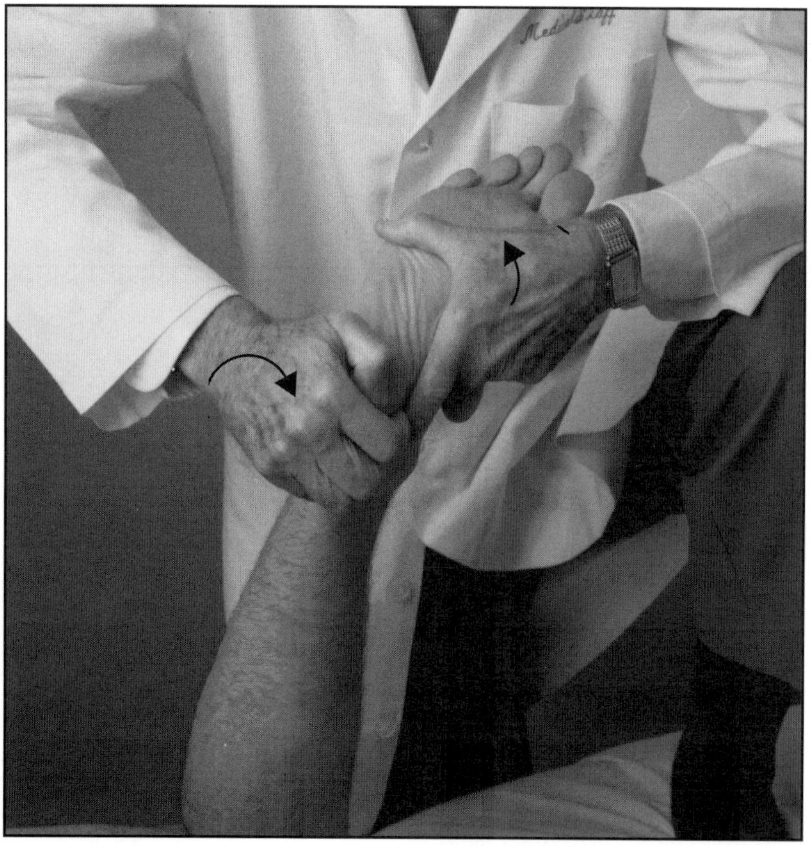

3. Medial Calcaneus

Treatment is just the opposite of Number 2 above.

EXTENDED FIFTH METATARSAL

One fairly common painful foot deformity is one where the front end of the fifth metatarsal and the fifth toe ride abnormally high in relation to the fourth metatarsal. This is found in a foot where the lateral half of the foot bears much more of the weight than it is designed for. The strong first metatarsal and great toe should be carrying most of the weight. The shoe should wear out first under the first metatarsal, but in this kind of a foot the center or even the lateral side of the shoe wears out. Usually there is a reversed transverse arch under the distal ends of the metatarsals that is convex below rather than concave. The cause may be an old chronic medial ankle. This is the main source of the so-called soft corn, between the fourth and fifth toes. Their relationship is bad enough that corners of toe bones press against each other so hard as to produce corns. Treatment includes further hyperextension of the fifth metatarsal so that it may return to a normal position and probably a correction of a medial ankle, if present. This produces the only lasting cure for this corn, for the strained metatarsal and for a plantar corn or callus on the fourth metatarsal.

Many painful feet may be traced to tight shoes or high heel shoes that make the foot look much smaller and prettier. For many years I had disappointing results, because women refused to wear shoes that would permit their feet to function normally. Finally I explained how essential normal foot function is to recovery and declined to treat those who were unwilling to give up the pretty shoes. I lived long enough to see great misery in these people as their trouble progressed, but it is a pretty hollow justification. Men seldom have this problem, although many of them wear shoes that are too narrow on the recommendation of shoe salesmen who often believe that feet should be supported by shoes.

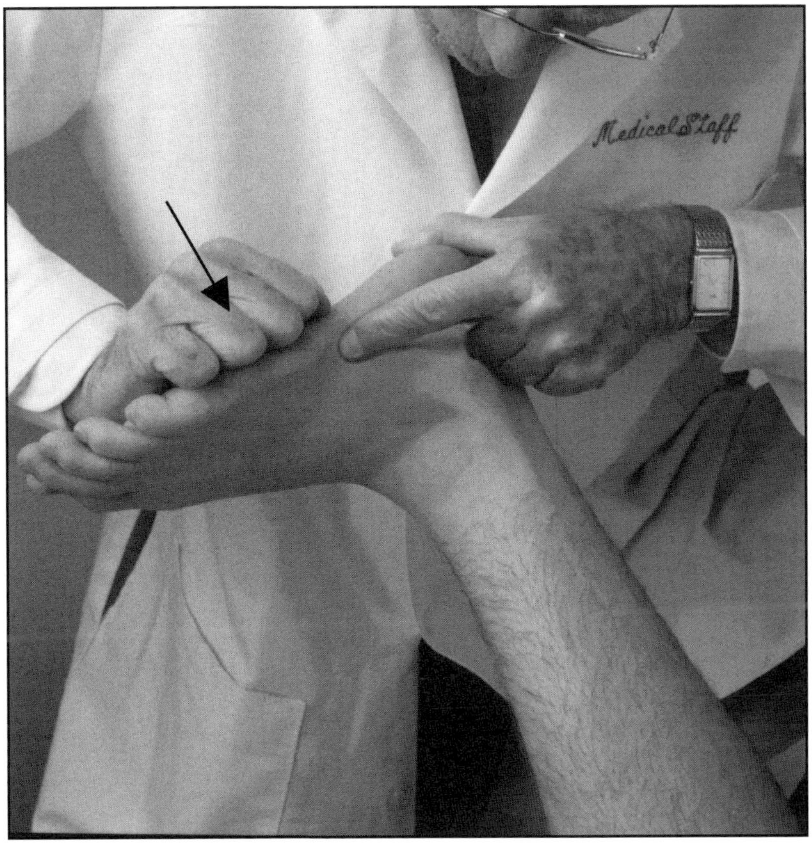

FLEXED METATARSALS

Most patients are aware of pain in the area at the distal ends of these bones, the site of many plantar callouses and corns. Success with these problems by manipulating the tarso-metatarsal joint has made me believe that all of these troubles arise as a result of too much pressure on some corners of bone pressing too hard against a shoe or another corner of bone. Most general treatment of these is as skin disorders and they are trimmed and padded to take the pressure off. The success of my treatment is because the source of these points of pressure is deformity of the way the metatarsals hit the shoe. If they lie flat, pressure is spread over an adequate surface, but if rotated, a corner of the front ends which strike the shoe can be tender for life. At the back ends of these metatarsals where I find the tenderpoints, they are off the ground because of the high arch. There is a procedure which relieves almost all of them. The operator places his thigh under the dorsum of the foot so that it rests upon his knee and thigh. This gives him enough power on the front of the tips of his fingers to grasp the front ends of the second, third, and fourth metatarsals, resting the back of his fingers on his thigh. Without this device we are likely to use the points of the tips of our fingers and that's painful. He makes a strong pull of the front of the foot into plantar flexion and external rotation of the metatarsals with equal amounts of force.

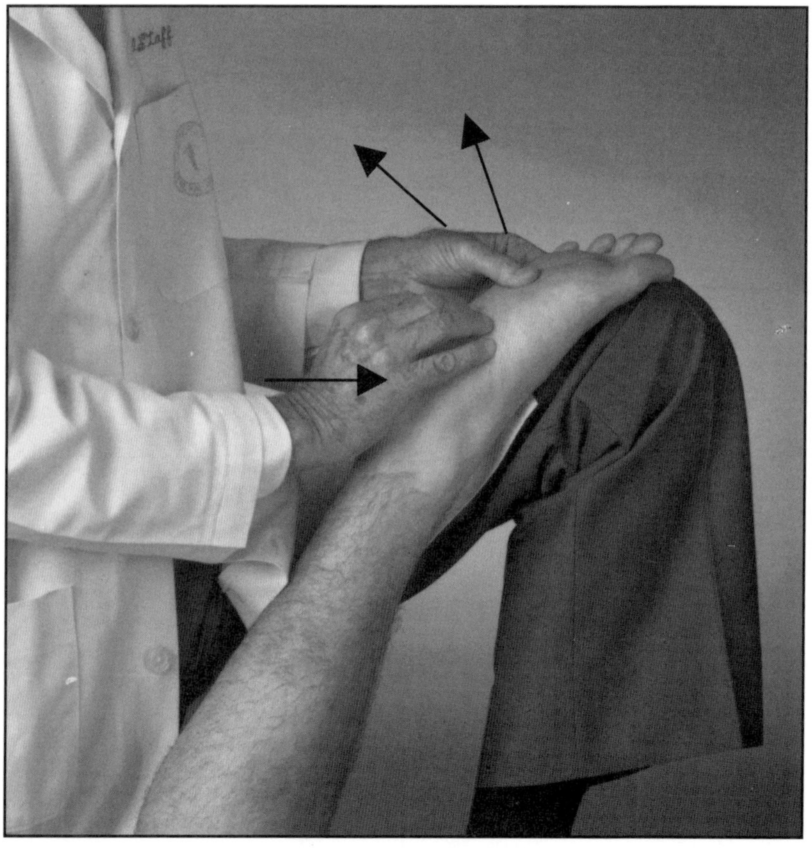

HAMMER TOES

This same dysfunction is, surprisingly, the culprit for a much different type of foot trouble that is equally common and poorly understood. Hammer toes have been considered to be due to a strange shortening of the extensor tendons of the toes. It causes a hyperextension of the metatarso-phalangeal joints. Not so strange. The knuckles of the toes strike the shoes too hard. In far advanced cases the tips of the toes strike the floor so hard on their points as to bleed. Many a sufferer has her roll of cotton under her toes to protect the toe tips. These toe extensors are too short because ***the arch of the foot is too high.*** This can be easily demonstrated in the prone position by pushing down on the plantar surface of the metarsals, making the foot relatively flat and watch the toes flex in the metatarso-phalangeal joints. Also a lasting recovery can be provided just by reducing the too high arch. Treatment is exactly the same as flexed metatarsals. Hyperflexed feet is very common, especially in females, and may be another of the bad results of high-heeled shoes. There is very much inflammation and it is almost impossible for patients to be off their feet enough to avoid aggravating their troubles, but except in very old patients with far advanced conditions, they can be cured. Patients must avoid high-heeled shoes. The hyperextended toe joints often join in with strains of their own. These are easily relieved with hyperextension. Tenderpoints are on top of the distal ends of the metatarsals. This fairly complicated concept of troubles in the front of the foot again seems illogical to many physicians. I can only say that the treatment has a high success rate.

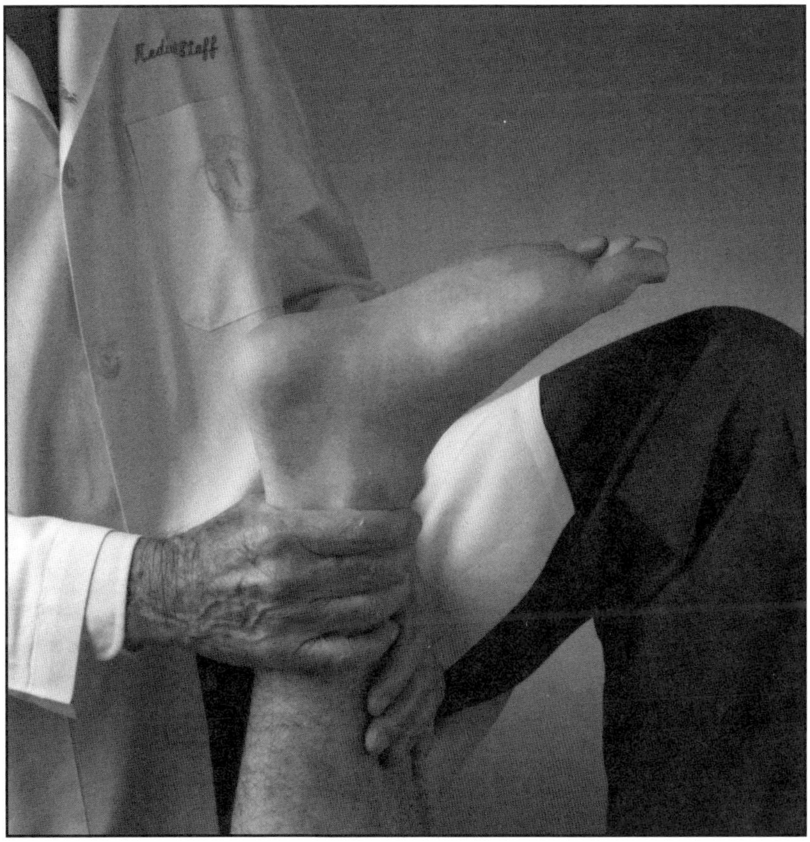

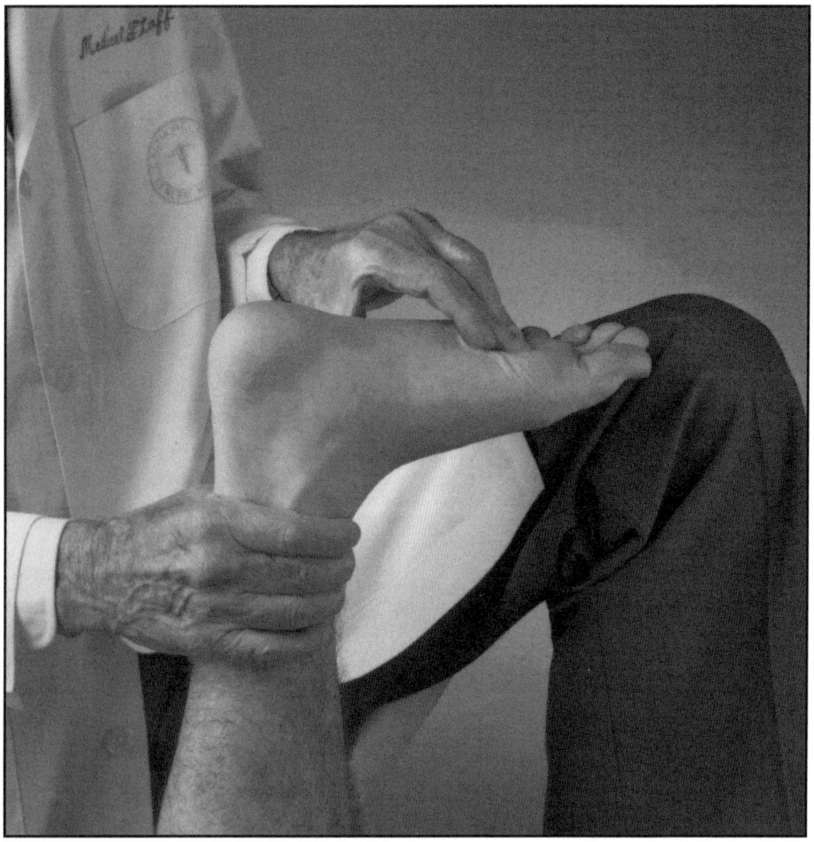

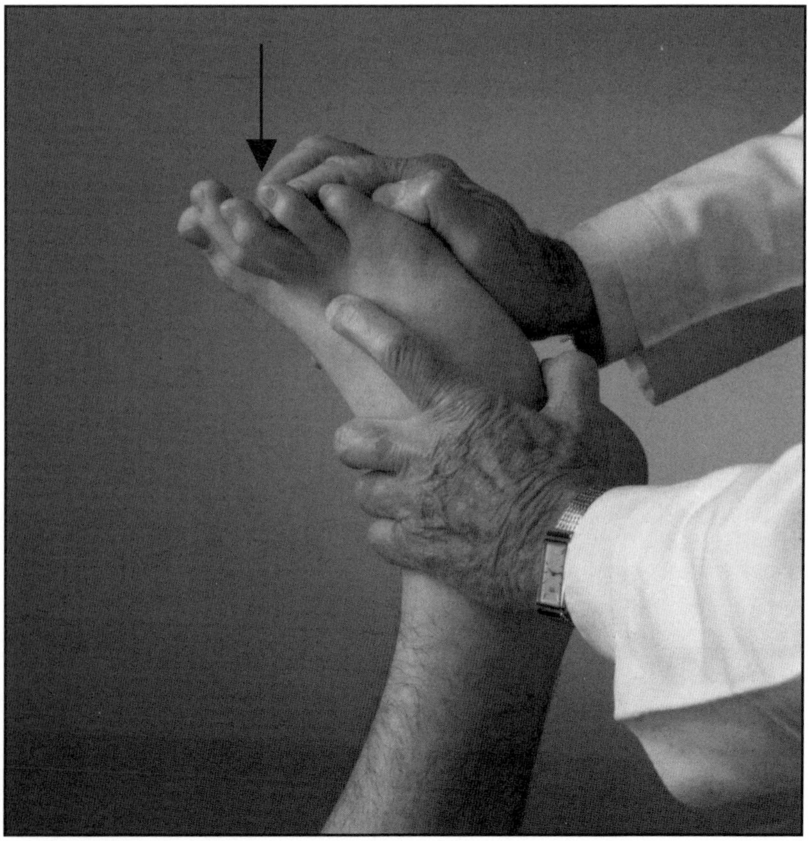

EXTENDED METATARSO-PHALANGES

FIRST METATARSAL

The big strong first metatarsal bone should be doing the bulk of the work of the front of the foot. It has one dysfunction much more common than any other. The tenderpoint for this is on the plantar surface but deep into the intermetatarsal area on the middle of the shaft of the bone. It is relieved by grasping the distal end of the metatarsal (not the toe) and twisting it into eversion. Fine tuning may involve internal or external rotation.

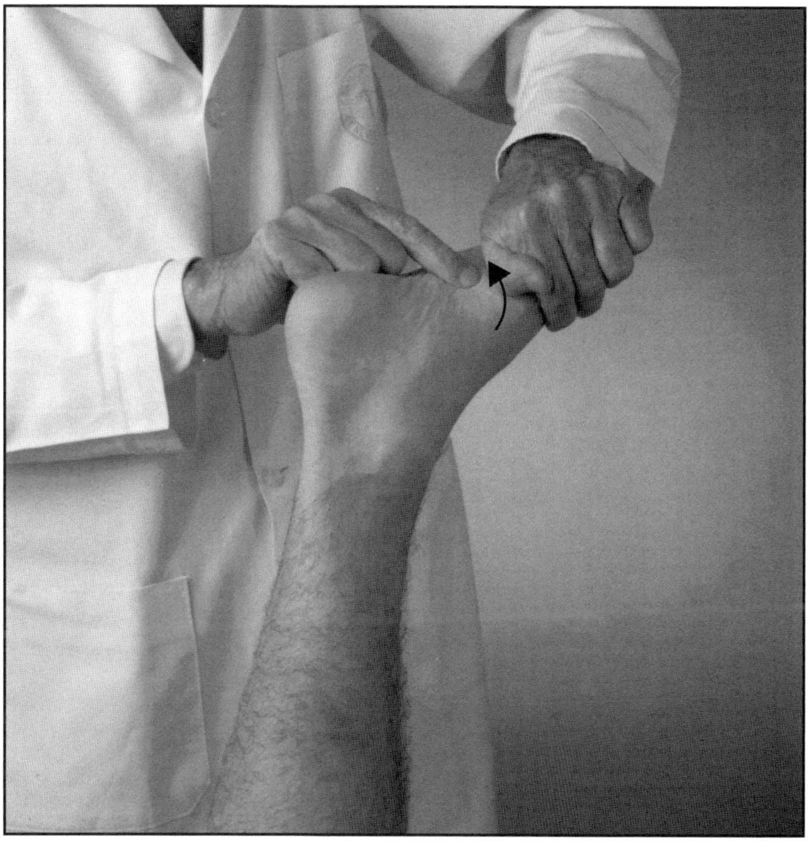

INCIPIENT BUNION

These again are diagnosable and treatable long before true bunion degeneration has set in. Foot problems' success demand a shoe that will permit the great toe to stop being forced into a sidebend that nature never meant for it to have. A surprising (to me) number of women flatly refuse to give up their pretty shoes, no matter how much pain they will suffer. By the time they hurt enough to listen they are beyond help from any treatment short of surgery. The great toe like all the other toes normally functions in extension and flexion. A shoe that pushes it far laterally will ruin the benefits of any treatment.

The tenderpoint is under the lateral sesamoid between the first and second metatarsals and toes. The toe is grasped and sidebent toward the center of the foot and rotate the toe in a plantar direction until comfort is achieved, again exaggerating the deformity to reduce it. With patient cooperation it can be cured.

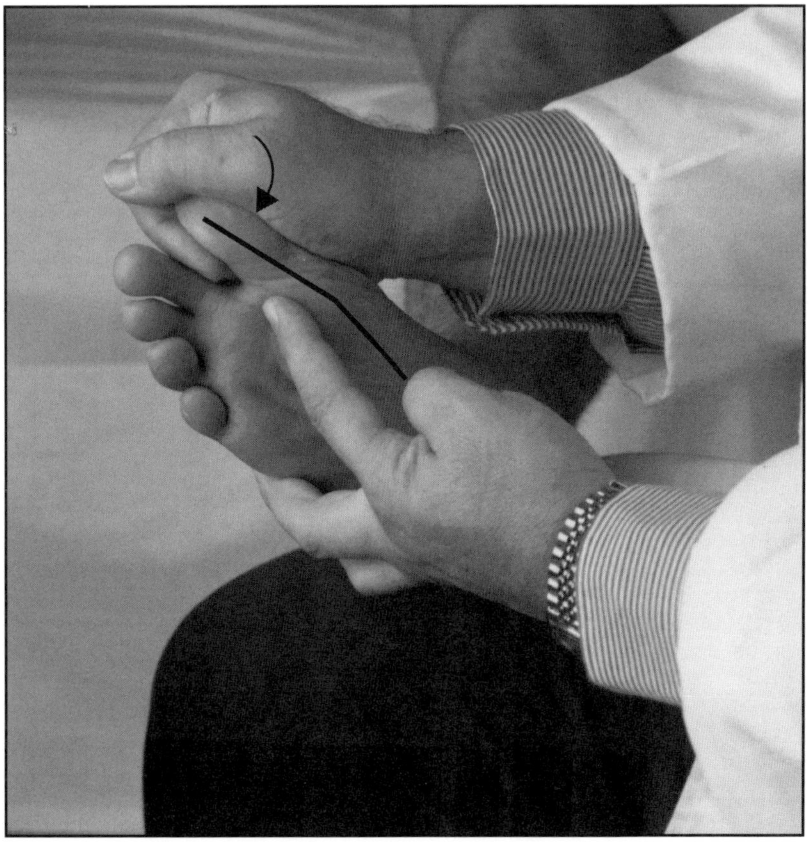

SHOULDER, ARM, AND HAND

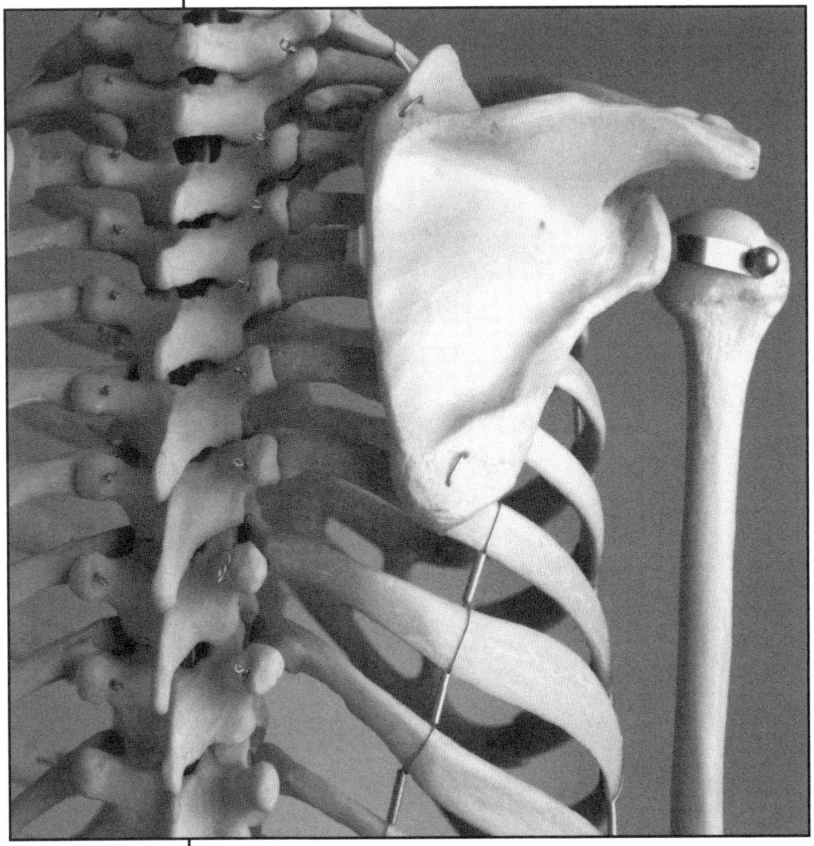

GENERAL

Aching or numb shoulders, arms and hands are the complaints. Many of them have troubles not recognized in the upper thoracic or rib areas. The top five thoracic segments must be corrected or the treatment for local upper extremity problems may be followed by many recurrences. This may be another surprise for beginners. The culprit has been thought to be the brachial plexus, but except for rare exceptions do I find the complicating dysfunctions in this area. Only after thorough care for the upper five thoracic inter-vertebral and costo-vertebral joints should local treatment be done. It often takes many disappointments before this becomes evident to the physician. As in other parts of the body, the patient will usually complain of pain in an area that does not have a tenderpoint. To satisfy him I always examine the site of the pain, but I expect to find my tenderpoint somewhere else.

Some of the common shoulder pains are found on the posterior surface of the scapula. They seem most easy to find with the patient lying supine. The patient may complain of pain in the front of the shoulder. Don't be misled. Although they do appear to occur in relationship to specific segments of the upper thoracic intervertebral joints and were described this way in the first issue, it seemed through the years of teaching that attempts to correlate them by students was more nuisance than help. For this issue, we are abandoning this to just indicate locations on the scapula of tenderpoints. For landmarks we use the borders and the spine of the scapula.

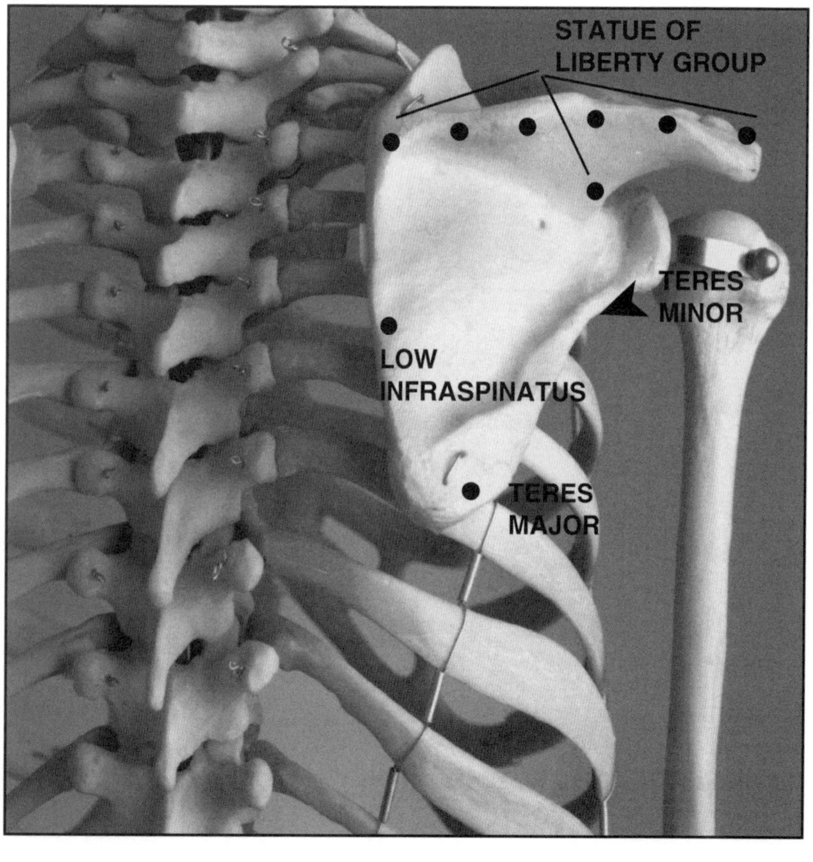

ANTERIOR ACROMIO-CLAVICULAR JOINTS

These are the most proximal important joints of the shoulder. They may suffer from two kinds of dysfunctions. The anterior has a tenderpoint slightly medial to the tip end of the clavicle in front. Treatment by drawing the arm across in front of the body and applying a little traction usually suffices. Similarly the uncommon posterior tenderpoint may be easily relieved with a pull behind the body.

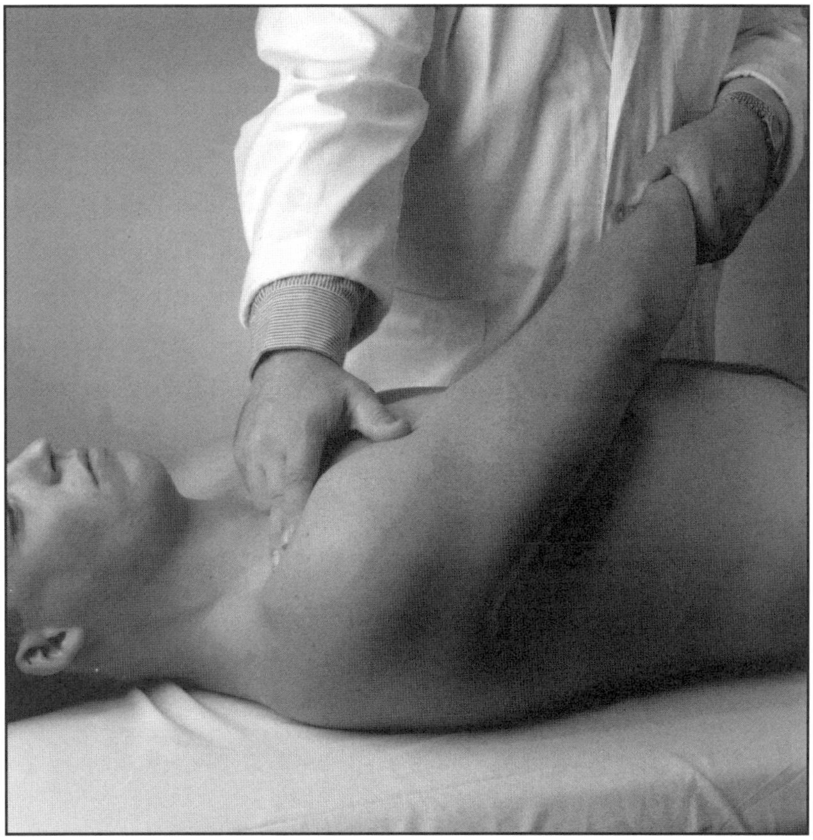

POSTERIOR ACROMIO-CLAVICULAR JOINTS

This strain between the lateral end of the clavicle and the scapula is relieved by a traction force on the arm which is held behind the back in an unstrained position with the hand about at the midline.

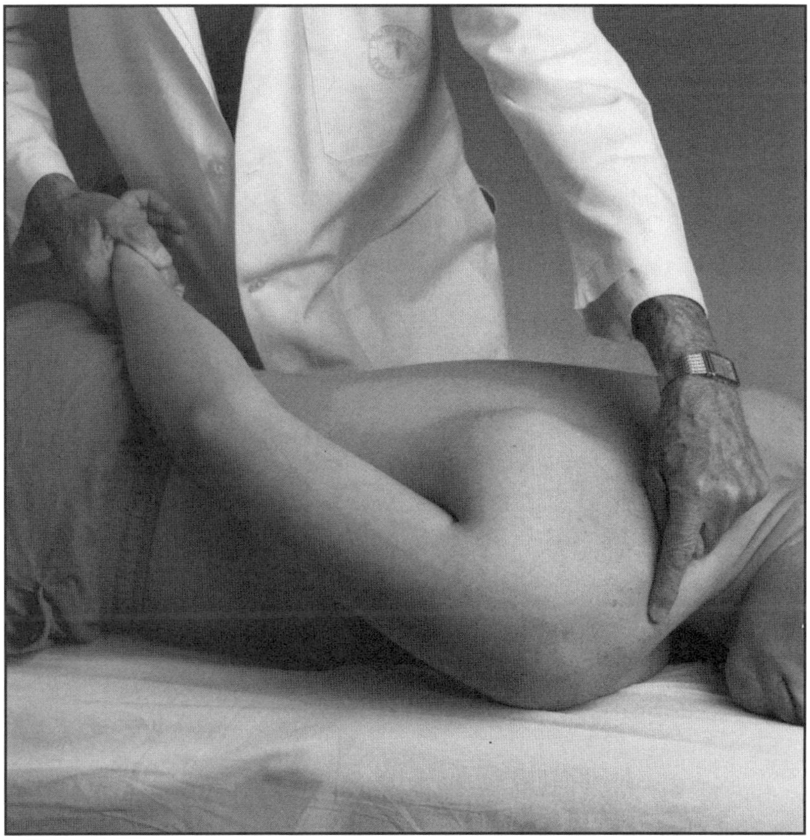

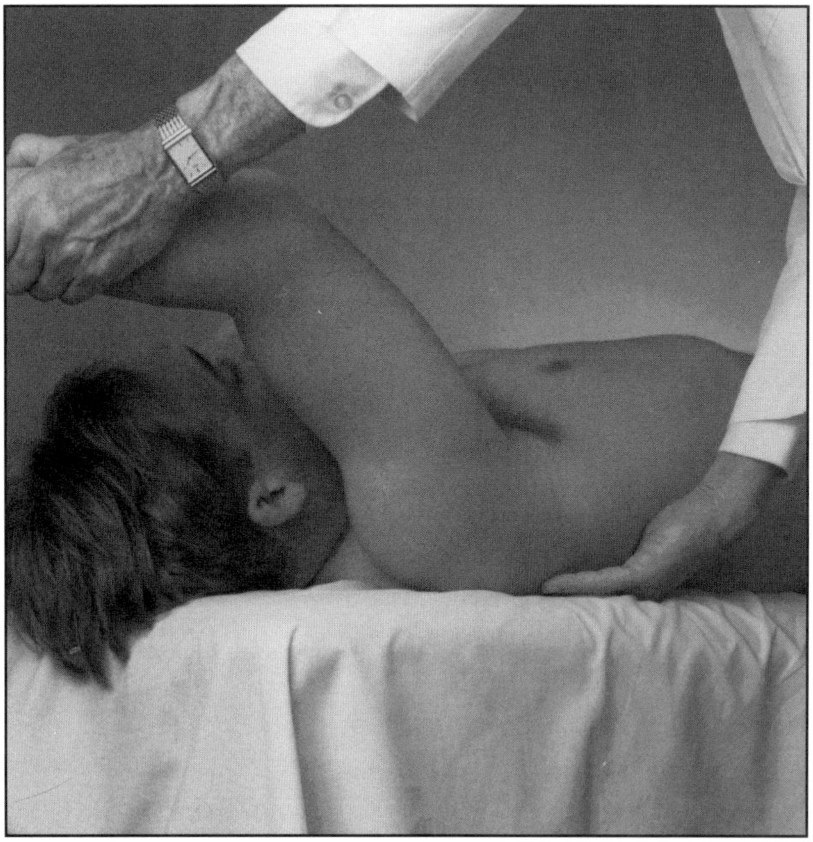

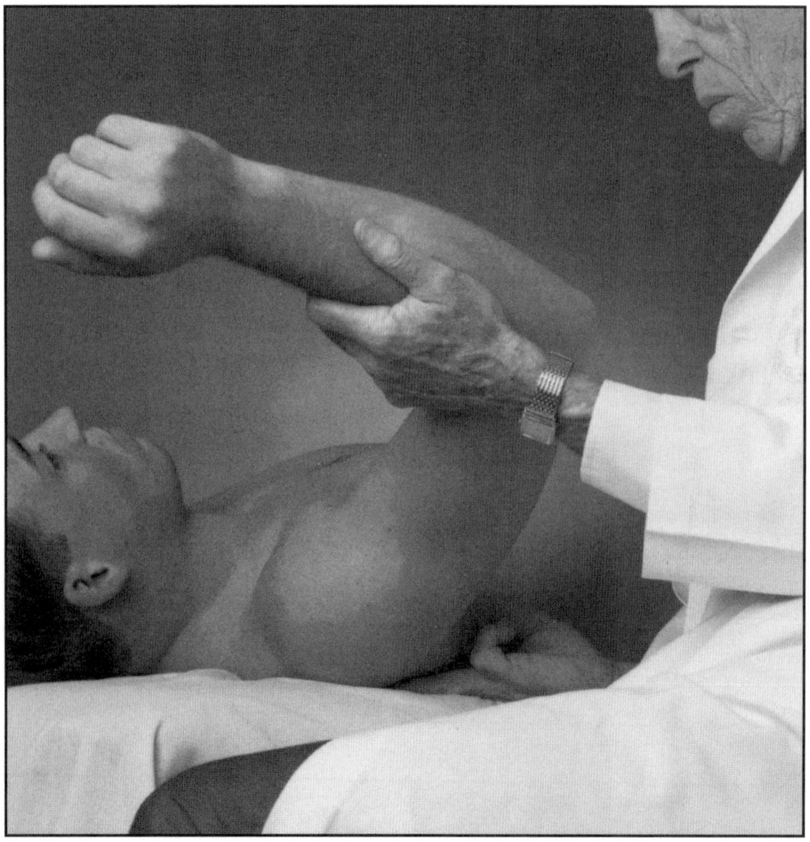

THE INFRASPINATUS MUSCLE

The infraspinatus muscle is fan-shaped so that different parts of it accomplish different things and need different treatments. A very common tenderpoint in it is out one centimenter from the medial margin and down from the spine (of the scapula) two inches. The operator should palpate seated beside the table, using the caudad hand in order to leave the cephalad hand free to place the arm up beside the patient's head. It is relatively easy to feel a tender, tense wisp of the flat muscle over a flat sheet of bone. It is now called the lower infraspinatus. Treatment is passively raising the arm straight forward until it is above the head. Fine tuning is mild adduction or abduction. The upper infraspinatus is found two or three centimenters below the spine and three centimeters more lateral than the lower one. This one is eased with the arm up but now not straight forward but also off to the side more in a 'statue of liberty' position.

THE TERES MINOR

This muscle stays behind for its insertion, arising from the posterior surface of the lateral edge of the scapula and inserting on the back of the greater tuberosity. To shorten and ease it, we need the humerus a little forward and outward with fairly marked external rotation. Patient can be supine or seated. Tenderpoint is on the lateral border of the scapula under the arm or in back of the head of the humerus.

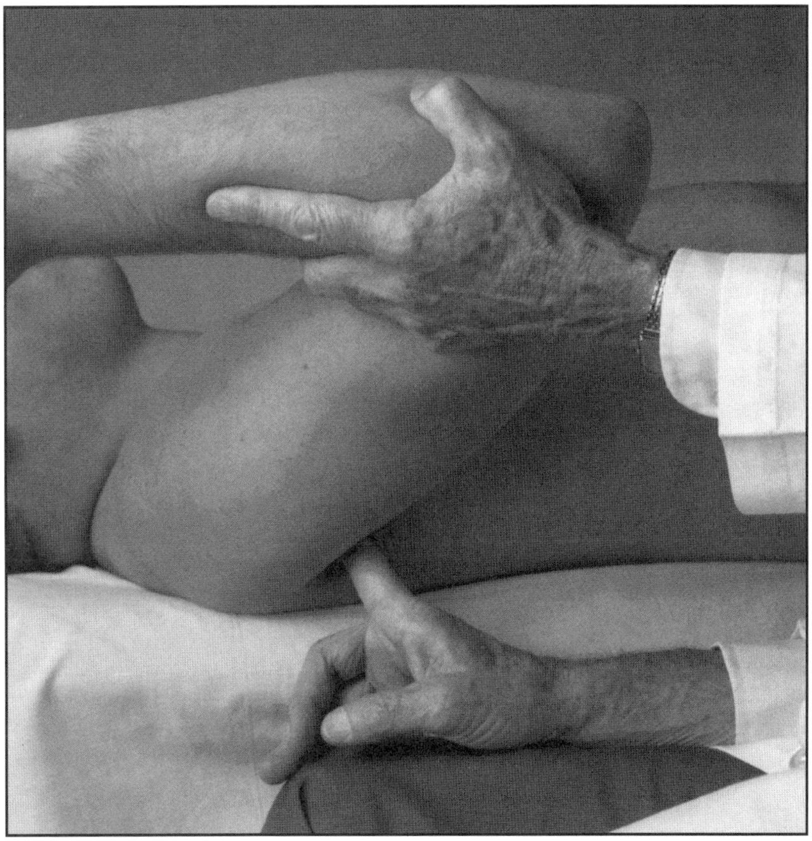

THE SUPRASPINATUS

This muscle is found in the fossa above the spine where it has its origin. From here it runs laterally and over the top of the greater tuberosity of the humerus to its anterior surface. It will ease with a combination of forty-five degree positions; forward, outward in abduction, and forty-five degrees of rotation outward. I sit beside my supine patient and lay his elbow over my shoulder. About the only confusion likely is that at the medial end its tenderpoint might be confused with a tenderpoint for an elevated second rib (which does not move with the shoulder as the supraspinatus does).

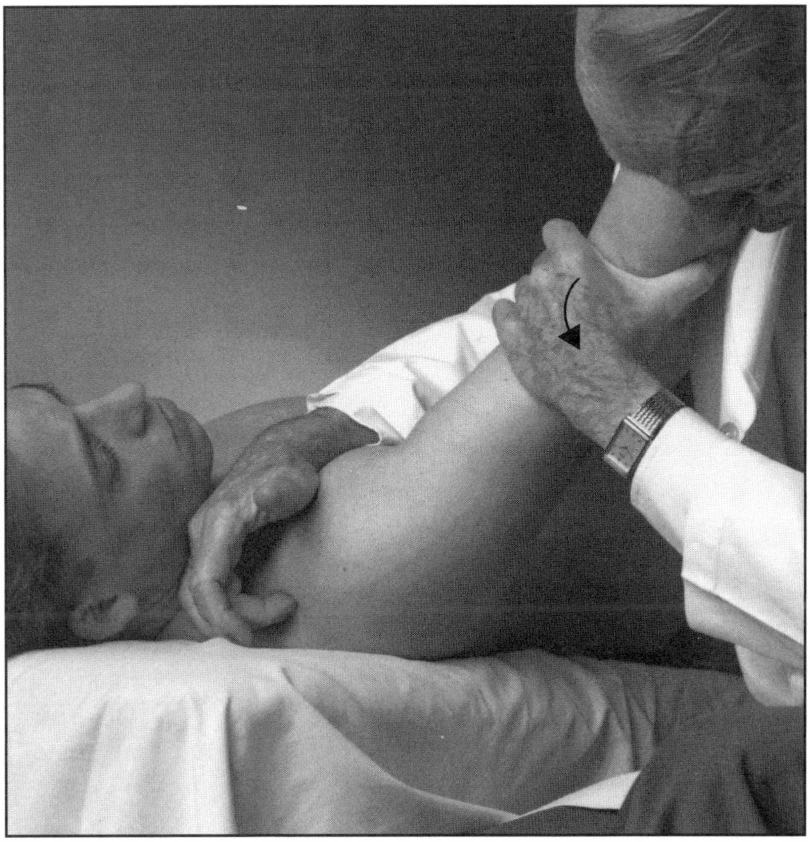

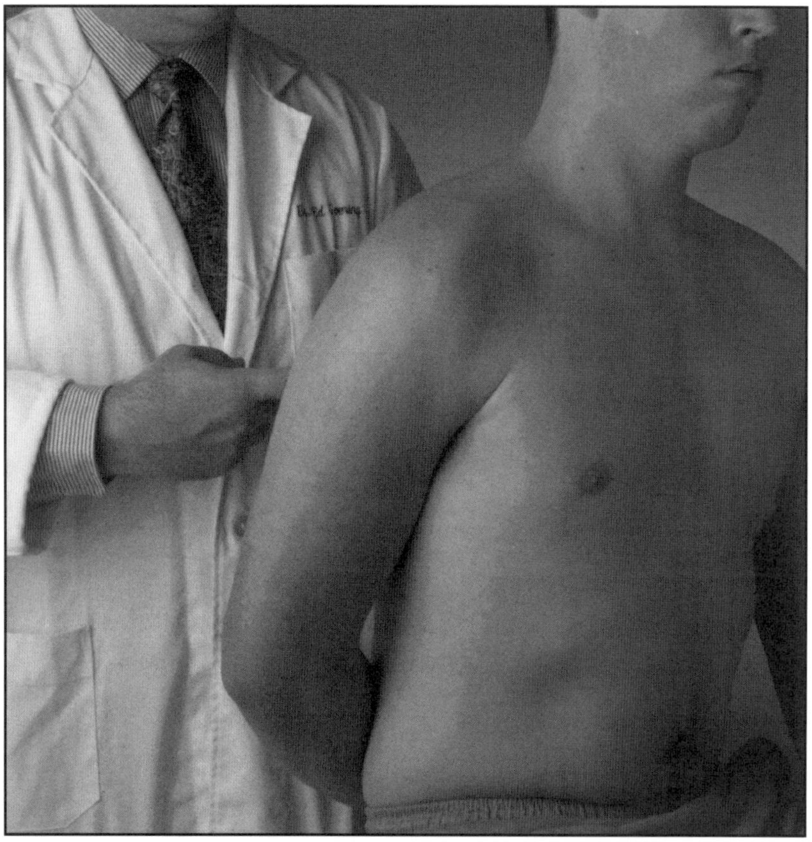

THE TERES MAJOR

The tenderpoint for this muscle starts on its origin at the lower lateral and posterior surface of the scapula, but it passes through the axilla to attach to the front of the upper humerus. Rotation is reversed from that of the minor, being a modified hammer-lock. The bent elbow is pulled back with the forearm also pulled back to produce marked internal rotation of the humerus. A little lift of the shoulder by a mild force up through the shaft of the humerus helps.

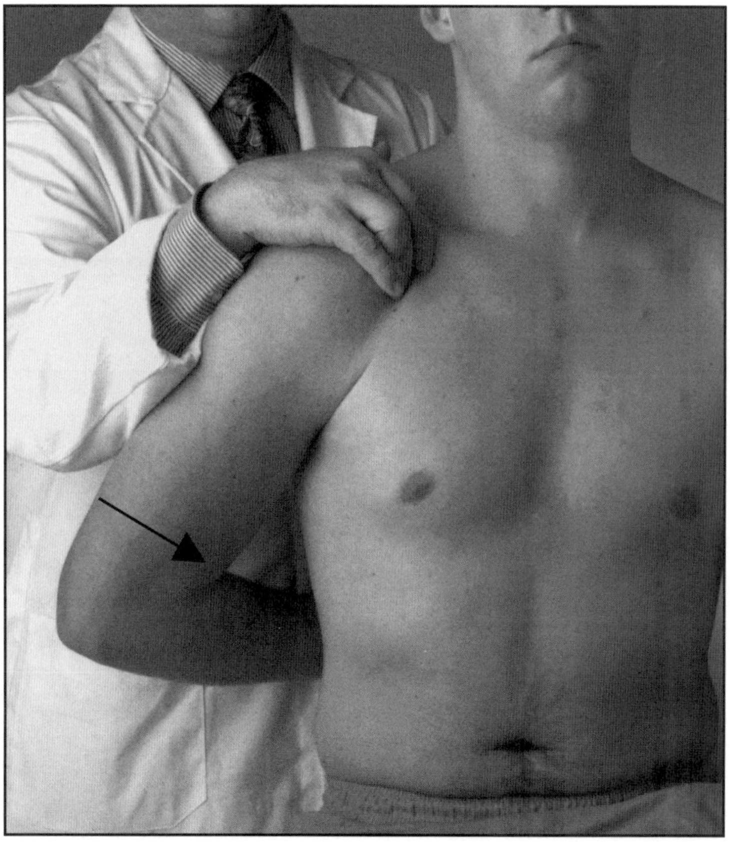

THE MEDIAL CORACOID

This superior medial surface of the front of the coracoid process of the scapula is the tenderpoint for one shoulder problem. It is found close up under the clavicle about two inches medial to the lateral end of the clavicle. According to my knowledge of this part of anatomy, the only muscle which might be involved would be the pectoralis minor, but I have trouble reasoning out any explanation for the treatment, which starts much like that for the teres major. Then the rotation is maintained, but the elbow is pushed forward. If you want to visualize this area, avoid looking at a skeleton. I have never seen one where the coracoid process is within less than a centimeter from the lower surface of the clavicle. Usually they show it to be down about an inch and a half. On a live one you can't insert a finger tip between them.

SUBSCAPULARIS AND LATISSIMUS DORSI

The former is the one I am interested in, but they are treated together. To find the subscapularis press fingers against the side of the chest and move them back and up till you strike something. That is the scapula and its subscapularis. It and the latissimus dorsi cross the axilla from back to front to insert on the front of the humerus. To relieve them the supine patient moves to the edge of the table and lets his arm hang down. The physician applies fairly strong internal rotation. I am less sure of the latissimus, but I suspect a spot on the front of the humerus a little medial to center might be its tender tendon. Both benefit from the internal rotation. The latissimus also likes traction.

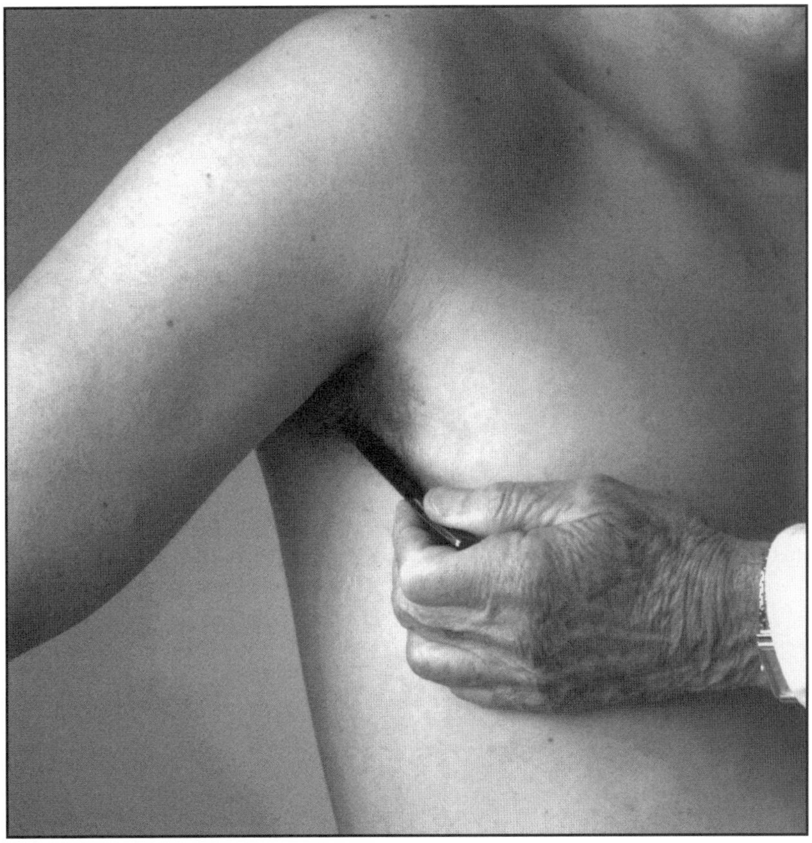

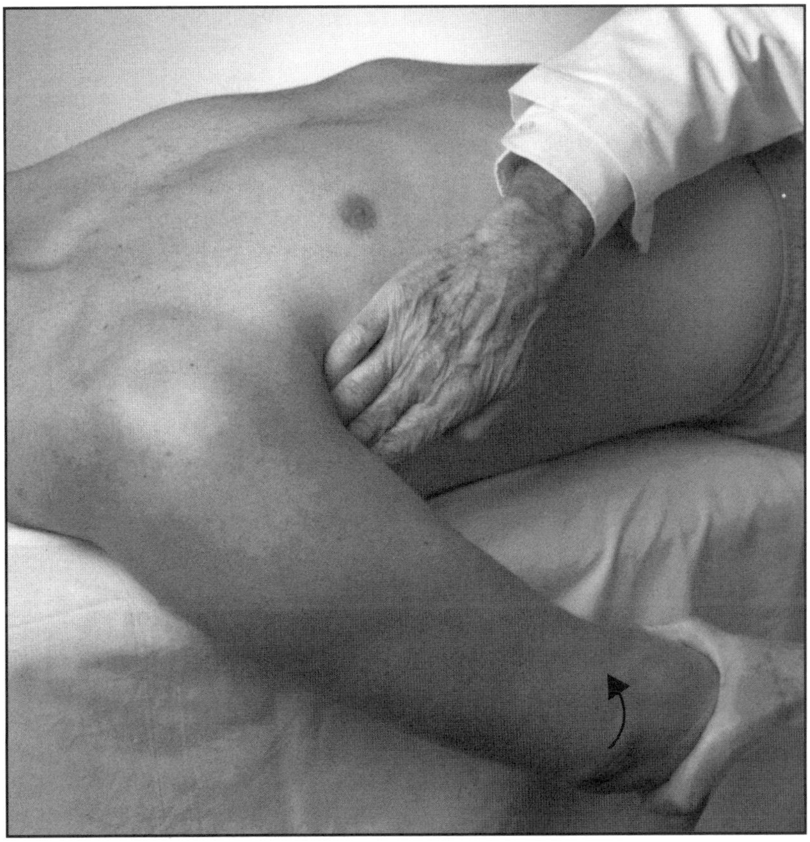

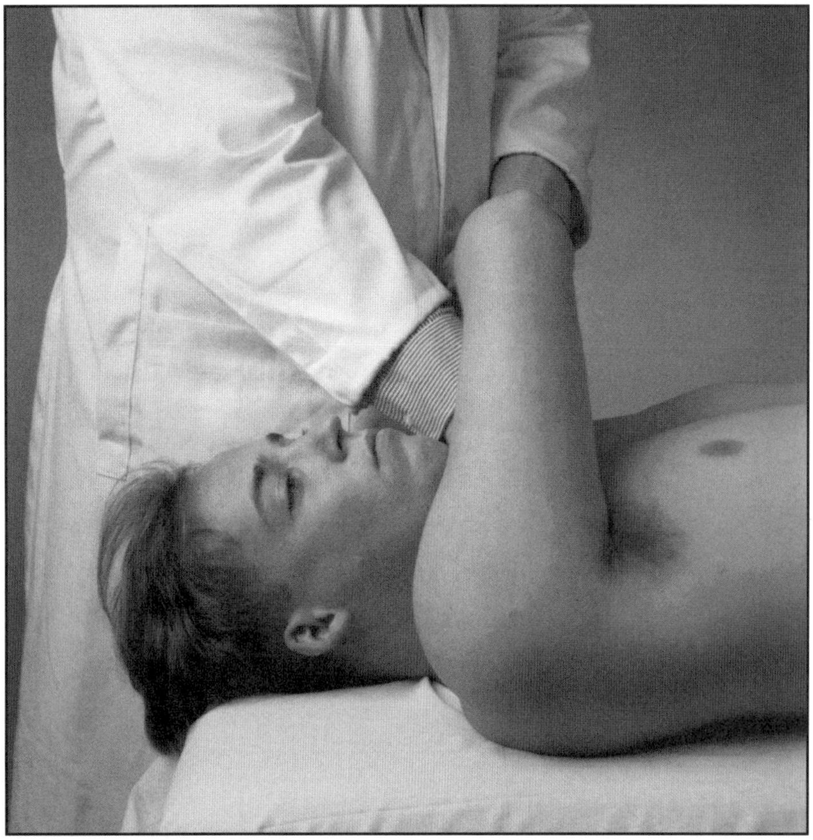

THE HEADS OF THE BICEPS MUSCLE

These have tenderpoints on the long head, *bottom photo,* in the bicipital groove, or the inferolateral surface of the coracoid process (short head), *top photo,* near their sites of origin. Relieved (long head) with wrist lying over the forehead of a supine patient. The short head needs more adduction of the humerus across the chest.

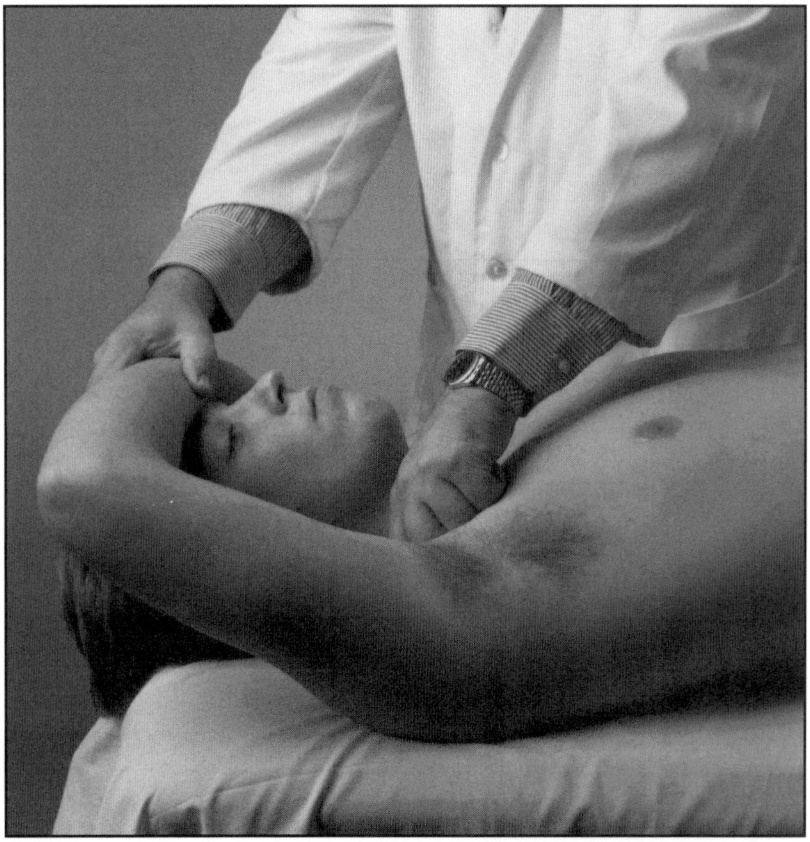

SUB DELTOID BURSA

It was not common in my opinion, but it had great publicity where I practiced. It was blamed for most shoulder problems, and the site for steroid injections (which sometimes worked). The tenderpoint is high on the anterolateral part of the humerus. To feel it the humerus must be brought forward enough to relax this portion of the deltoid. If at this time it is found to be tender, simply raising the humerus a little further will ease it.

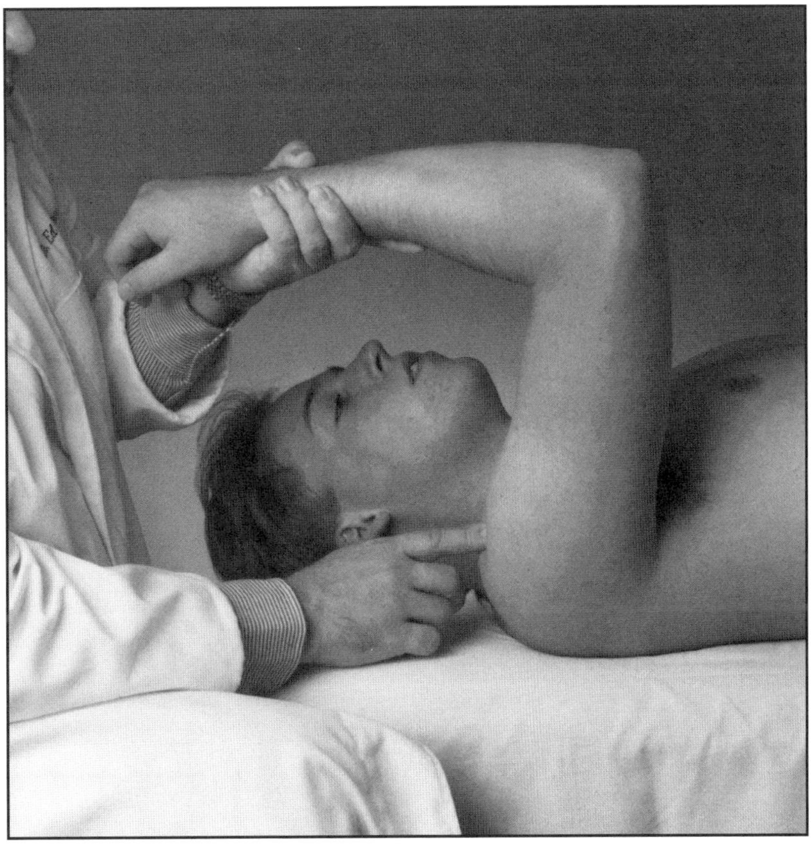

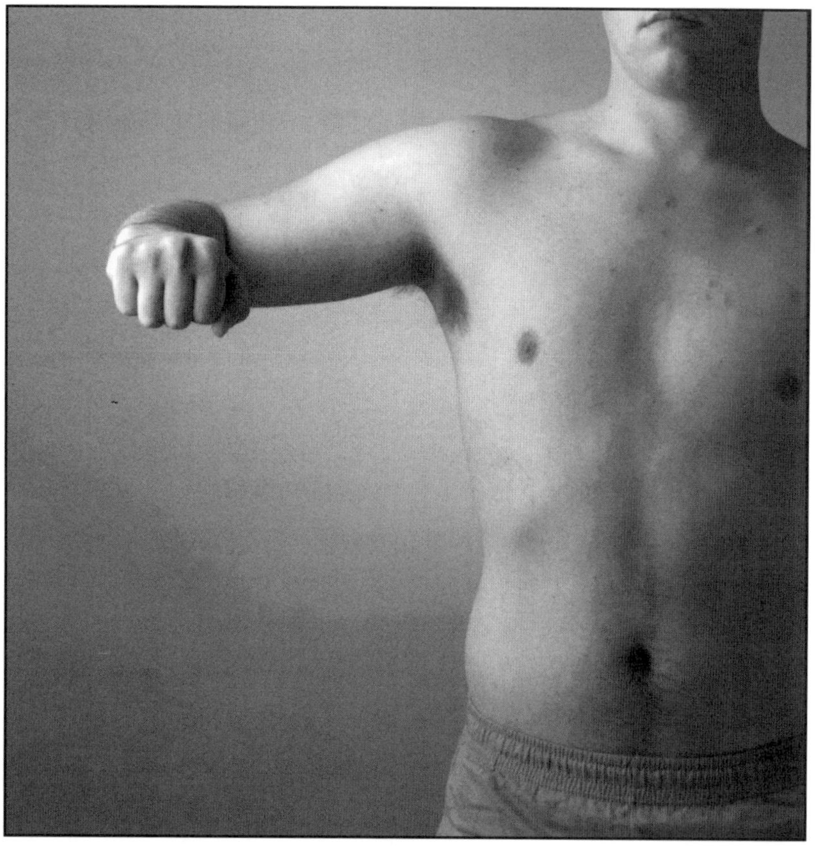

TWO NON-SHOULDER PROBLEMS

These can make the shoulder painful and stiff, but shoulder structures seem not to be involved.

Second Rib Depressed—This one is diagnosed by the complaint characteristic of this problem. The patient stands and shows the action which hurts; straight abduction. This is a result of a depressed second rib. Abduction of the humerus lifts it against its better judgement. Typical depressed rib treatment is effective.

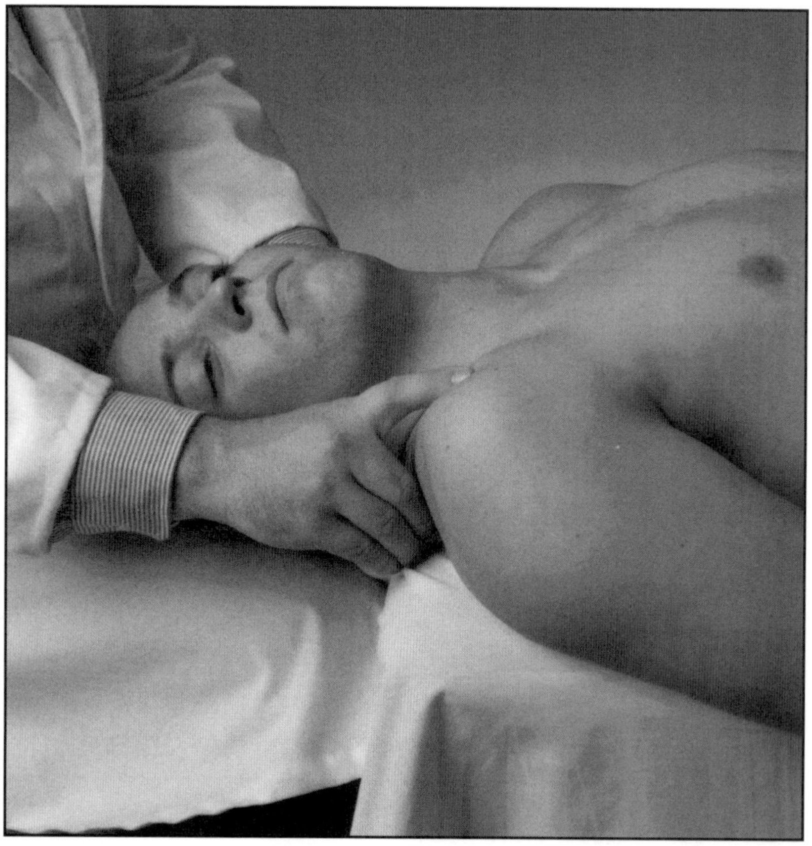

Lateral Coracoid Process—The other was even more confusing to me. The tenderpoint is on the supero-lateral part of the coracoid process of the scapula. Nothing I did to the shoulder influenced it, but it ceased when I suspended the head and neck of the supine patient off the end of the table, extended the neck, sidebent it away from the tender side and rotated toward or away from it.

FROZEN SHOULDER

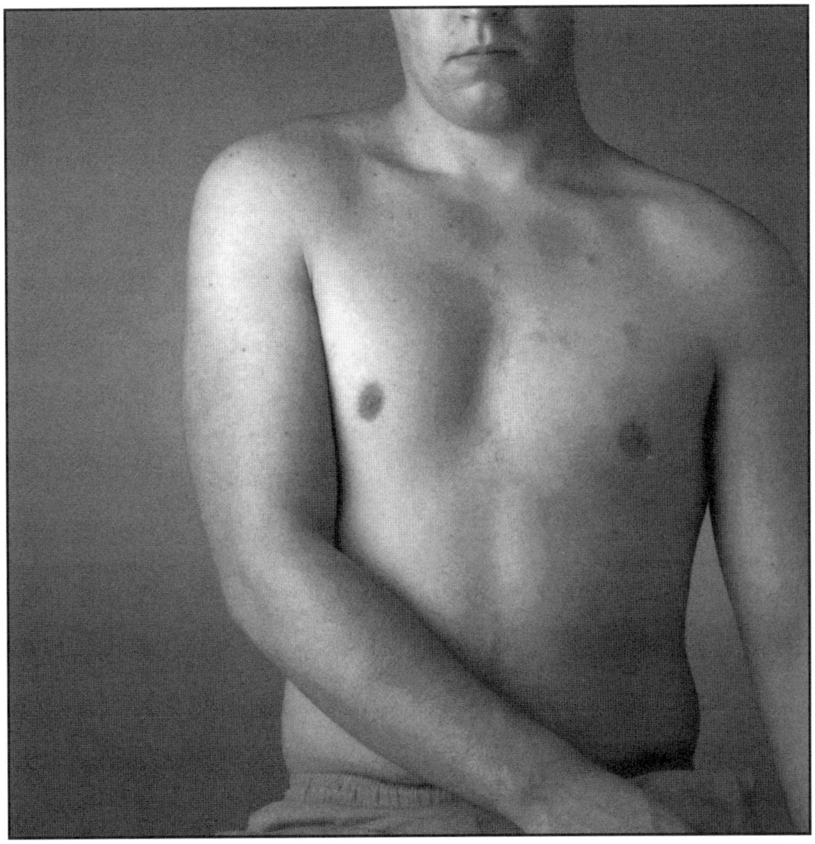

Top photo shows frozen shoulder posture. Pulling down aggravates a frosted shoulder. (A frosted shoulder is just a mild frozen shoulder.)

This very painful condition when severe can be diagnosed many yards away. The patient clutches his arm as close to his chest as possible and can't bear to have it abducted. He would like to adduct more but his chest is in the way. He can be hyperadducted by a device which makes use of the remarkable ability of the scapula to rotate outward. To accomplish this, the elbow is left compressed against the side of the chest. Force is applied on the elbow directly up the shaft of the humerus, pushing the shoulder high. This raises the shoulder and rotates the scapula outward. The outward rotation serves to produce the needed hyperadduction of the humeral joint. This is about the only move that is not painful. The patient can learn to sit by a low table and place his elbow on it. Then by lowering his trunk he can force his shoulder into the position. There is a milder form of this that is not so obvious. It can easily be diagnosed by pain from pulling down on the humerus.

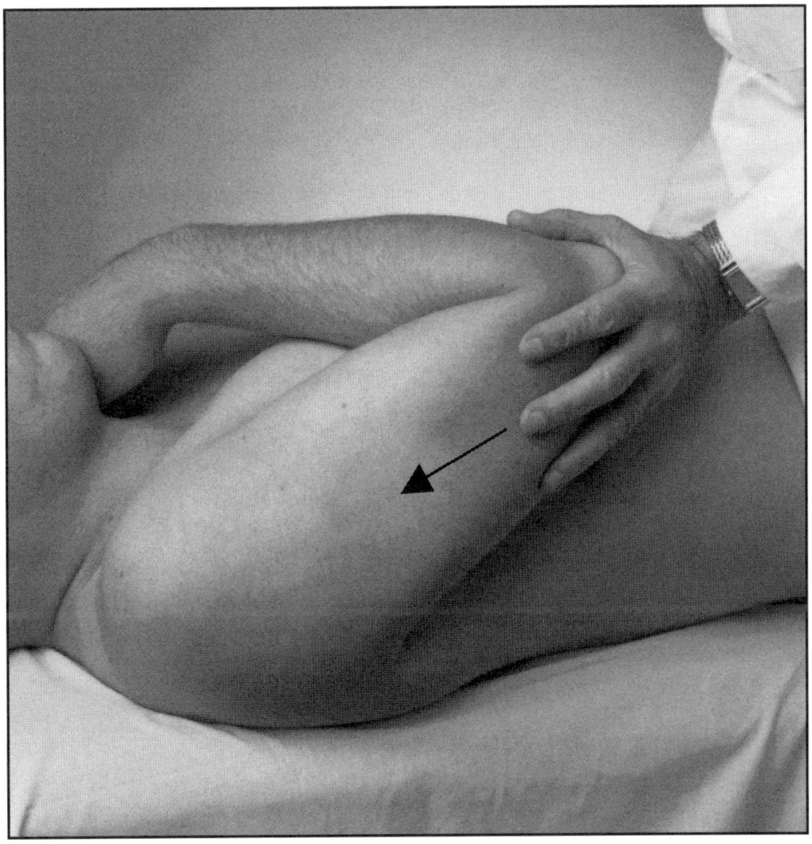

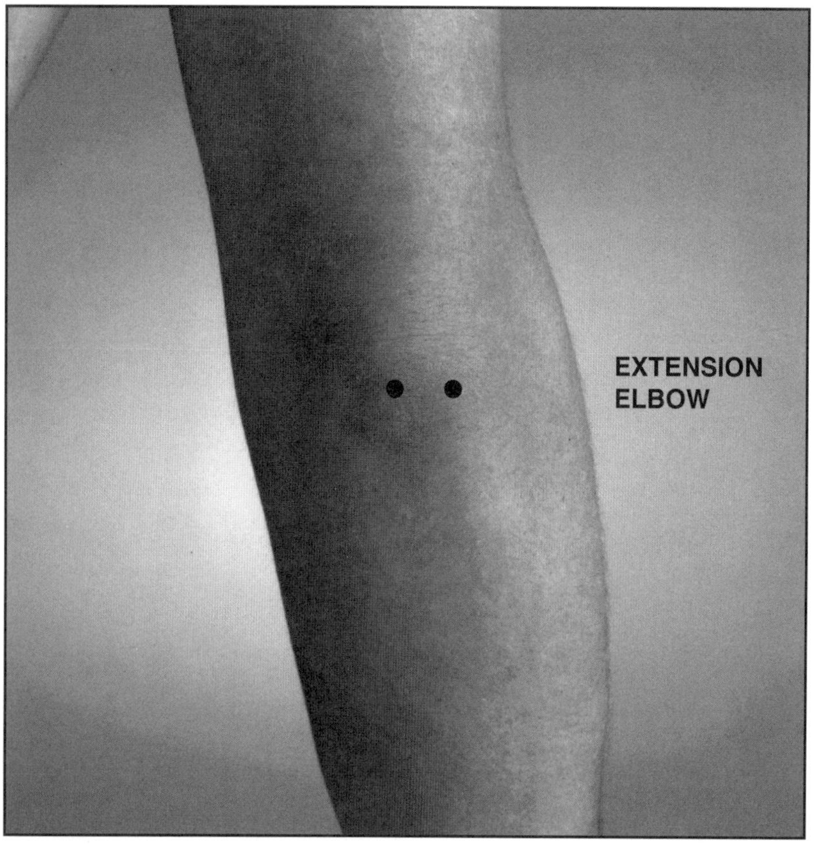

The Elbow

This remarkable joint, capable of combining a bending and rotary ability both in the amount of about 180 degrees seems to offer relatively little trouble for a joint so sophisticated and apparently vulnerable.

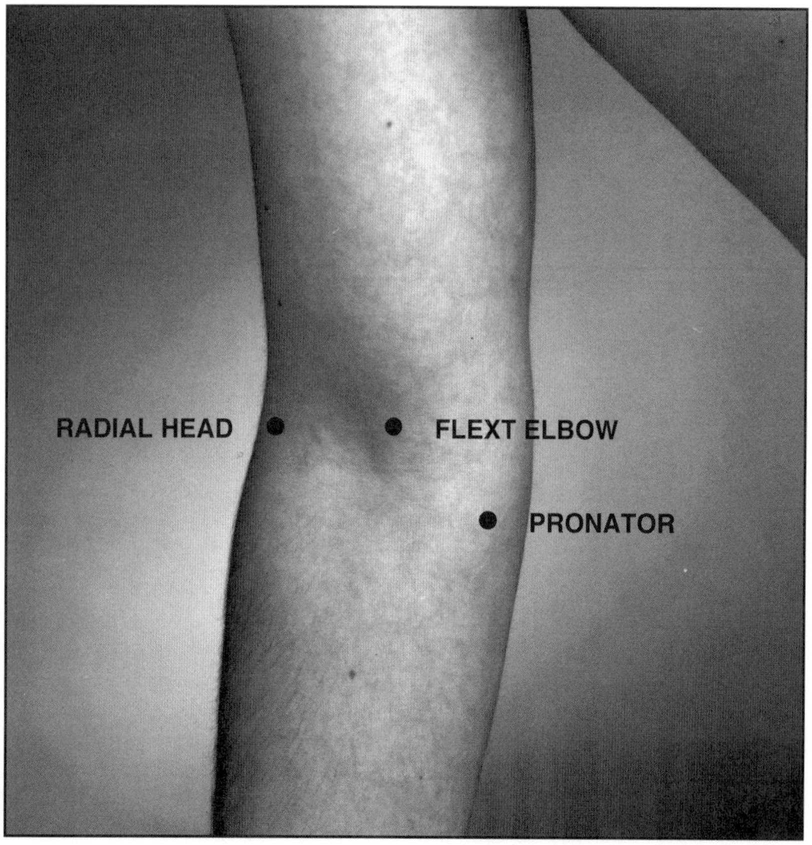

THE RADIAL HEAD

This dysfunction is the most important one of the elbow. After searching and working alone I finally began to realize that the problem I called radial head was the same as the one the orthopedic surgeons called epycondylitis. I found the tip of the epicondyle to be as tender as the radial head, and they found the opposite. The anterior lateral part of the head of the radius is sharply tender. Treatment is full extension of the elbow, but not hyperextension, fairly marked supination. Fine tune with abduction or adduction.

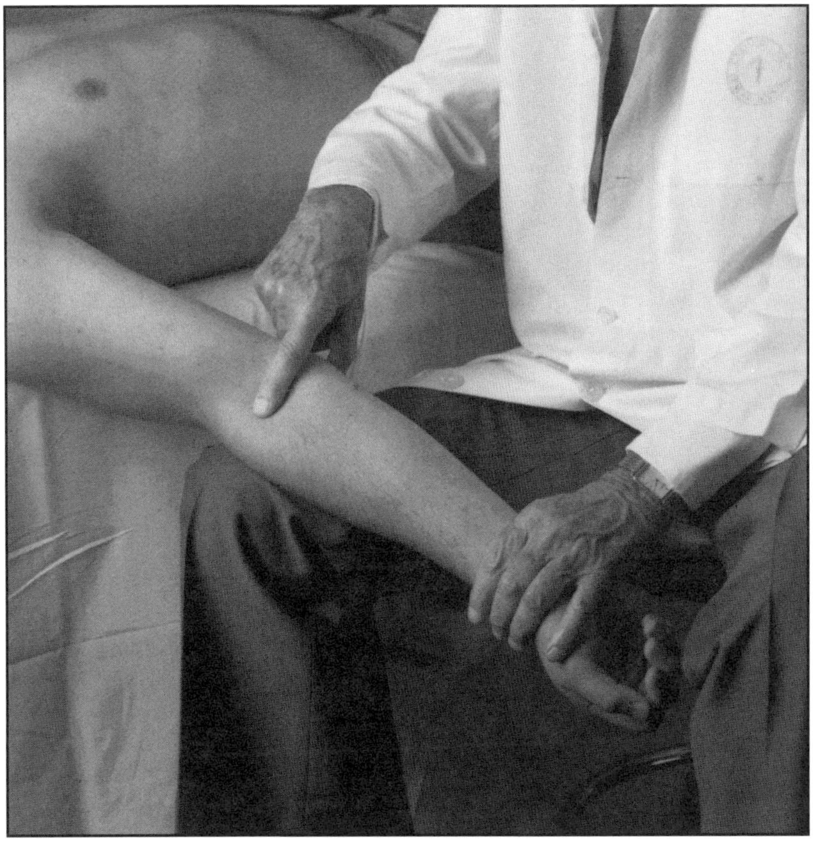

PRONATOR

Tenderness for this is on the medial part of the front of the elbow from the epicondyle forward nearly to the anticubital fossa. Relief comes with flexion to ninety degrees turning the forearm in to place back of the hand against the chest (picture fails to show this), about ninety degrees, and pronation of the wrist.

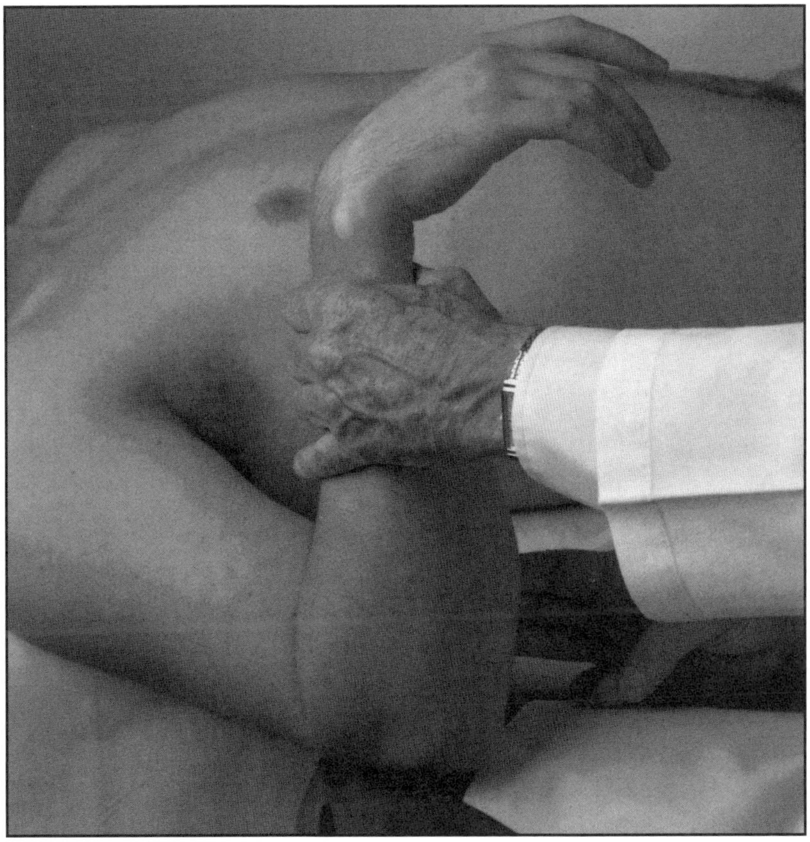

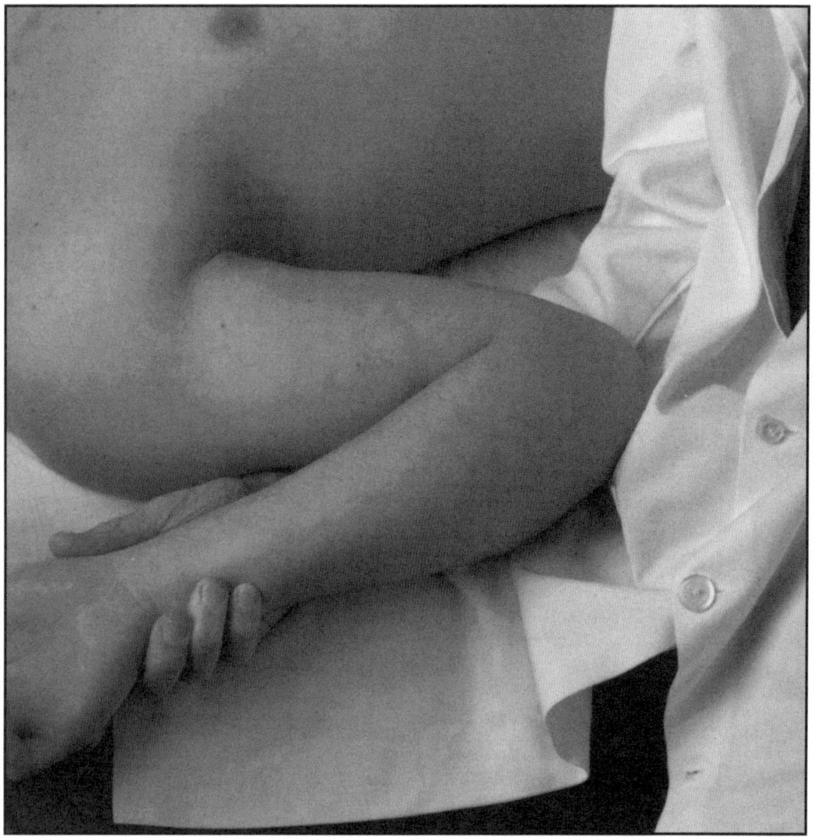

FLEXION ELBOW

This is not nearly so common. Tenderness is on the coronoid process of the ulna. If severe, the patient comes in with elbow flexed. Treatment is marked flexion usually with the forearm pulled a little out to the side and with the palm forward. In full flexion there is no room for your palpating finger tip. Treat it and straighten enough to feel it. Most will ease.

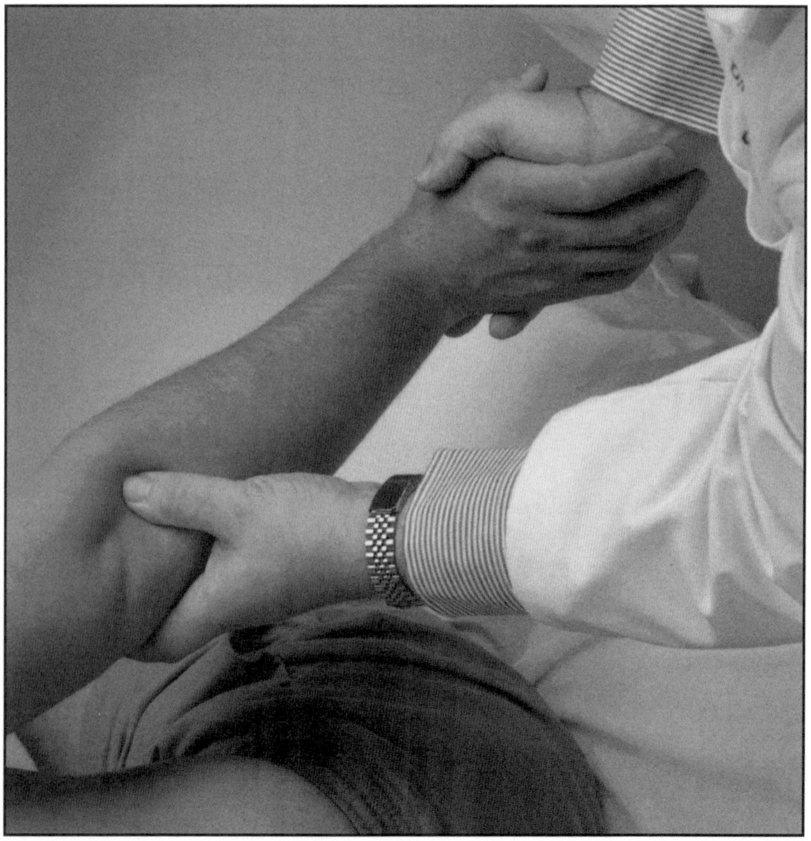

EXTENSION ELBOW

Pain and weakness are reported in the biceps, but the tenderpoint is at the side of the olecranon process of the ulna near a triceps tendon. Treatment is hyperextension of elbow with fine tuning of adduction or abduction.

There are other rare elbow problems. Since movements are gross, it is relatively easy to fumble your way to a successful treatment.

Wrist and Hand

GENERAL

Because there are eight bones in the wrist, I had visions of very complicated manouvers being necessary. I was surprised how easy wrist treatment usually is. I treat it as if it were just one joint and still expect good success. If wrist is tender on the dorsal side, I extend and rotate. If it is on the palmar side, I flex and rotate. Occasionally fine tune with sidebending. There are many with tender spots on the flexor tendons that have been diagnosed carpal tunnel syndrome, which respond to this type of treatment. I can only guess that they had been misdiagnosed. Patients usually can treat themselves, if I show them. Remember most of the wrist bones are in the 'heel' of the hand, not above it. Remember, even though the wrist is the site of pain, be sure to check out the elbow. Often this is the source of wrist pain without any elbow pain.

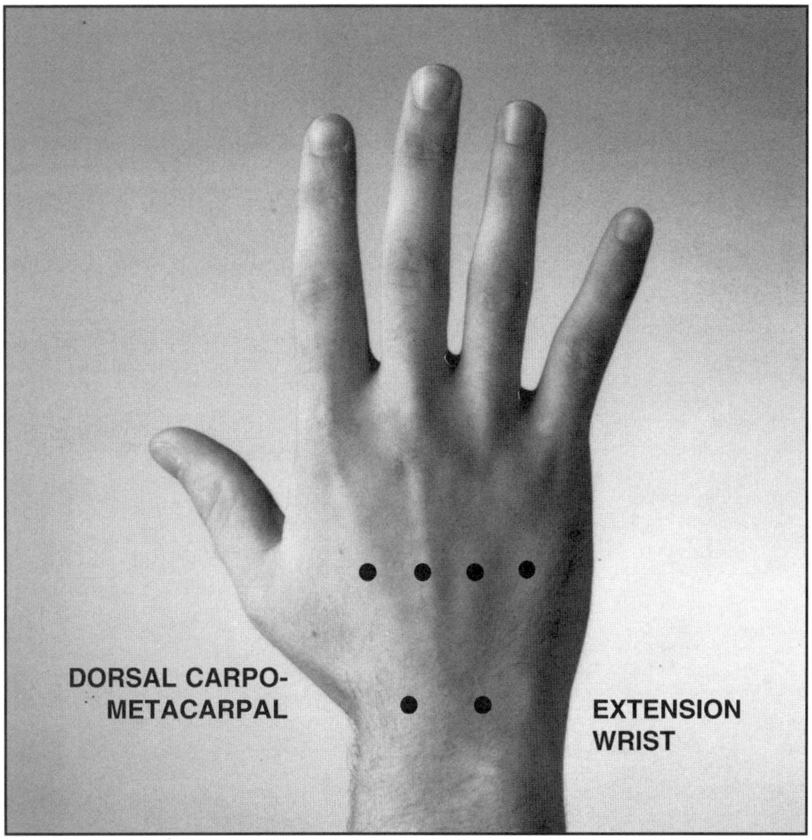

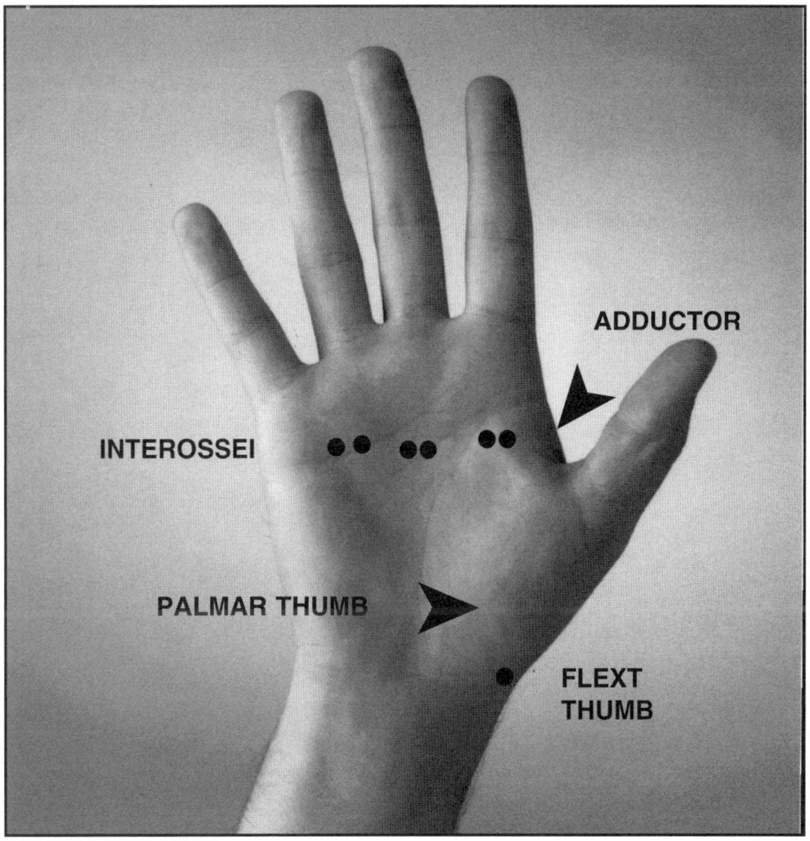

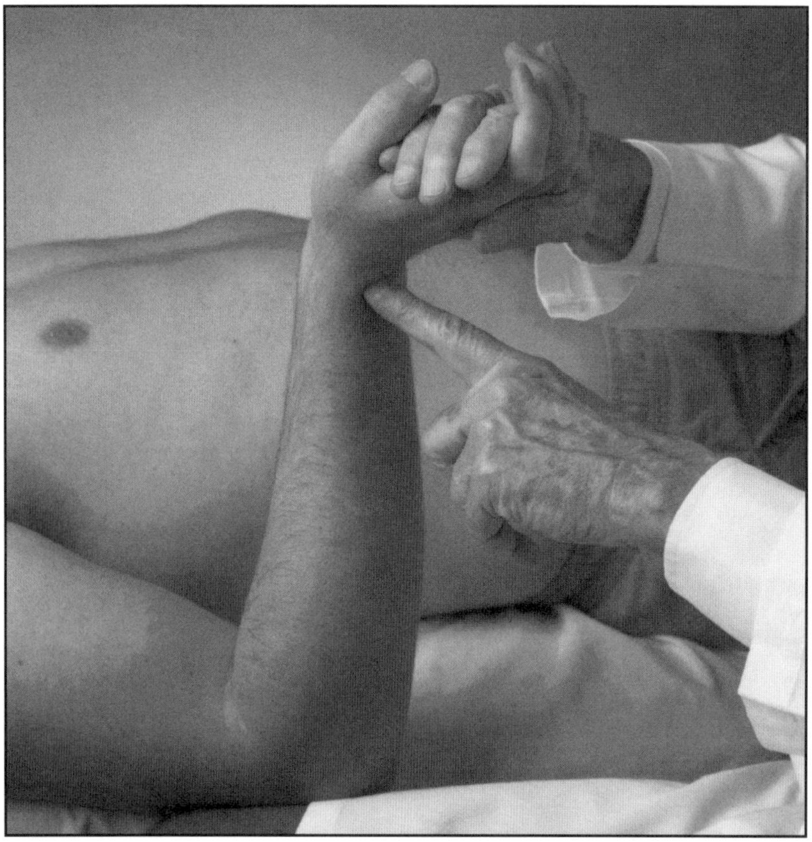

EXTENSION WRIST

The many small bones of the wrist tend to make it appear complicated, but experience shows it to work as one joint except in rare cases. It follows the rule of thumb that tenderness on the dorsal side is relieved by folding the hand over it in extension.

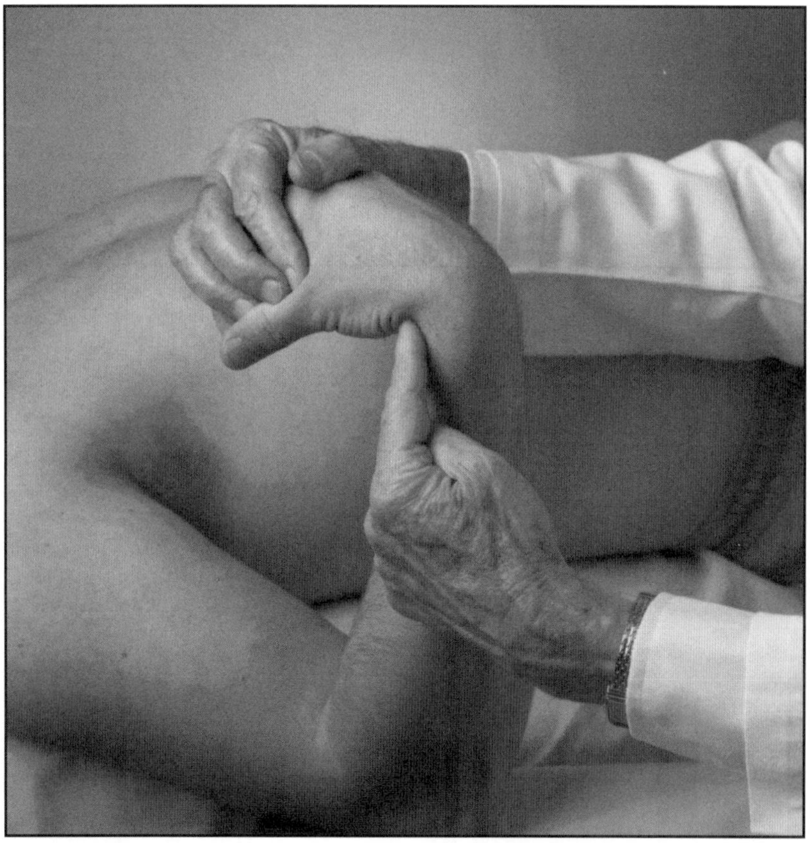

THE THUMB

The most important part of the hand is the apposing thumb. Without a working thumb, fifty per cent of the hand use is lost. Many older women have painful, weak thumbs that they have lived with many years, because they never had any treatment that helped it. It can be relieved and cured. There are three types.

1. Flexion Wrist and Thumb—Tender on the flexor side of the base of the first metacarpal or a little more lateral. Treatment needs flexion of entire wrist with an excess added by mild pressure on the thumb. Fine tune with rotation of the wrist. This is very common.

2. Palmar Thumb—Tender in palm pushing deep in the palmar side of the head of the first metacarpal, probing from the opposite side of the hand on the medial side of the first carpo-metacarpal joint. This is relieved by pulling the thumb across the palm and internally rotating it. Like many other hand problems, the patient can be taught to treat herself.

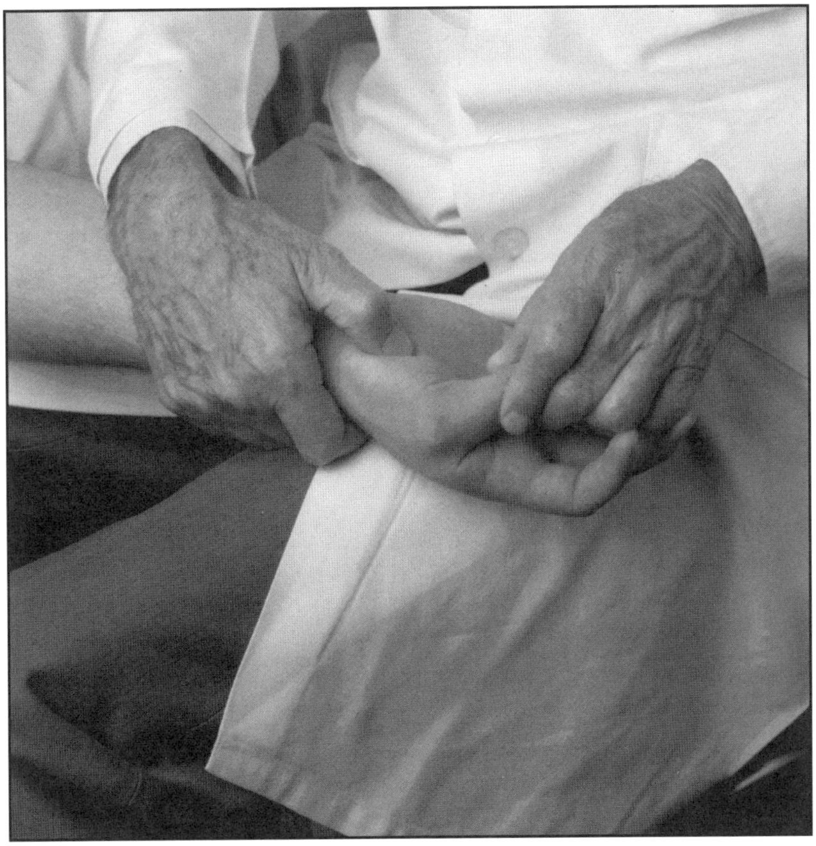

3. Adductor Pollicis—This is uncommon. Thumb is pushed between index and third fingers of the hand and compressed by doctor's hand. Tenderpoint is in the web. There was a recent fad for treating headaches by stimulating this, but I just used it for the thumb.

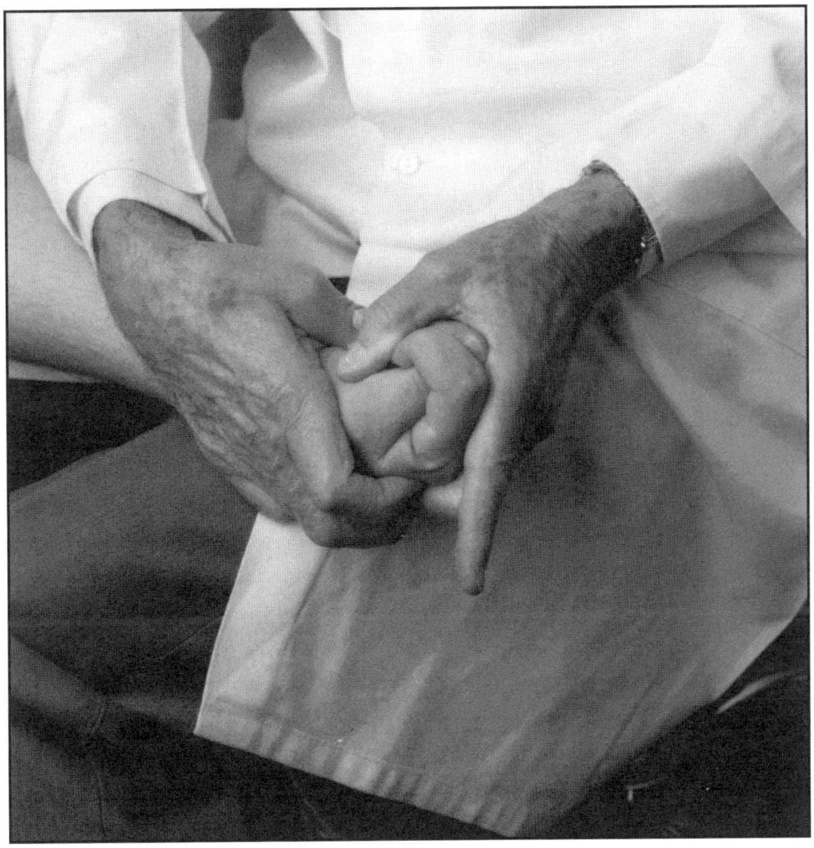

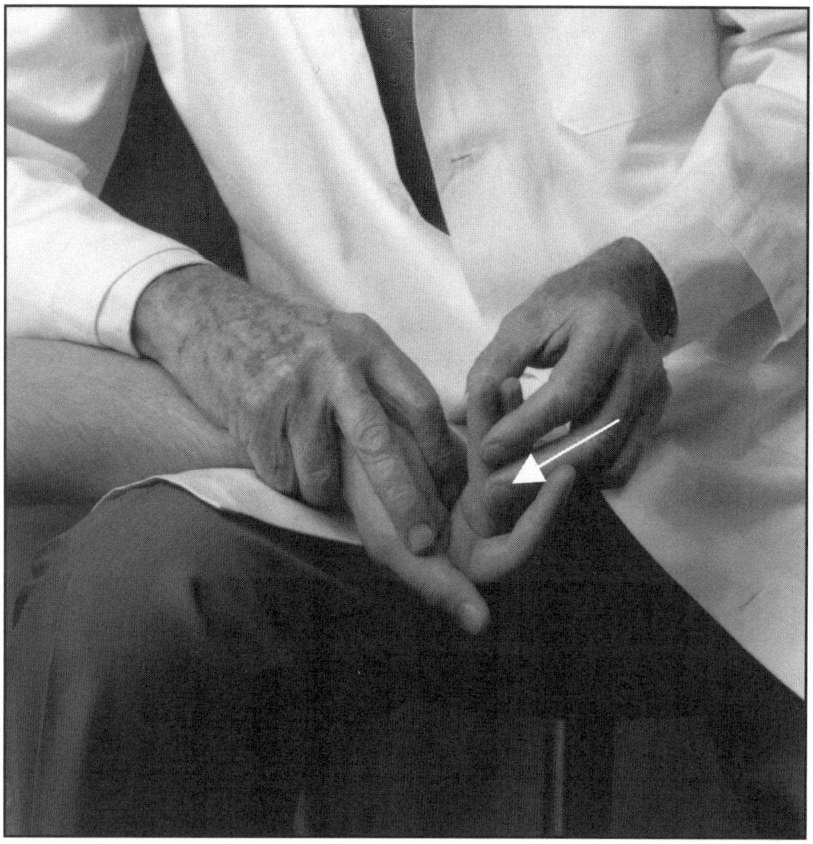

FINGERS THAT LOCK IN FLEXION

These especially affect the index or third finger. They hang-up in flexion at the first interphalangeal joint, but the treatment is forced flexion of the metacarpo-phalangeal joint with the finger pulled slightly laterally toward the tender side of the metacarpal bone. Tenderpoint is in the palm on one interossius muscle of the affected finger.

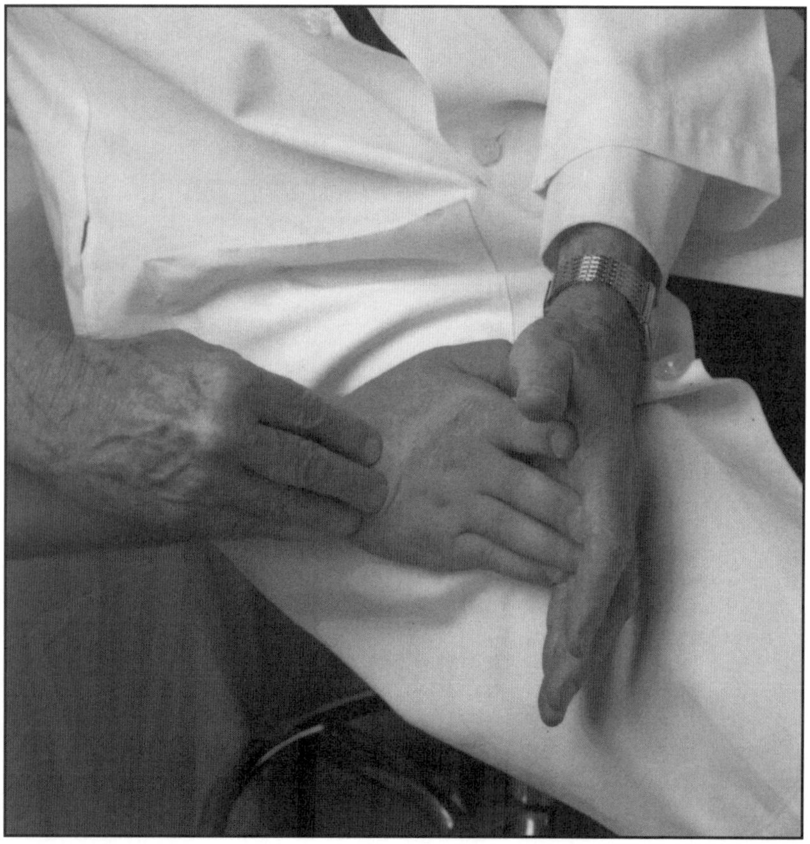

DORSAL CARPO-METACARPAL AND METACARPO PHALANGEAL

Complaint is loss of gripping strength: "I can't lift my suitcase." Again the tenderpoint is on the opposite side of the supposedly weak muscles of the hand, usually heads of the metacarpal bones in the back of the hand.

Treatment is extension of the fingers and wrist. Strength returns before they leave.

DUPUYTRON'S CONTRACTURE

I have been assured this cannot be as labeled. It is a hard, chronic, fibrous feeling contraction of almost all the palmar muscles, disfiguring the hand. I didn't have much hope for the first one. It didn't seem any better after my treatment of forced flexion, but the patient returned three days later with a nearly normal hand. I was more astonished than he. I have only seen one other, but results were equally good.

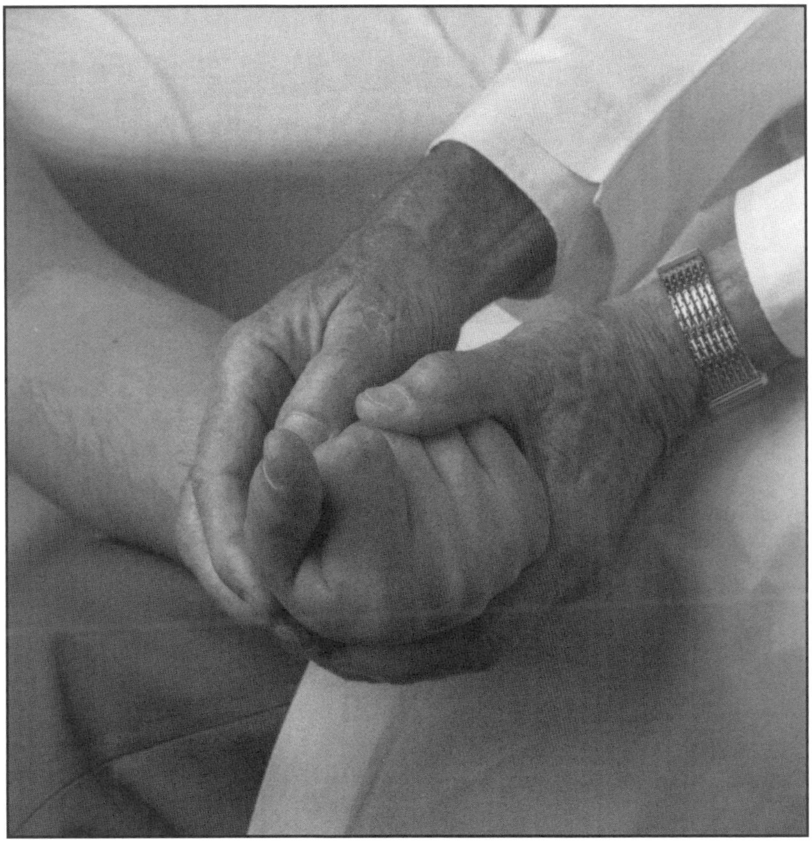

CRANIO-FACIAL DYSFUNCTIONS

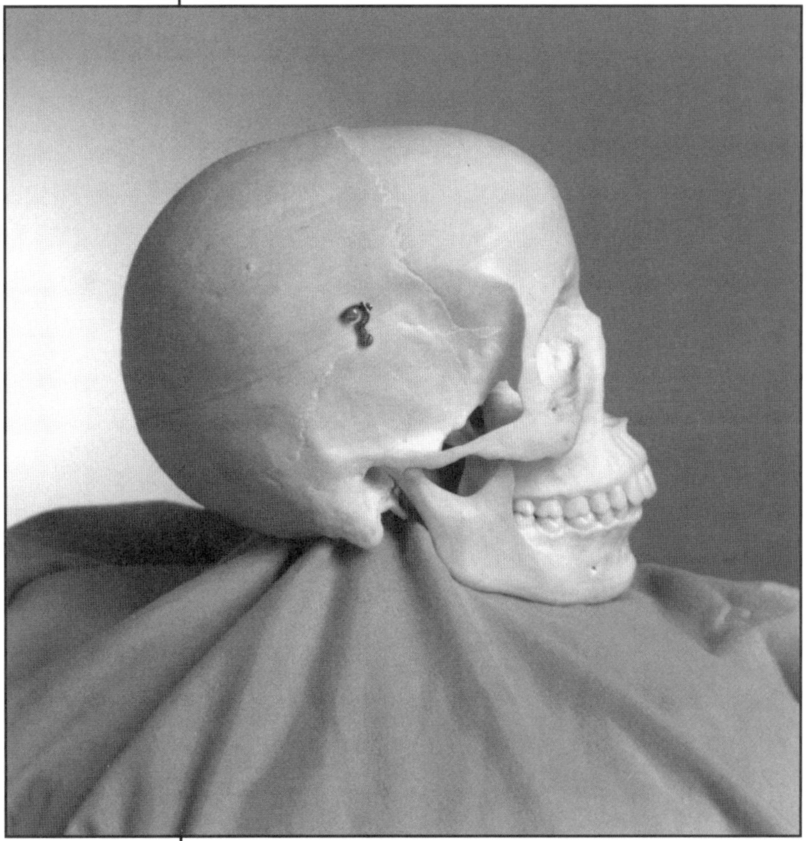

GENERAL

Treatment of the cranium had been developed by an enterprising physician, William Garner Sutherland, DO. He advanced the ideas of the movement in the skull, then believed to be immovable, and a distinct respiratory mechanism of the cerebrospinal fluid. As well as I understand his methods, he aided and balanced this cranial respiratory function by using very subtle forces, with much benefit to the head. Many of his faithful followers are highly skilled cranio-sacral manipulators who have done some wonderful things for heads. Realizing that it would take me years to develop the highly sophisticated skills of the Sutherland cranial treatment, not to mention trying to teach it in my book, I started with the idea that, if counterstrain is a valid approach to the rest of the body, it should be valid for the skull too.

Sutherland used indirect treatment. In other words an indirect treatment is one which moved parts in the way they moved easily to release them so they could also move easily in the opposite direction too. Counterstrain uses indirect treatment too. By using the same body responses that had kept me doing the right things on the rest of the body, I could safely treat something I knew as little about as the skull. I didn't have to understand what the skull needed; the skull, itself, knew and could tell me. If the patient understands that the physician is depending on him to say what feels good and what hurts, he can insure that everything that is done is beneficial. He can start easing the skull's dysfunctions the first day.

After thirty some years of practice, I make no claim to knowing all the changes I make in a skull with any treatment. The body tells me so well that I can with confidence use stronger forces than Sutherland practitioners use. The cranio-facial dysfunctions have seemed especially important to me, because the cranium contains the brain, the thalamus, and the pituitary gland, and could be expected to have important influences on them. Some of the Sutherland practitioners in their zeal have come to regard the cranial treatment as all important to the point of neglecting treatment of the rest of the body. To me it is just another part of the body I hope to keep functioning well.

Like any other part of the body the skull presents tenderpoints which help me to know about what to do. Some of the terms I use I borrowed from the Sutherland practitioners, because they seem to explain what I think I am doing.

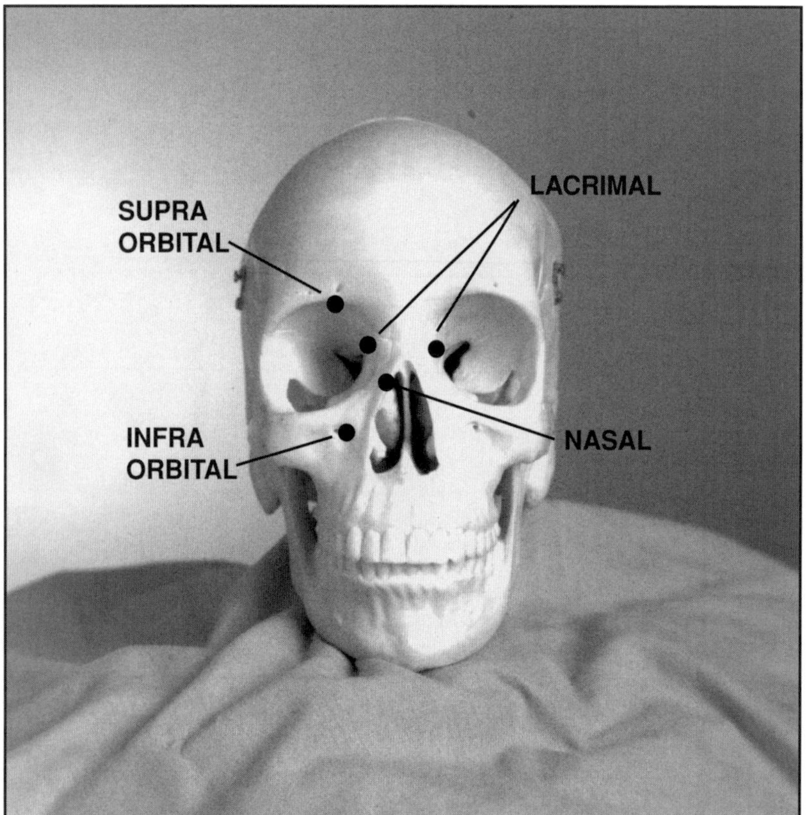

THE OCCIPITAL BONE

If we consider the cranium to be another structural appendage of the body, it is reasonable to proceed first from its most proximal part, the occipital bone, as it articulates with the top of the neck.

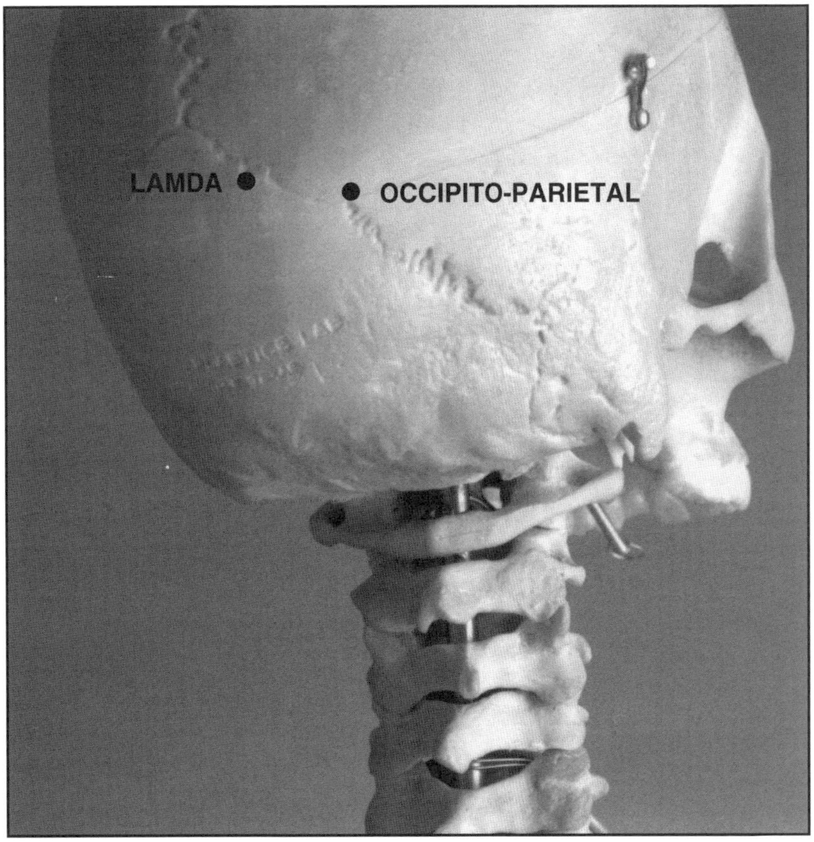

LATERAL SKULL

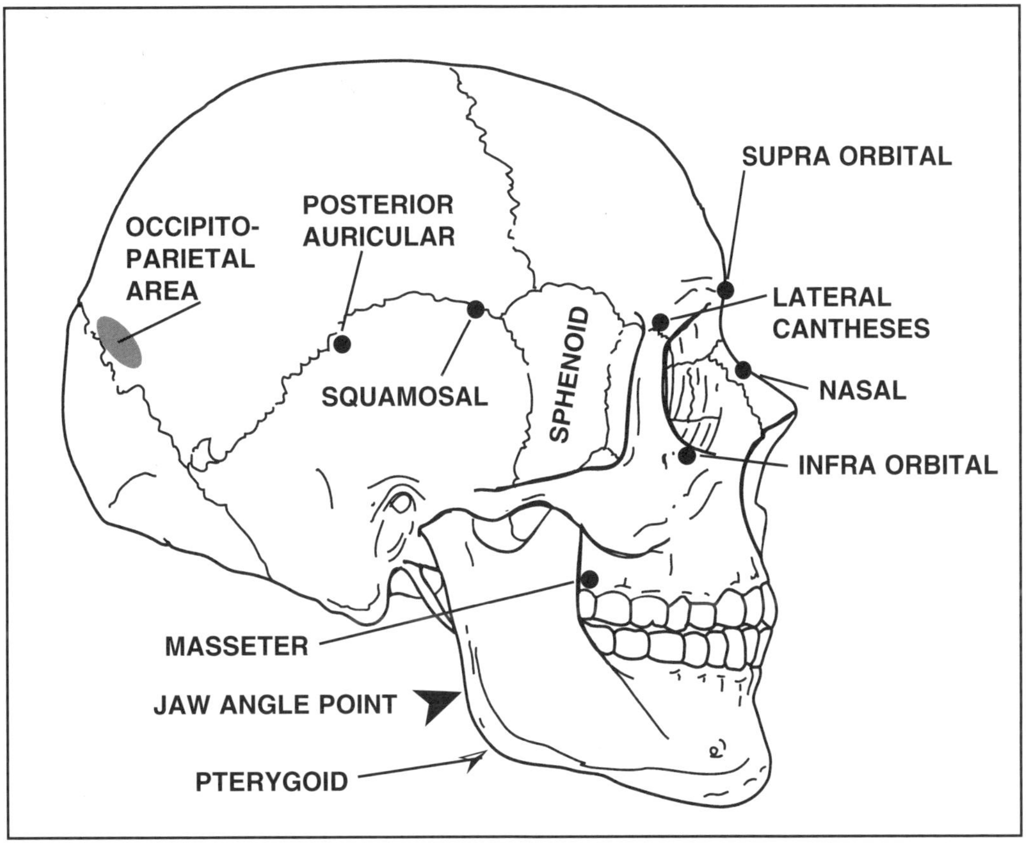

SPHENOBASILAR TORSION

Perhaps the most important union with another key bone seems to be subject to torsion. The inion is our landmark. Three centimeters lateral usually on the right may be a tenderpoint. One hand grasps the whole occiput; the other grasps the front of the head including the cheek bones and twists the occiput up on the tender side and the face down on that side. In addition to this pull, the front end is slightly side bent away over a vertical axis. If it is right, it feels good to the patient. Motion felt here is minimal, but as increasing torsion force is applied, the skull shows a lull in its resistance to resume again immediately. This lull I interpret as a point of mobility.

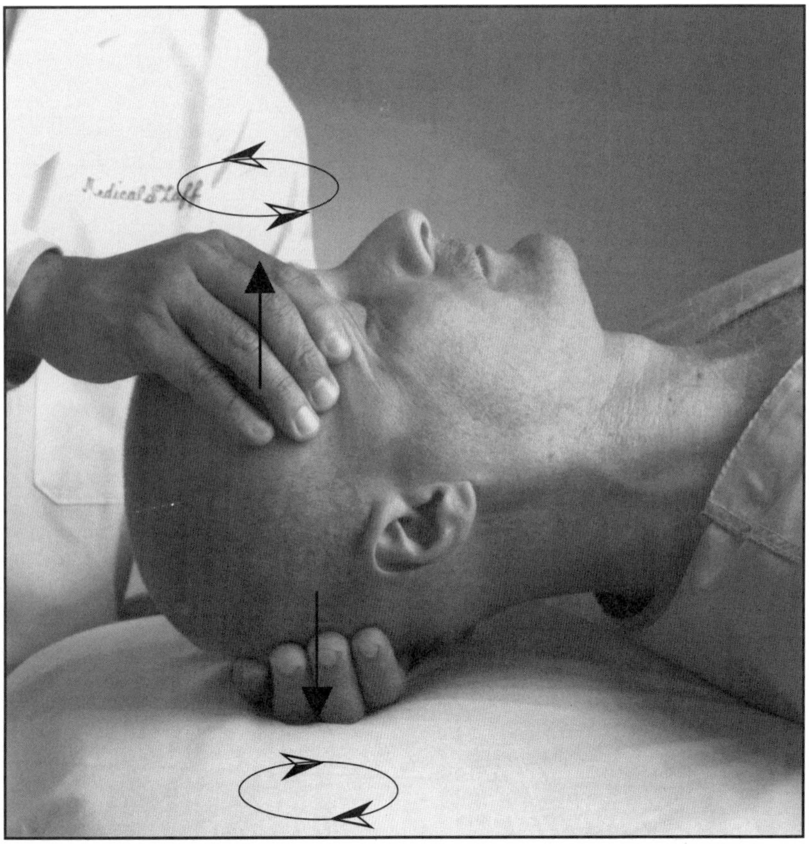

LATERAL STRAIN

This imagines a sideward shearing strain between the basilar part of the occiput and the back of the sphenoid bone. This is one of the few for which I have found no tenderpoint. Treatment is pressure on one side of the frontal and cheek bones and the opposite side of the occiput. It is then repeated using opposite sides. If there is no good or bad feeling, we assume there is no strain. If one way feels good, treat it that way.

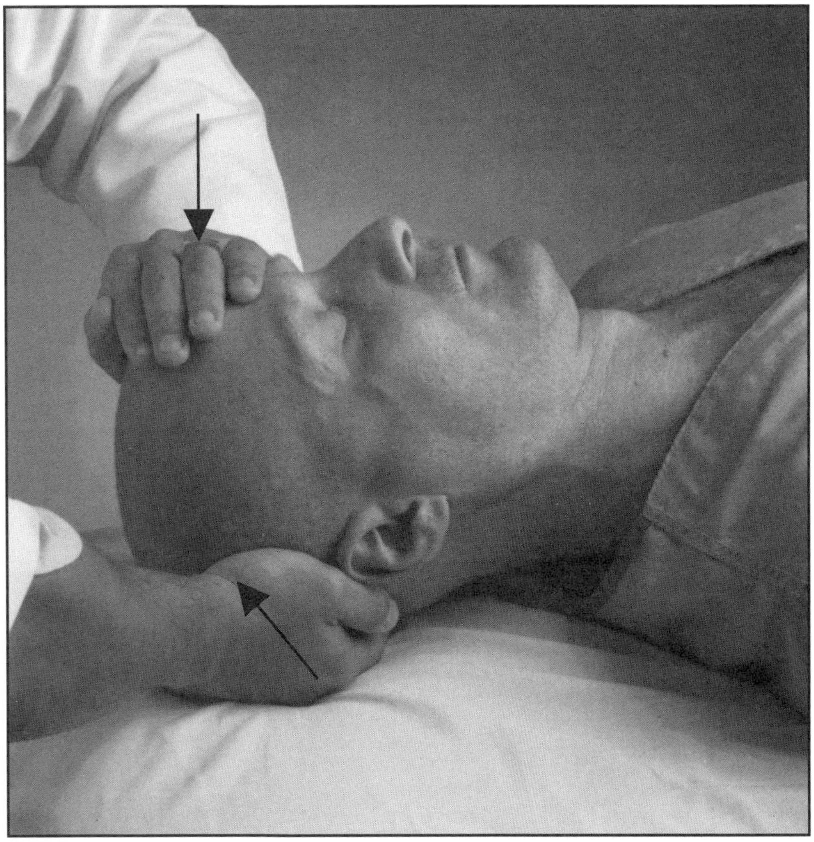

OCCIPITO-MASTOID

For the tenderpoint, start at the tip of the mastoid process. There is a shallow valley that runs up medial to and behind the mastoid ridge. Move up along it three or four centimeters where it may be tender. Treatment involves pressure on the sides of the head enough to prevent the hands slipping. If the operator's palms cover the ears, it is about right. Again the forces are torsion; clockwise bilaterally or counter-clockwise around a transverse axis. One direction feels much better than the other and decreases the tenderpoint, if the physician isn't too busy to monitor it.

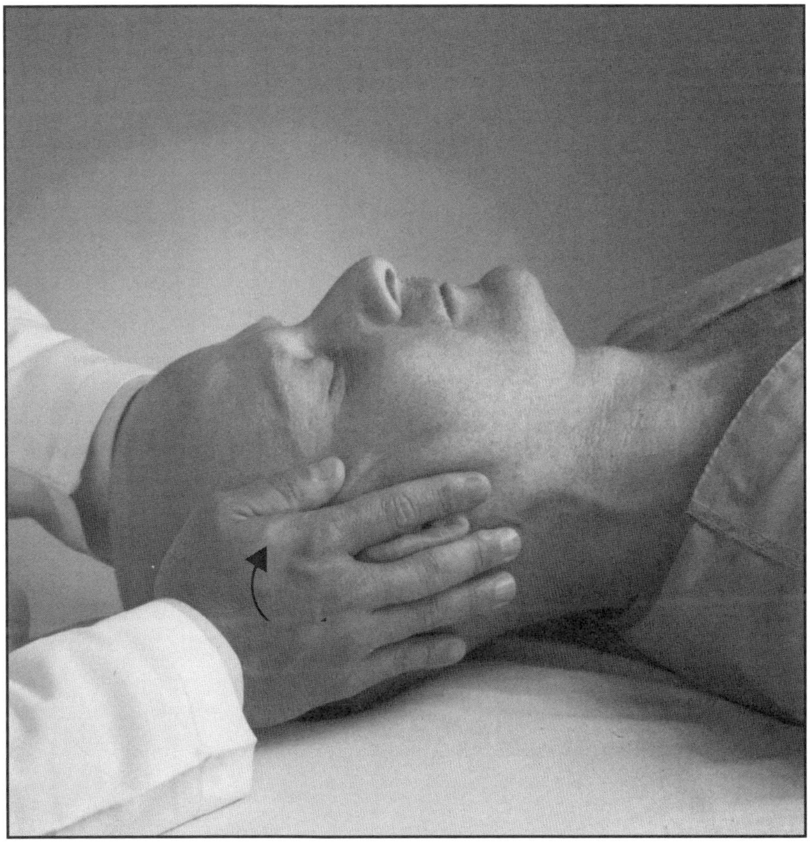

OCCIPITO-PARIETAL

The lambdoid suture is easier to palpate than most beginners think. Probe deeply over the smooth surface of the occiput, moving laterally; the surface becomes rough at the lambdoid suture so that it can be traced up to the lambda. In spite of its late discovery it is fairly common. The tenderpoint and skull pain are out three inches on the suture from the central lambda and usually on the parietal side. A force with the fingertips pressed about an inch further forward, pulling the parietal bone forward and toward the midline is effective. A few of these weren't eased until pressure on the front edge of the parietal bone was used. The patient is well aware of a good relief when placement of fingers and the force is right. He can coach you.

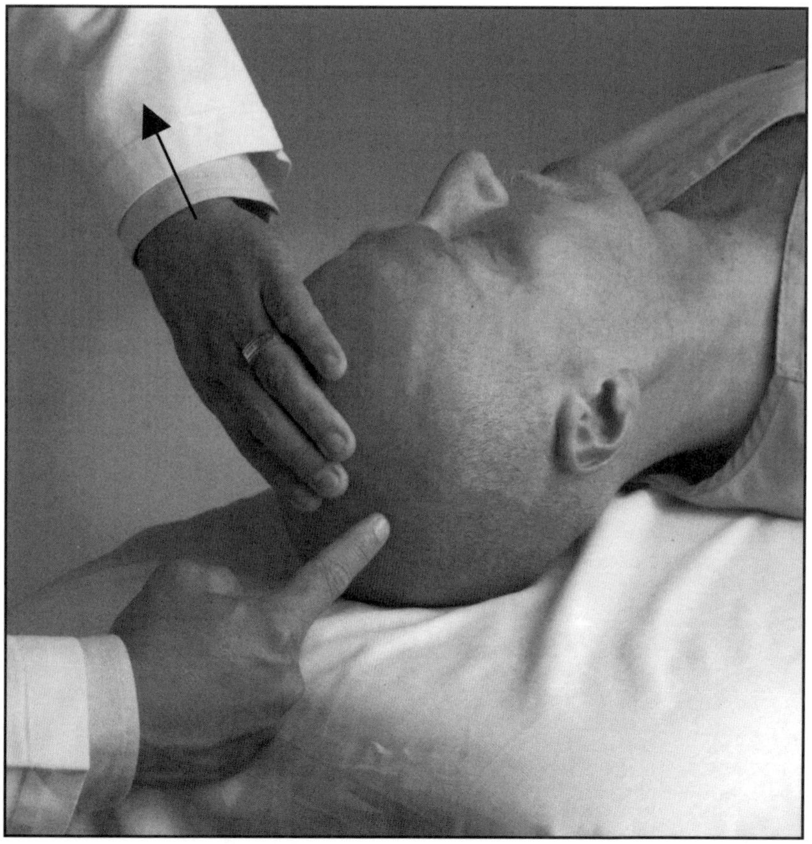

OCCIPITAL

This posterior cranial tenderpoint is found halfway between the tenderpoints for the posterior first cervical and the occipito mastoid. Relief may be obtained in two ways. One is transverse compression of the posterior skull performed with the thenar eminence of the palm pressing medially over the mastoid process and counterforce from the finger tips on the back of the other side of the occiput. This isn't always effective. The other method involves oblique compression of the skull between the occiput tenderpoint and the coronal suture on the top of the head. This is the only treatment using pressure over the tenderpoint.

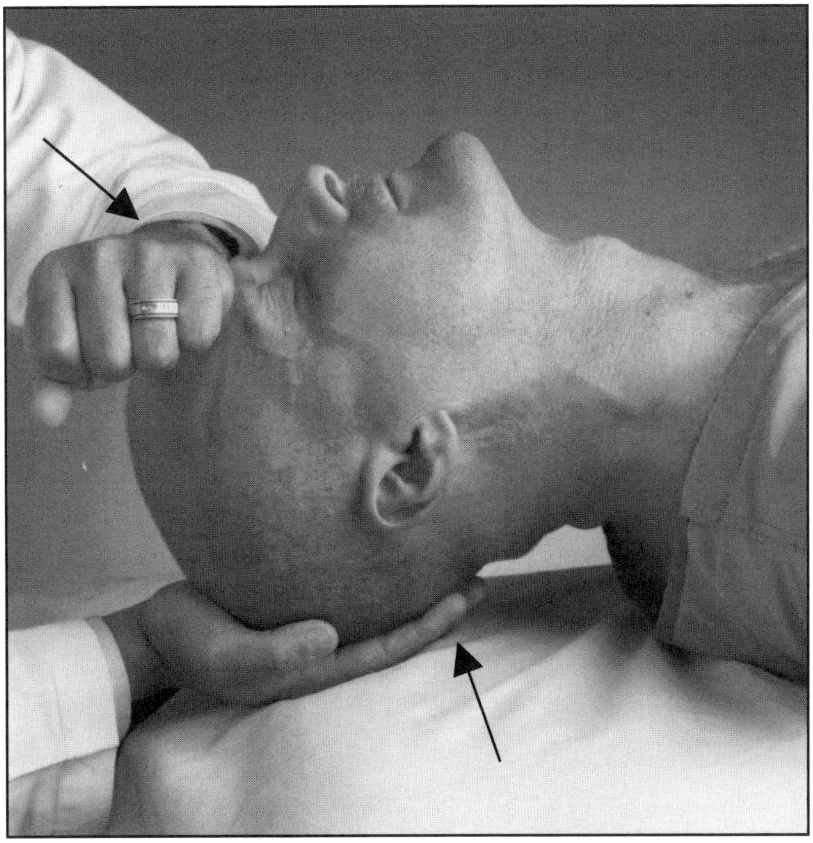

LAMBDOID

This is a relatively uncommon tender spot on the edge of the occipital bone within three centimeters of the lambda. Simply press on the same area on the opposite side from the tender side for relief.

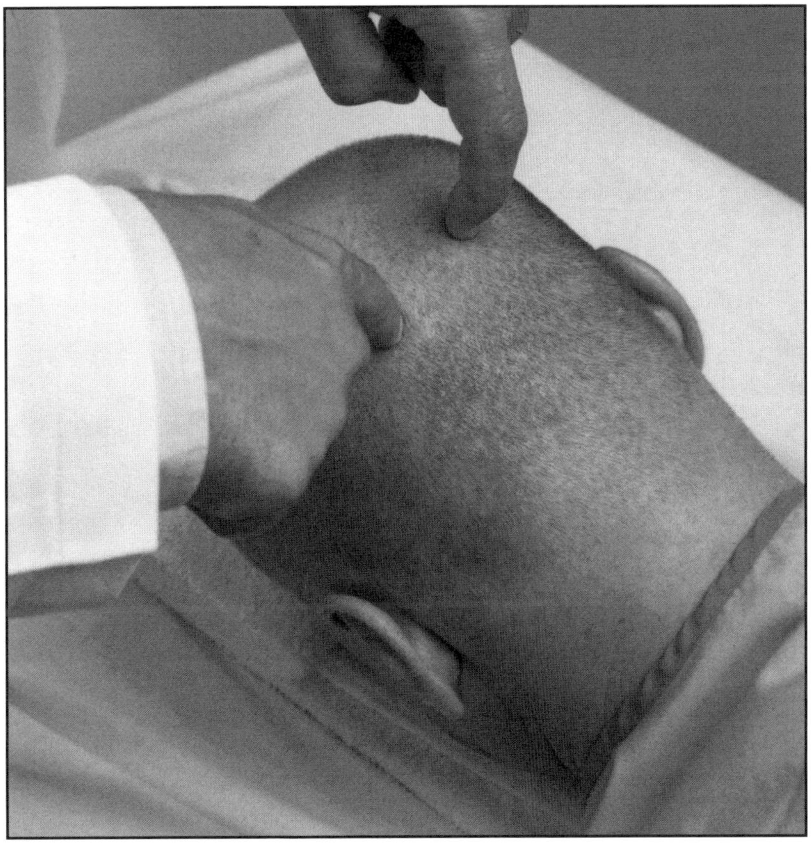

THE SPHENOID BONE

Since it articulates with most of the other bones and forms most of the base of the skull in front of the occiput, it seems to be involved to some extent with everything done to the cranium, but only on the greater wing in the temple behind the ridge of the orbit of the eye can it be palpated externally.

The greater wings are palpated together for comparison. If one is tender, it is likely also to be less concave than its opposite. It seems impossible that it could be displaced laterally, but that is the impression I get when I feel this. On this assumption and with our policy that any deformity can best be reduced indirectly by first making it more deformed, we press on the well, concave side with the heel of one hand. Counterforce is applied by the palm of the other hand on the side of the frontal bone, leaving one finger free to monitor tenderness at the sore greater wing. Whether our reasoning is right or not, this produces good relief routinely and does reduce the deformity. Except for residual edema on the tender wing, the concavities appear more equal.

As I consider the occipital bone the most proximal and the sphenoid the key bone of the skull, all my cranial treatments start with them in mind. Everything else is more distal.

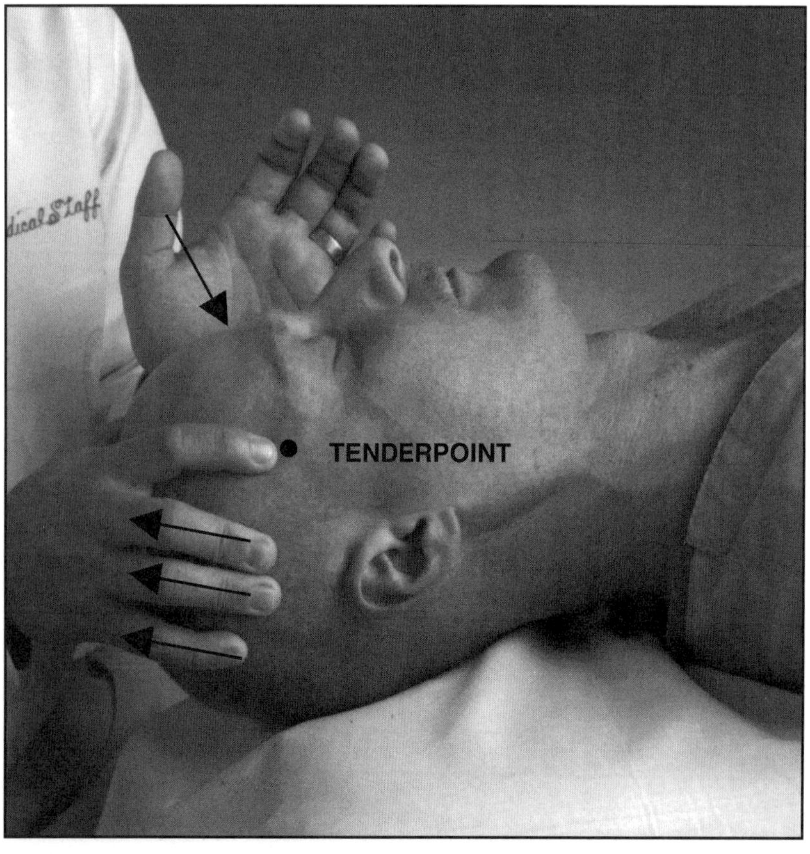

POSTERIOR AURICULAR AND SQUAMOSAL

One centimeter behind the top of the pinna of the ear is a depression the size of a finger-tip. I call it posterior auricular and think it must be due to strain in the back part of the squamosal suture. Also two centimenters forward from the top of the pinna the suture can be palpated. I call it the squamosal. These two may be relieved similarly. Patient lies on the well side with a rolled towel under his zygomatic arch, running from front to back. The force is upward pressure on the lower part of the parietal bone at the place where pulling cephalad and medially on the skin makes the skin over the tenderpoint move the most. This pull, applied more deeply while a tenderpoint is monitored will relieve either one. If these are found bilaterally or just because many people like it, pressure on the temporal bones with the ear cupped beneath the palms of both hands provides good relief.

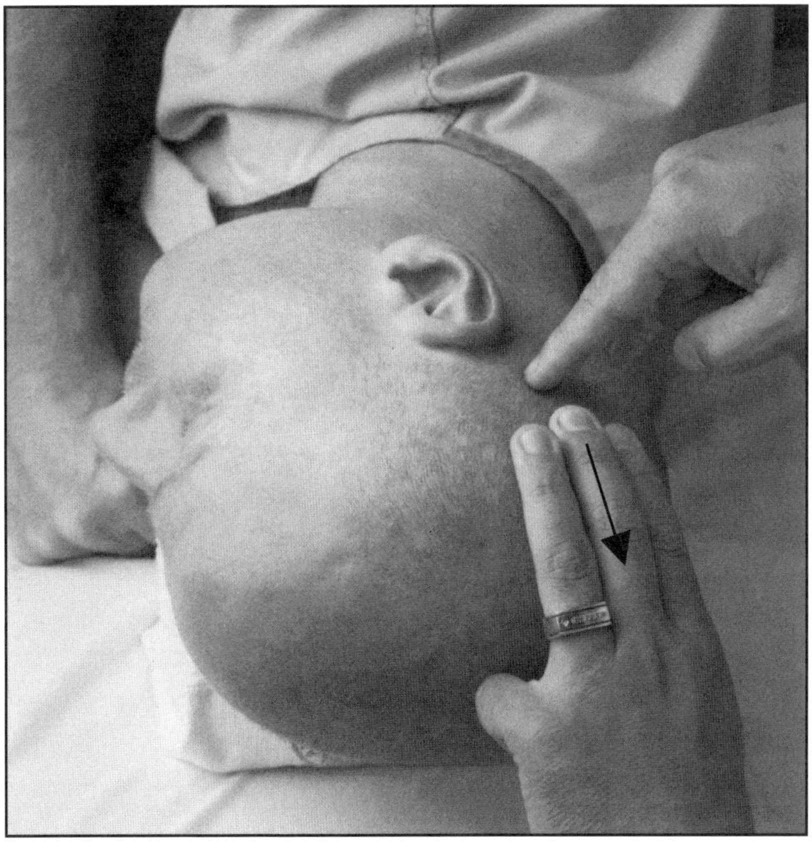

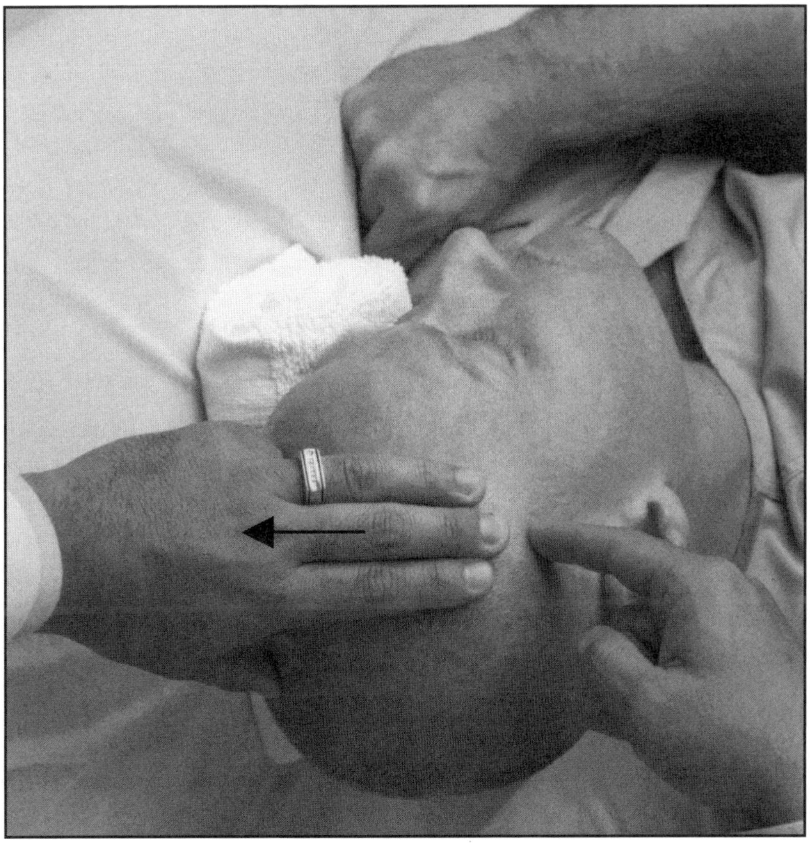

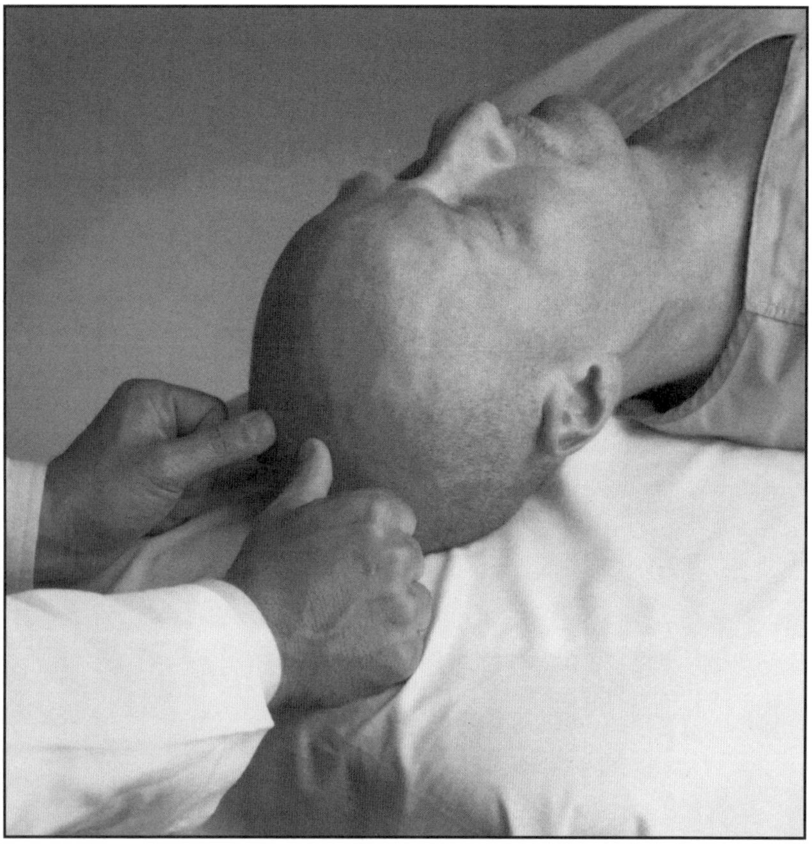

CORONAL

The medial anterior corner of the parietal bone may be tender just behind the coronal suture. It is relatively high. Move across and press on the low one.

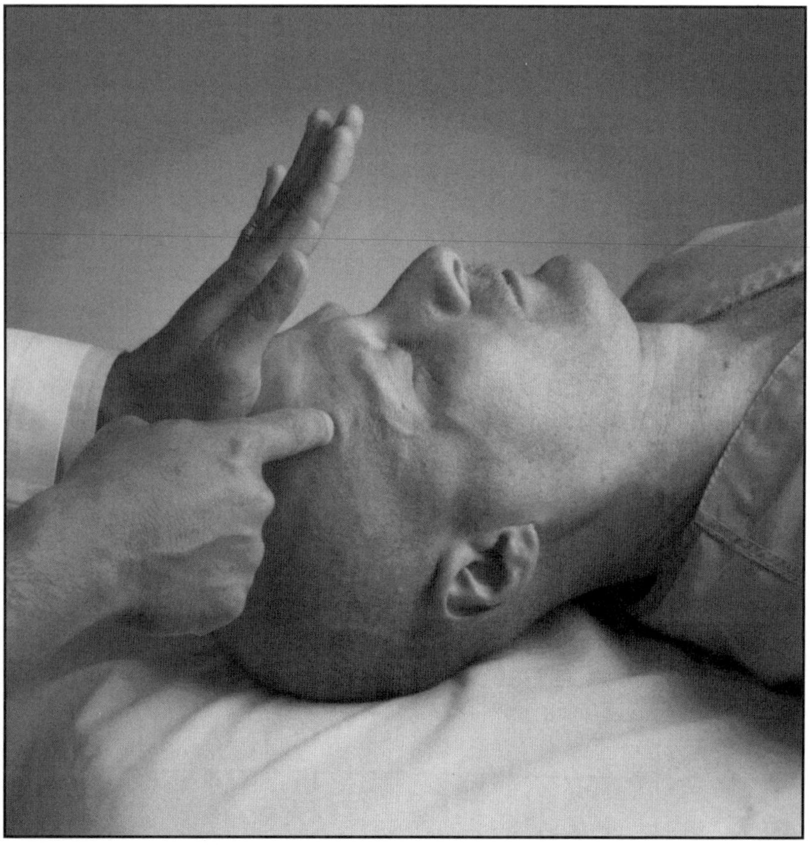

FRONTAL

Another spot just on the front side of the coronal suture on the central back edge of the frontal bone is a place to push to help ease headache above the eye.

LATERAL CANTHUS

These are different because we need to fold the skull over the tenderpoint. The common one, lateral canthus, is on the orbital ridge just back of the lateral canthus of the eye. Pressure below the zygomatic bone and pulling the frontal bone toward it, gives relief.

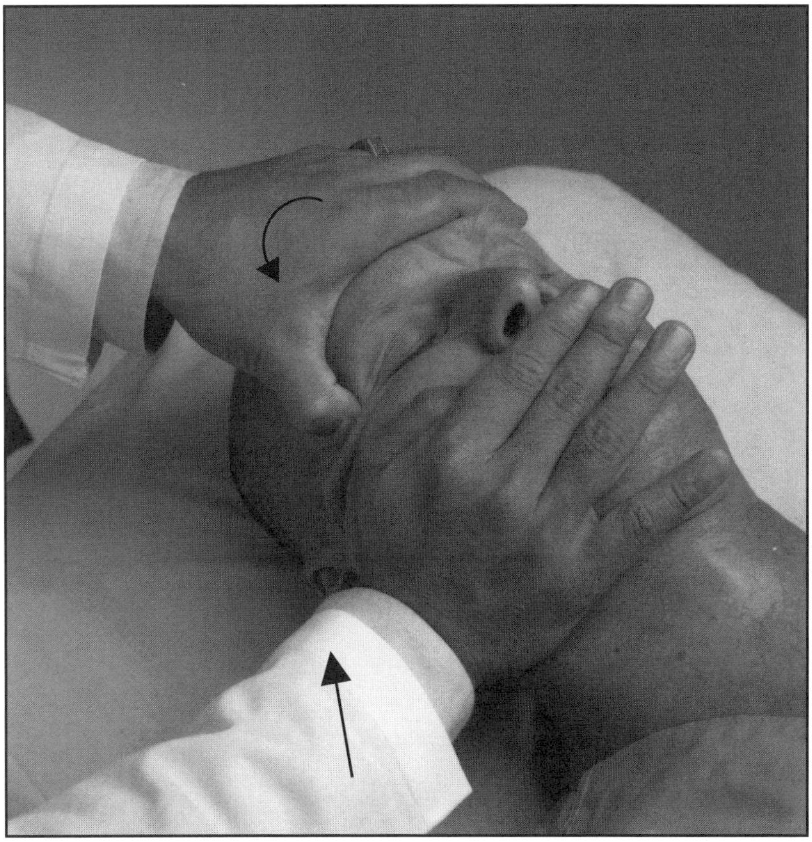

ZYGOMATIC

The same type of pull for a tenderpoint just above the zygomatic arch of the temporal bone, pulling the temporal and parietal toward each other is good. Rare.

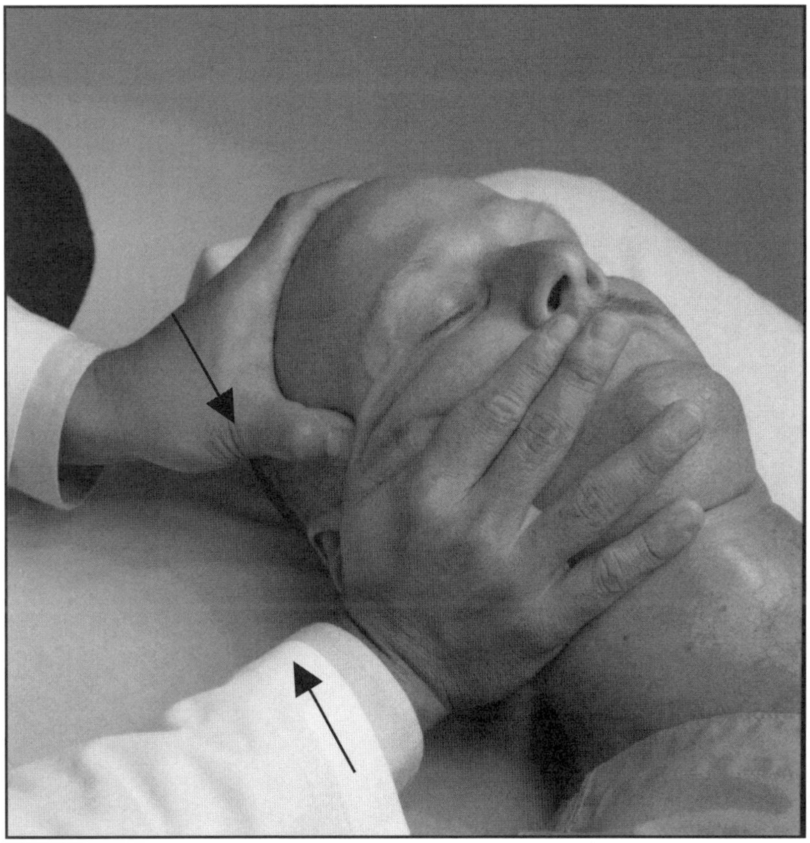

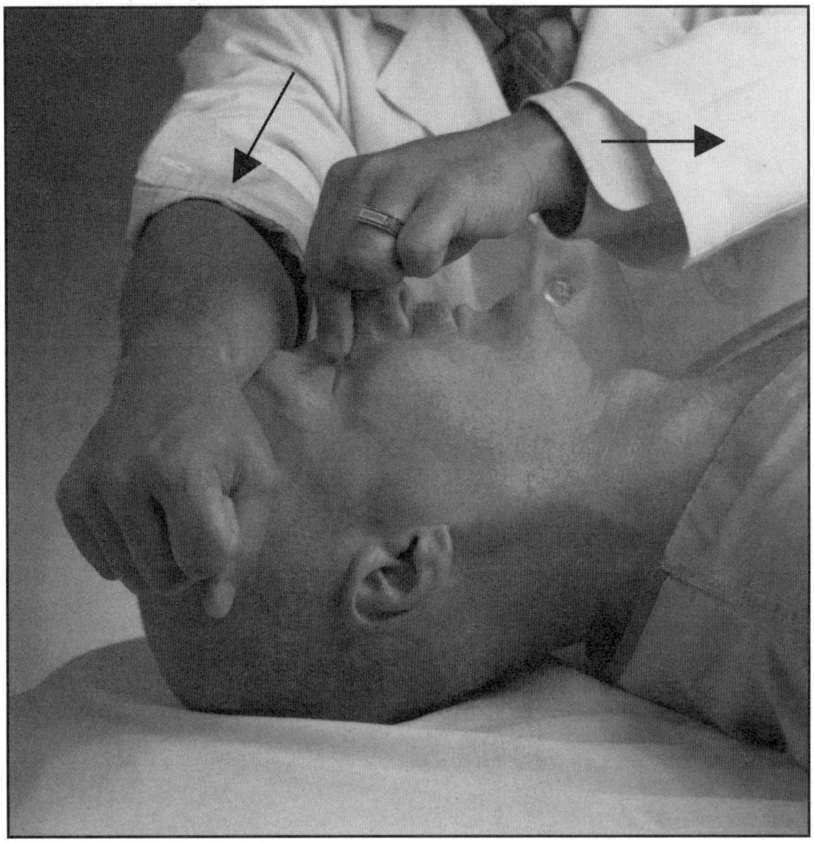

OPHTHALMIC OR SUPRA ORBITAL NERVE

Tenderpoint is on inner edge of orbit near supraorbital foramen. Treatment is traction down from the frontal, pinching the nasal bones between thumb and finger. Counterforce is up on the frontal with a forearm. Sometimes it also needs lateral force pressing from the well side.

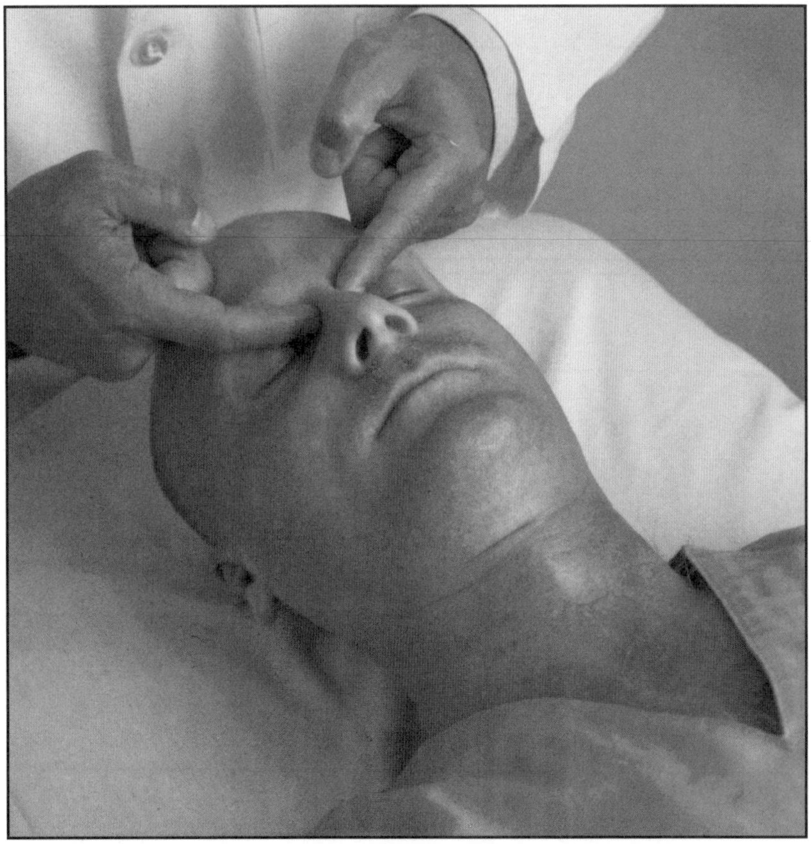

NASAL

One side of the bridge of the nose is tender. It is relieved by pressure on the opposite side. This makes the nose feel and work better. One important thing this relieves is chronic tearing. The nasolacrymal duct seems to get occluded. This must make the duct patent again. My reputation was along other lines so I wasn't consulted for this problem. The ones I found were incidental to something else and formed a very short series. The one I failed on had a history of having probes passed down the nasolacrymal duct for years.

INFRAORBITAL

So named because the tenderpoint is close to the infraorbital foramen. Force is applied with the palms of both hands pressing obliquely backward and medialward. If the operator's palmar fascia is tensed by finger extension, the discomfort over the zygomatic bone where it is being pressed is mild. When done correctly, the patient still has a little pressure pain on the zygomatic bone that is being compressed and a good feeling at the back of his nose that he didn't know was hurting. Patients suffering chronic rhinitis or 'sinus' trouble swear by this one. Very common and important.

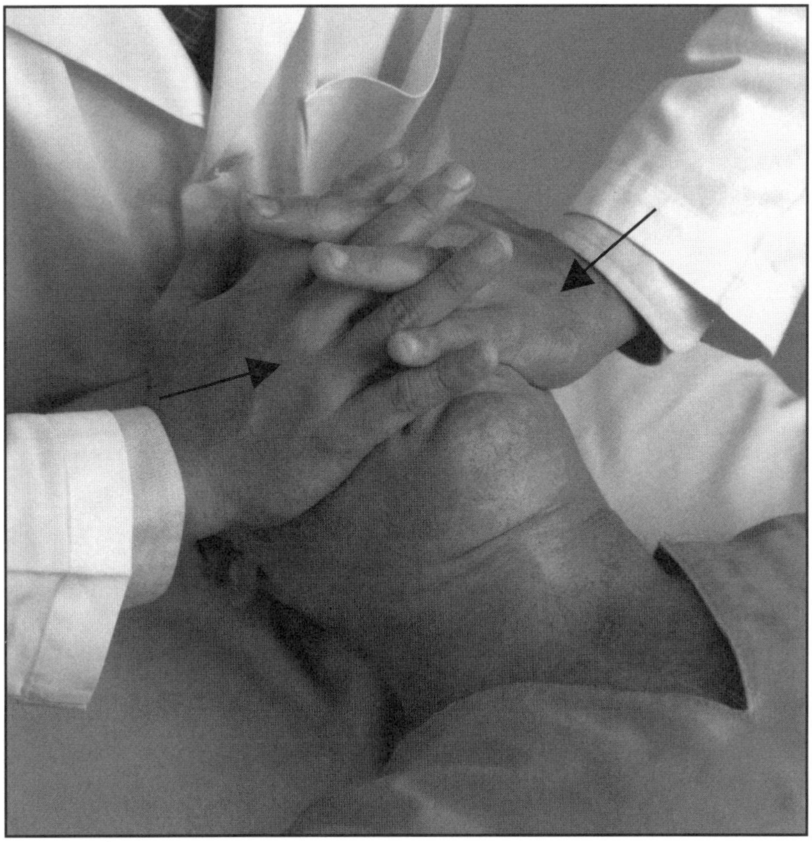

BILATERAL COMPRESSION

Like many other cranial treatments, this is done if the pressure feels good to the patient. It is performed by compression medially with the palms of the hands covering the pinna of the ears.

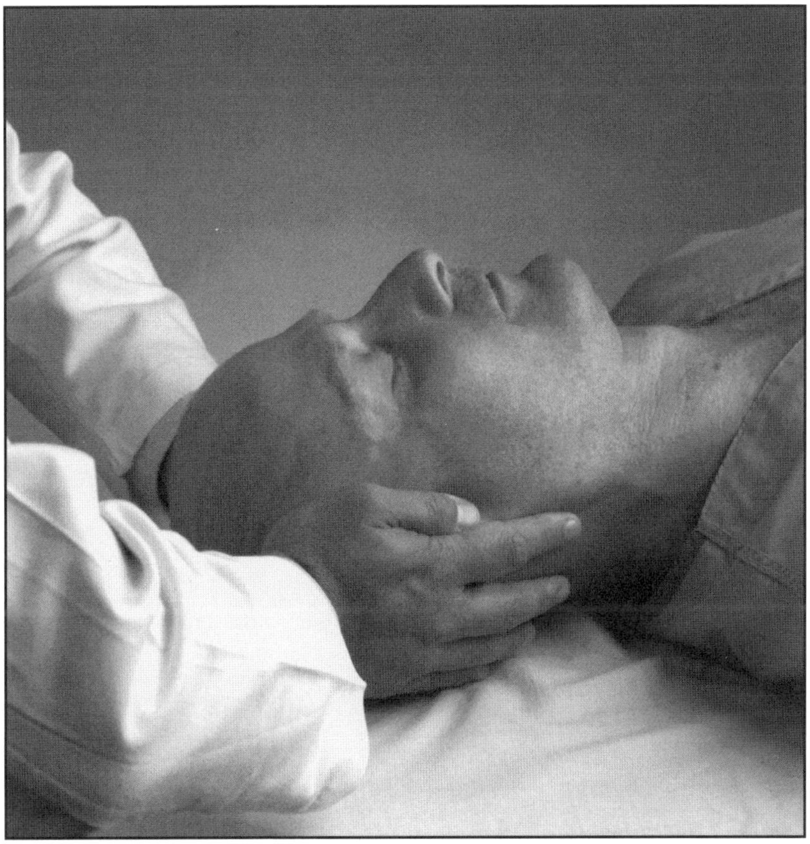

LACRIMAL

This is done by pressing the thumb and index fingers deep in the medial side of the orbit. It takes a little practice to know just how far in on the eyelid to start the push. If it is too far out over the eyeball, there will be pressure on the eyeball. If it is started too far medially, it will be difficult to go deep enough to reach the lacrimal bone. Gentle pressure on the lacrimals often frees up their ability to move.

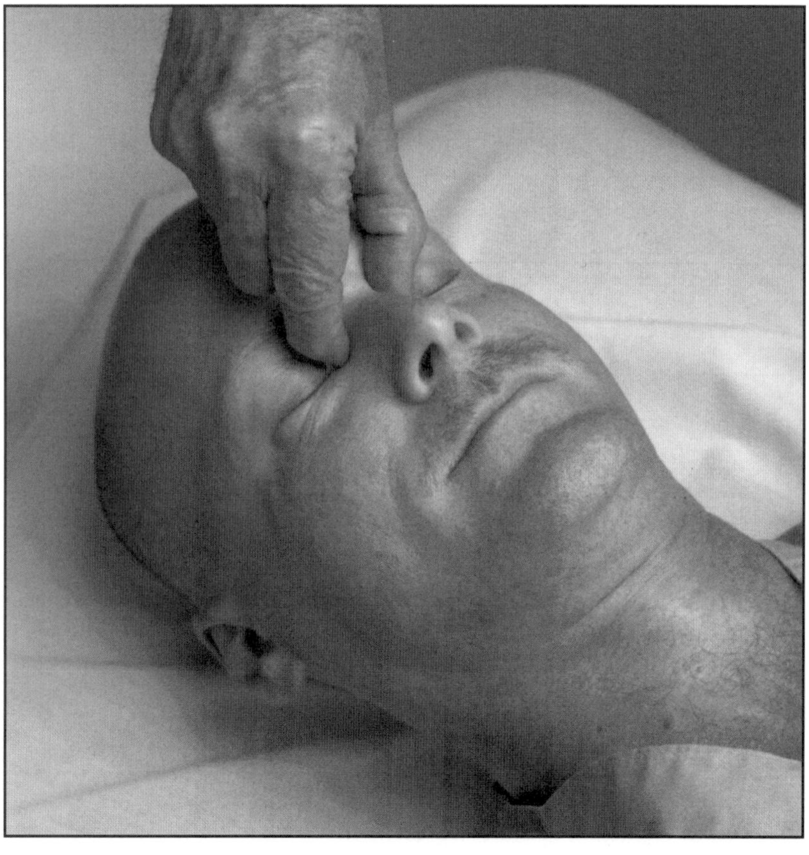

The Temporo-Mandibular Joint

GENERAL

This obviously important joint can have several problems, most of them unilateral. When the jaw is opened slowly it can be seen to deviate to one side and then return to the midline. There must be more than one mechanism involved, because there are two tenderpoints on opposite sides of the jaw that are found with the same deviation.

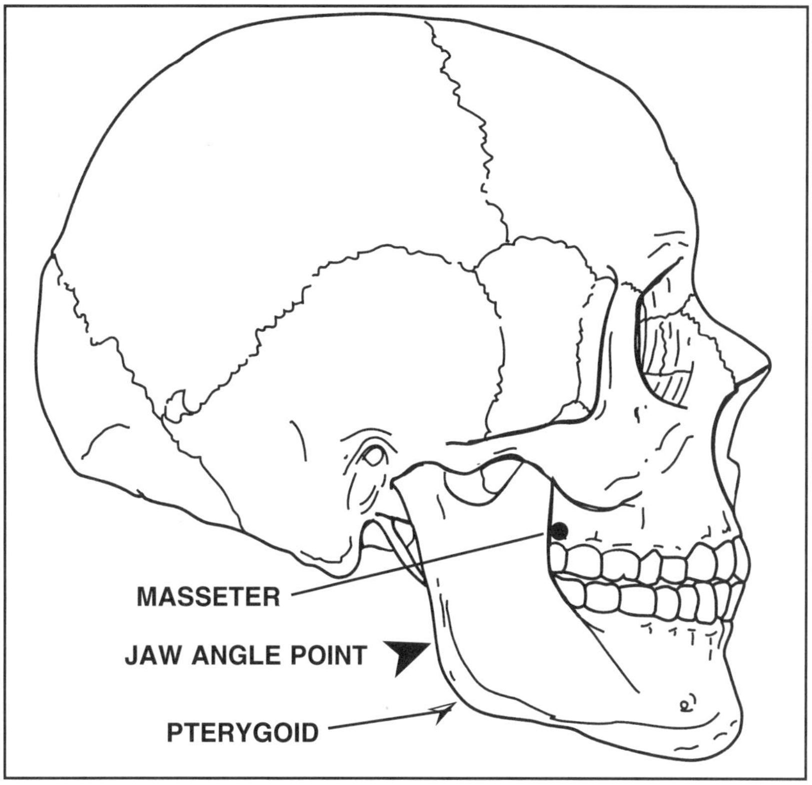

MASSETER

In both cases, treatment involves pushing the slightly open jaw toward the side of the deviation. The tenderpoint on the side toward the deviation seems to be in the masseter near front of the ascending ramus of the mandible.

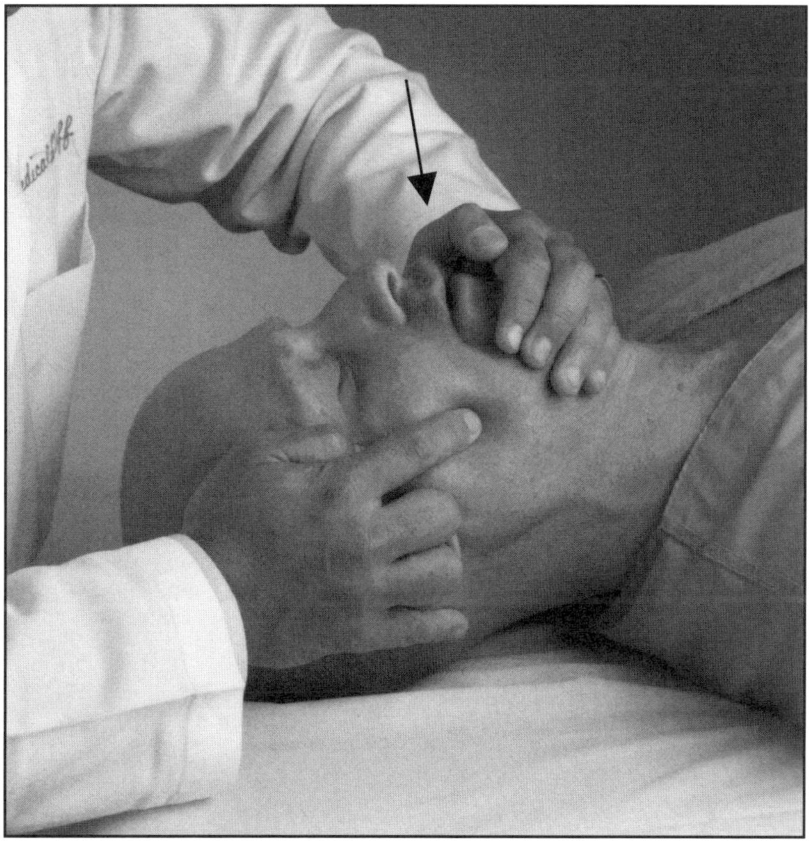

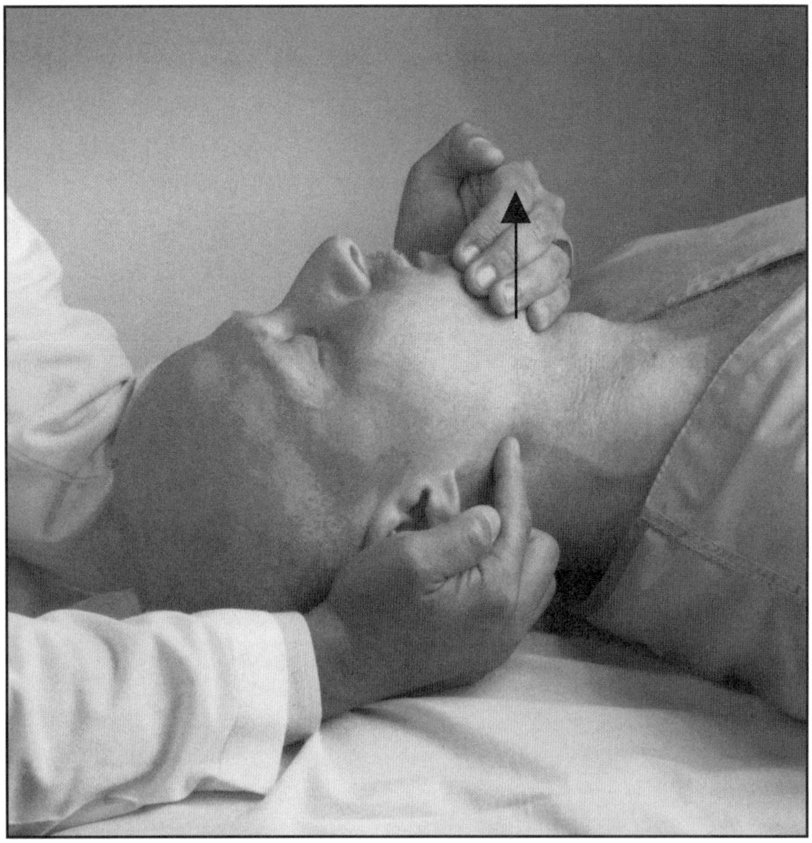

JAW ANGLE

The other point is on the back of the jaw on the opposite side behind the ascending ramus, less than two centimenters above the angle of the mandible and not to be confused with the point for the very common anterior first cervical which is up at the lobe of the ear. Force is applied near the point of the chin to move it laterally and rotate it. A counterforce is applied on the cheekbone.

Again, the tenderpoint high on the back edge of the ascending ramus, in spite of being so close is not a temporomandibular point, because it is relieved simply by rotating the head on the neck.

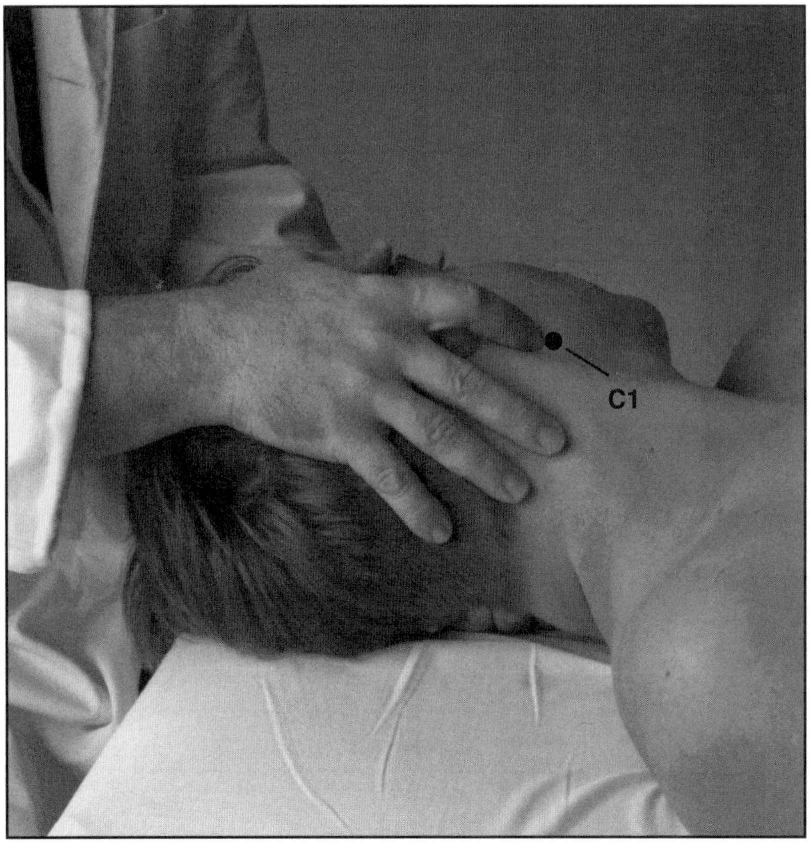

C1 is not a jaw point. Another case where things that must be so—are not. C1 point is very close to the TMJ, but is not from this joint but from the first cervical.

INTERNAL PTERYGOID

Another tenderpoint is on the medial side of the ascending ramus. It can best be palpated by a finger in the back of the mouth. The best success I have had is from a lateral force on the side of the ascending ramus on the affected side. This would seem to apply lateral force, shortening the internal pterygoid muscle without any rotation. Also this may be relieved with the jaw wide open and forced toward the sore pterygoid side.

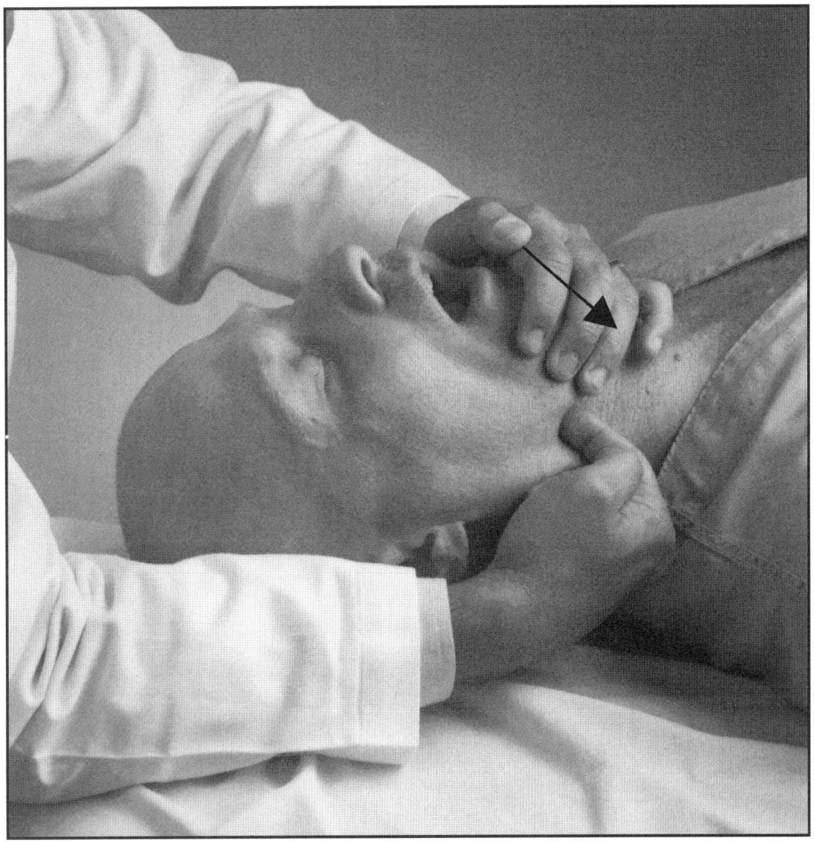

LOCKED CLOSED MANDIBLE

Another jaw problem that seems not to be well understood by anyone is the jaw that can open only slightly. My efforts to ease this by holding the patient's jaw tightly closed weren't helpful until I asked him to try to open against my force until he was tired. About three sessions of about twenty seconds each of this has given good results.

One thing more I have observed in anyone with any kind of jaw pain is the high percent of them that have a dysfunction in the fourth cervical joint. If present, it should be treated first.

As said before there are many rare dysfunctions not included that the experienced operator can usually work out for himself.

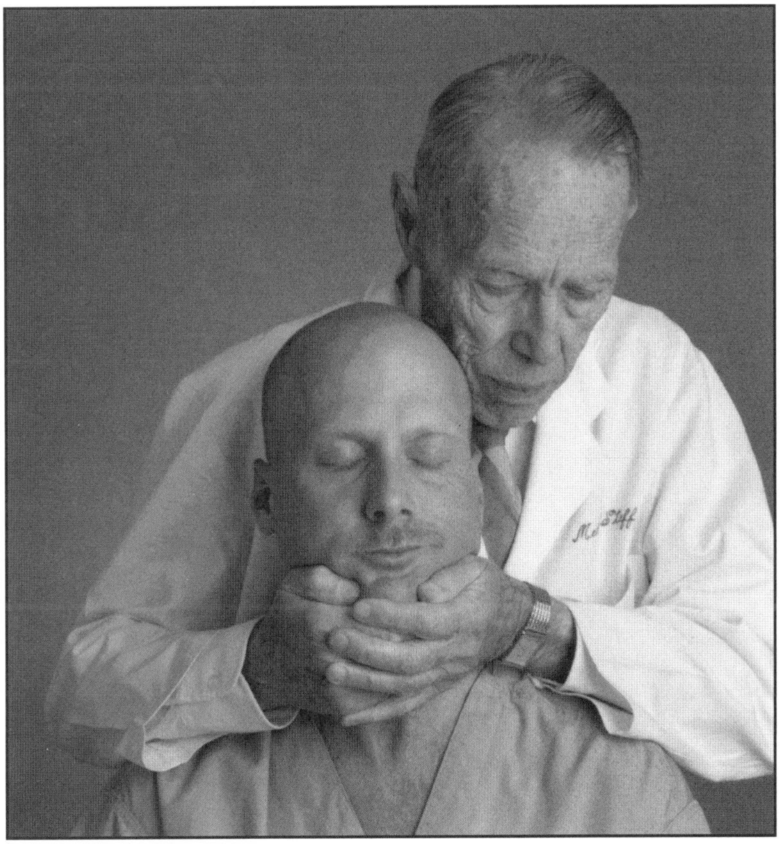

REFERENCES

PREFACE:

1. Korr, I.M. "Proprioceptors and Somatic Dysfunction." *JAOA* 74: 638-50 Mar 75.
2. Northup, G.W. *Osteopathic Medicine. An American Reformation.* Chicago: American Osteopathic Association, 1966, p16.
3. Sutherland,W.G. "The Cranial Bowl." *JAOA* 43:348–53 Apr 44.
4. Hoover, H.V. "Functional Technique." *Yearbook.* Carmel, CA: Academy Applied Osteopathy, 1958, pp 47–51.
5. Jones, L.H. "Spontaneous Release by Positioning." *DO* 4: 109–16 Jan 64.
6. Ruddy, T.J. "Osteopathic Rhythmic Resistive Duction Therapy." *Yearbook.* Carmel, CA: Academy of Applied Osteopathy, 1961, pp 58–68.
7. Mitchel, F.L. Personal communication.

PHYSIOLOGY OF MANIPULATION

1. Wyke, B.D., P. Polecek. "Structural and Functional Characteristics of the Joint Receptor Apparatus." Acta Chir. orthop. Traum. Cech. 40 (1973) 489 and Wyke, B.D., P. Polecek. "Articular Neurology—The Present Position." *Journal of Bone and Joint Surgery,* 57-b (1975) 401.
2. Freeman, M.A.R., B.D. Wyke. "The Innervation of the Knee Joint. An Anatomical and Histological Study in the Cat." *Journal of Anatomy,* (Longon) 101 (1967) 505.
3. Vrettos, X.C., B.D. Wyke. "Articular Reflexogenic Systems in the Costovertebral Joints." *Journal of Bone and Joint Surgery.* 56-B (1979) 382.
4. Freeman, M.A.R., B.D. Wyke. "The Innervation of the Knee Joint. An Anatomical and Histological Study in the Cat." *Journal of Anatomy,* (Longon) 101 (1967) 505.
5. Wyke, B.D. "Neurological Mechanisms in the Experience of Pain." *Acupuncture and Electro-Ther. Research.* 4 (1979a) 27.
6. Bonica, J.D., D. Albe-Fessard. *Advances in Pain Research and Therapy.* NY: Raven Press, 1980.
7. Wyke, B.D. "Neurological Mechanisms in the Experience of Pain." *Acupuncture and Electro-Ther. Research.* 4 (1979a) 27.
8. Sato, A. "The Somato-Sympathetic Reflexes; their Physiologic and Clinical Significance." 1975 National Institute of Neurological and Communicative Disorders and Stroke. Monograph No. 15, 163–172.
9. Beal, M.D., J. Dvorak. "Palpatory Examination of the Spine: A Comparison of the results of two methods. Relationship of Segmental (Somatic) Disfunction to Visceral Disease." *Journal of Manual Medicine,* 2 (1984).
10. Larson, J.N. "Summary of Side and Occurrence of Patients in the Intensive Care Unit." *Journal of the American Osteopathic Association,* 75 (1976) 840–842.
11. Korr, I.M. "Proprioceptors and Somatic Dysfunction." *Journal of the American Osteopathic Association,* 74 (1975) 638.
12. Dvorak, J., V. Dvorak. *Manual Medicine,* (1990) 40.
13. Richmond, F.J., V.C. Abrahams. "What are the Proprioceptors of the Neck?" *Progress of Brain Research.* 50 (1979) 245.
14. Richmond, F.J., V.C. Abrahams. "What are the Proprioceptors of the Neck?" *Progress of Brain Research.* 50 (1979) 245.
15. Granit, R. *Receptors and Sensory Perception.* New Haven: Yale University Press, 1955, p118–119.
16. Granit, R. "The Functional Role of Muscle Spindles—Facts and Hypothesis." *Brain* 98 (1975) 531–556.
17. Hassler, R. Neuronale Grundlagen der spastichen Tonussteigerung. In Bauer, H.J., W.P. Koella, A. Struppler Therapie der Spastik. Verlag fur angwandte Wissenschafter, Muchen 1981.
18. Dvorak, J., V. Dvorak. *Manual Medicine,* (1990) 40.
19. Groves, P.M., D. Lee and R.F. Thompson. "Effects of Stimulus and Intensity on Habituation and Sensitization in Acute Spinal Cat." *Psychology and Behavior,* Vol. 4, (1968) 383–388.
20. Groves, P. and R.F. Thompson: Habituation. "A Dual-Process Theory." *Psychological Review* 1970, Vol. 77, No. 5, 419–451.
21. Patterson, M.M., and J.E. Steinmetz. "Long-Lasting Alterations of Spinal Reflexes: A Potential Basis for Somatic Dysfunction." *Manual Medicine* (1986) 2:38–42.
22. Beal, M.D., J. Dvorak. "Palpatory Examination of the Spine: A Comparison of the results of two methods. Relationship of Segmental (Somatic) Disfunction to Visceral Disease." *Journal of Manual Medicine,* 2 (1984).
23. Mense, S. "Nervous Outflow from Sceletal Muscle Following Chemical Noxious Stimulation." *Journal of Physiology* (London) 267 (1977) 75–88.
24. Schmidt, R.F., K.D. Kniffki, E.D.

Schomburg. Der Einfluss kleinkalibriger Muskelafferenzen auf den Muskeltonus. In Bauer, H.J., W.P. Koella, A. Struppier. Therapie der Spastik. Verlag fur angewandte Wissenschaften, Munchen, 1981.

25. Fassbender, H.G. Der Rheumatische Schmerz, Med. Welt 36 (1980) 1263.

26. Schmidt, R.F., K.D. Kniffki, E.D. Schomburg. Der Einfluss kleinkalibriger Muskelafferenzen auf den Muskeltonus. In Bauer, H.J., W.P. Koella, A. Struppier: Therapie der Spastik. Verlag fur angewandte Wissenschaften, Munchen, 1981.

27. Dvorak, J., V. Dvorak. *Manual Medicine,* (1990) 40.

28. Wyke, B.D. "Neurological Mechanisms in the Experience of Pain." *Acupuncture and Electro-Ther. Research.* 4 (1979a) 27.

ADDITIONAL REFERENCES

Jones, L.H. "Foot Treatment Without Hand Trauma." *JAOA* 72: 481–9 Jan 73.

Jones, L.H. "Missed Anterior Spinal Lesions. A Preliminary Report." *DO* 6:75–9 Mar 66.

Owens, C. *An Endocrine Interpretation of Chapman's Reflexes.* Second Edition. Chatanooga, TN: Chatanooga Printing and Engraving, 1937.

Rumney, I.C. "Structural Diagnosis and Manipulative Therapy." *J Osteopathy* 70: 21–33 Jan 63. Revised Version D.O. 4:135–42 Sep 63.

"Strain and Counterstrain. Rationale of Manipulation" Address given at the Fourth Annual Post-Graduate Seminar of the American Academy of Osteopathy. Colorado Springs, May 25–27,1972.

Travell, J. "Basis of the Multiple Uses of Local Block of Somatic Trigger Areas. Procaine Infiltration and Ethyl Chloride Spray." *Mississippi Valley Med J* 71:13–21 Jan 49.

INDEX